Drugs
for the Heart

Drugs for the Heart

Second Expanded Edition

Edited by

Lionel H. Opie, M.D., D. Phil., F.R.C.P.
Professor of Medicine
University of Cape Town
Cape Town, South Africa;
Consultant Professor
Division of Cardiology
Stanford University Medical Center
Stanford, California

With the collaboration of

Kanu Chatterjee, M.B., F.R.C.P.

Bernard J. Gersh, M.B., Ch.B., D. Phil., M.R.C.P.

Donald C. Harrison, M.D.

Norman M. Kaplan, M.D.

Frank I. Marcus, M.D.

Bramah N. Singh, M.D., D. Phil., F.R.C.P.

Edmund H. Sonnenblick, M.D.

Udho Thadani, M.B.B.S., M.R.C.P., F.R.C.P. (C.)

Foreword by

Eugene Braunwald, M.D.

G&S

Grune & Stratton, Inc.
Harcourt Brace Jovanovich, Publishers
Orlando   New York   San Diego   Boston   London
San Francisco   Tokyo   Sydney   Toronto

Library of Congress Cataloging-in-Publication Data

Drugs for the heart.

"Adapted from Drugs and the heart by L.H. Opie"—T.p. verso.
Includes bibliographies and index.
1. Cardiovascular agents.   I. Opie, Lionel H.
II. Chatterjee, Kanu.   III. Opie, Lionel, H.   Drugs and
the heart. [DNLM: 1. Cardiovascular Agents—adverse
effects.   2. Cardiovascular Agents—therapeutic use.
3. Heart—drug effects.   QV 150 D7938]
RM345.D784   1987   616.1'2061   86-22927
ISBN 0-8089-1840-0

Grune & Stratton, Inc.
Orlando, Florida 32887

Distributed in the United Kingdom by
Grune & Stratton, Ltd.
24/28 Oval Road, London NW 1

Library of Congress Catalog Number 86-22927
International Standard Book Number 0-8089-1840-0
Printed in the United States of America
86 87 88 89   10 9 8 7 6 5 4 3 2 1

Contents

Foreword

During the past decade, an extraordinary array of new cardio-vascular drugs has become available and both students and practitioners of medicine have difficulty in making a decision on how to choose the proper drugs for their patients. Professor Opie's book provides a rational approach to this most important medical decision. This marvelous book is a concise yet complete presentation of cardiac pharmacology. It presents, in a very readable and eminently understandable fashion, an extraordinary amount of important information on the effects of drugs on the heart and circulation. Professor Opie has the unique ability to explain in a straightforward manner the mechanism of action of drugs without oversimplifying these complex matters. Simultaneously his book provides important practical information to the clinician. This concise volume should be of value and interest to anyone who wishes to gain a clear understanding of cardiovascular therapeutics.

Eugene Braunwald, M.D.
Physician-in-Chief
Brigham and Beth Israel Hospitals
Harvard Medical School
Boston, Massachusetts

Preface

This updated and substantially revised edition has been expanded and comes in a new format. Four new chapters highlight recent advances in the constantly expanding areas of cardiovascular pharmacology: diuretics, angiotensin-converting enzyme inhibitors, thrombolytic agents, and lipid-lowering agents.

Our aim is to produce a pocket-size compendium, designed specifically to meet the needs of the hard-pressed resident or the equally busy practicing cardiologist needing to identify the best drug, its dose, and its side-effects at a moment's notice. Special care has therefore been given to the selection of new material. Extensive indexing and cross-referencing aim to make the information readily accessible. Each page has a summary heading. Variations in typeface highlight important information, new drugs, and new uses for old drugs. References have been completely updated to mid-1986.

This edition has departed from the concept of a distinctly "American edition" to incorporate the wider approach that made the first Lancet edition so popular. The European practice of today may become the American practice of tomorrow (and vice versa), so that a global view is necessary. However, meticulous attention has been paid to indicate clearly which drugs and indications have been approved in the USA by the Food and Drug Administration (FDA), whose recommendations are becoming increasingly stringent and reflect excellent judgment.

The best way to use this book is obvious—carry it with you, always! Don't hesitate to consult it in front of your patients, they appreciate your desire to be exact and to use the best possible drug in the optimal dose for their complaint.

Preface to the First American Edition

Cardiovascular pharmacology is a very active scene. A plethora of new agents are now offered to the clinician—to say nothing of the new indications that are being found for old agents. Every agent seems to have several actions that are often apparently unconnected. Confusion is rife.

In this book, we hope to restore some order by examining six groups of drugs: β-blockers, nitrates, calcium antagonists, antiarrhythmics, digitalis and sympathomimetics, and vasodilators. We will discuss what is known of their actions at both the cellular and the clinical levels. A knowledge of cellular mechanisms may help to avoid a serious hazard in polypharmacy. Information on clinical results will equally discourage adoption of the large number of drugs that should work but do not, or that have never been properly tested. We will speak often of "usual" or "average" or "maximum" doses, and some readers may protest that such terms are utterly not helpful. They are intended largely to allow some comparison of costs; it is not enough to know that one tablet is cheaper than another.

The ready availability of so many agents means that the physician has great power for poor as well as for good results. Not all cardiac illness steadily progresses. Some patients with angina spontaneously improve. Cardiac failure may be temporarily worsened by intercurrent illness while postinfarct arrhythmias come and go. We must constantly be asking ourselves whether the therapy can be simplified or stopped; and, conversely, whether the time has come for one of the more vigorous regimens described in these articles.

So, on to β-blockers.

Acknowledgments

The rapid appearance of this completely revised edition has been made possible by the willing and unstinting cooperation of many people. First, I would like to thank my coauthors for generously sharing their expertise and clinical skills on which this book is based and for undertaking their meticulous updating of the earlier text. We extend a special welcome to Kanu Chatterjee and to Eugene Braunwald, joining us for the first time. Second, we thank the staff of Grune & Stratton for so efficiently dealing with the deadline and preparing such a well produced book. The figures (specifically my copyright unless otherwise stated) are based chiefly on the artistic skills of Jeanne Walker with Jean Powell, and Linda Coetzee providing excellent help. And, last but not least, my secretary June Chambers is thanked for prodigious patience and unfailing skills.

Contributors

Eugene Braunwald, M.D. (Foreword)
Physician-in-Chief, Brigham and Beth Israel Hospitals, Harvard Medical School, Boston, Massachusetts

Kanu Chatterjee, M.B., F.R.C.P.
Professor of Medicine, Lucie Stern Professor of Cardiology, University of California, San Francisco, California

Bernard J. Gersh, M.B., Ch.B., D. Phil., M.R.C.P.
Consultant in Cardiovascular Diseases and Internal Medicine, Mayo Clinic and Mayo Foundation; Professor of Medicine, Mayo Medical School, Rochester, Minnesota

Donald C. Harrison, M.D.
Chief of Cardiology, Cardiology Division, Stanford University Medical Center; William G. Irwin Professor of Medicine, Stanford University School of Medicine, Stanford, California

Norman M. Kaplan, M.D.
Professor of Internal Medicine, University of Texas Health Sciences Center at Dallas; Southwestern Medical School, Dallas, Texas

Frank I. Marcus, M.D.
Distinguished Professor of Medicine, Cardiology Section, University of Arizona, Tucson, Arizona

Lionel H. Opie, M.D., D. Phil., F.R.C.P.
Professor of Medicine, University of Cape Town, Cape Town, South Africa; Consultant Professor, Division of Cardiology, Stanford University Medical Center, Stanford, California

Bramah N. Singh, M.D., D. Phil., F.R.C.P.
Professor of Medicine, University of California at Los Angeles; Director, Cardiovascular Research, Wadsworth Veterans Administration Hospital, Los Angeles, California

Edmund H. Sonnenblick, M.D.
Chief, Division of Cardiology; Olson Professor of Medicine, Albert Einstein College of Medicine, Bronx, New York

Udho Thadani, M.B.B.S., M.R.C.P., F.R.C.P. (C)
Professor of Medicine, University of Oklahoma Health Sciences Center; Director of Clinical Cardiology, Oklahoma Memorial Hospital and Veterans Administration Medical Center, Oklahoma City, Oklahoma

Drugs
for the Heart

L. H. Opie, E. H. Sonnenblick
N. M. Kaplan, U. Thadani

1

β-Blocking Agents

β-Adrenergic receptor antagonist agents remain a cornerstone in the therapy of angina pectoris and hypertension, although now increasingly challenged by the calcium antagonists. β-Blockers also retain their position amongst the basic therapies for numerous other conditions including arrhythmias and hypertrophic cardiomyopathy.

The β-Adrenoceptor

Our understanding of adrenergic effects is based on Ahlquist's original classification of adrenoceptors into α and β types. The β-receptors are classically divided into the β_1-receptors found in heart muscle and the β_2-receptors of bronchial and vascular smooth muscle; it is now known that there also are sizeable populations of β_2-receptors in the myocardium. Some metabolic β-receptors cannot easily be classified. Situated on the cell membrane, the β-receptor is probably part of the adenylate cyclase system (Fig. 1-1). There are several receptor sites for adenylate cyclase: one for β-agonists, one for glucagon, one for thyroid hormone, and one for histamine. Each agonist, acting on its receptor site, can activate adenylate cyclase to produce cyclic AMP from ATP. Cyclic AMP is the intracellular messenger of β-stimulation; among its actions is the "opening" of calcium channels to promote a positive inotropic effect. In the sinus node the pacemaker current is increased (positive chronotropic effect). The effect of a given β-blocking agent depends not only on the way it is absorbed, bound to plasma proteins, and on its metabolites, but also on the extent to which it inhibits the β-receptor (lock and key fit).

ANGINA PECTORIS

β-Blockade reduces the oxygen demand of the heart in several ways (Fig. 1-2)—notably, by reducing the double product (heart rate × blood pressure) and depressing contractility. The list of contraindications and side-effects is formidable (Table 1-1). **The most important contraindication is asthma or a past history of asthma;** several fatalities or near fatalities have been reported with the first dose of noncardioselective agents and even selective agents can only be given under supervision.

All β-blockers are potentially equally effective in angina pectoris (Table 1-2) and the choice of drug matters little except that ultralong-acting compounds such as nadolol[33] need only be given once daily. But about 20 percent of patients do not respond to any β-blocker,[48] possibly because of: (1) a significant role for coronary artery spasm in the production of angina; (2) an underlying severe obstructive coronary artery disease, responsible for angina at a low level of exertion and at heart rates of 100 beats/min or lower; or (3) an abnor-

Drugs for the Heart, Second Expanded Edition
Copyright © 1987 by Grune & Stratton, Inc.

1

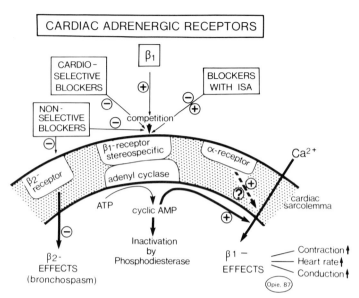

Fig. 1-1. Cardiac adrenergic receptors. β_1-Agonists act on the β_1-selective receptor in the heart cell membrane. Nonselective blockade by propranolol gives β_1 plus β_2-blockade. Cardioselective blockers at low doses are relatively β_1-specific. Agents with ISA (intrinsic sympathomimetic activity, Fig. 1-6) simultaneously block and stimulate the receptor with the blockade dominating during states of enhanced sympathetic tone.

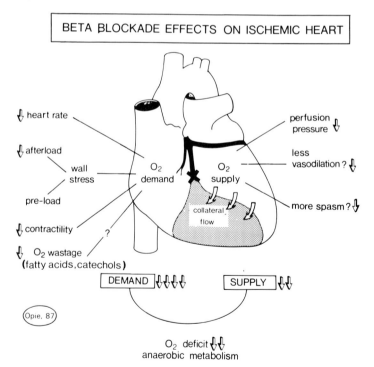

Fig. 1-2. Effects of β-blockade on ischemic heart. β-blockade has a beneficial effect on the ischemic myocardium, unless (1) the preload rises substantially as in left heart failure or (2) there is vasospastic angina when spasm may be promoted in some patients.

TABLE 1-1
β-BLOCKADE: CONTRAINDICATIONS

Cardiac
Absolute: *Severe bradycardia, high-degree heart block, left ventricular failure* (exception: some cardiomyopathies), acute myocardial infarction unless monitored.
Relative: Treated heart failure, cardiomegaly without clinical failure (not a contraindication in hypertensive heart disease), Prinzmetal's angina (unopposed α-spasm), high doses of other agents depressing SA or AV nodes (verapamil, diltiazem, digitalis, antiarrhythmic agents); in angina, avoid sudden withdrawal, danger in unreliable patient.

Pulmonary
Absolute: *Severe asthma or bronchospasm.* No patient may be given a β-blocker without questions for past or present asthma. Fatalities have resulted when this rule is ignored.
Relative: Mild asthma or bronchospasm or chronic airways disease. Use agents with cardioselectivity plus β_2-stimulants (by inhalation). High ISA also protects, but loss of sensitivity to β_2-stimulation.

Central Nervous
Absolute: *Severe depression* (avoid propranolol).
Relative: Vivid dreams: avoid highly lipid-soluble agents (propranolol, alprenolol) and pindolol; avoid evening dose or try timolol. Visual hallucinations: change from propranolol. Fatigue (all agents; try change of agent). Impotence: rare unless added α-blockade (try change of agent). Psychotropic drugs (with adrenergic augmentation) may adversely interact with β-blockers.

Peripheral Vascular
Absolute: *Active disease:* gangrene, skin necrosis, severe or worsening claudication.
Relative: Cold extremities, absent pulses, Raynaud's phenomenon. Avoid nonselective agents without ISA* (propranolol, sotalol, nadolol); prefer high ISA* (pindolol) or cardioselectivity.

Diabetes Mellitus
Relative: Insulin-requiring diabetes: nonselective agents decrease reaction to hypoglycemia; use selective agents—atenolol, metoprolol (acebutolol more doubtful). β-Blockers may increase blood sugar by 1.0–1.5 mmol/L. Adjust control accordingly.

Renal Failure
Relative: In general, renal blood flow falls. Reduce doses of all except pindolol.

Liver Disease
Relative: Avoid agents with high hepatic clearance (propranolol, oxprenolol, timolol, acebutolol, metoprolol). Use agents with low clearance (atenolol, nadolol, sotalol, or pindolol). If plasma proteins low, reduce dose of highly bound agents (propranolol, pindolol).

Pregnancy Hypertension
β-Blockade increasingly used but may depress vital signs in neonate and cause uterine vasoconstriction. Labetalol and atenolol best tested. Avoid diuretics—low blood volume.

Surgical Operations
β-Blockade may be maintained throughout, provided indication is not trivial; otherwise stop 24–48 hours beforehand. May protect against anesthetic arrhythmias. Use atropine for bradycardia, β-agonist for severe hypotension.

Age
β-Blockade, possibly less effective in hypertension in the elderly, can still be used especially in combination with diuretics. Watch pharmacokinetics and side-effects.

Smoking
In hypertension, β-blockade is not effective in reducing coronary events in smoking men.

*ISA = intrinsic sympathomimetic activity

mal increase in left ventricular (LV) end-diastolic pressure resulting from an excess negative inotropic effect and a resultant decrease in subendocardial blood flow. Although it is conventional to adjust the dose of a β-blocker to secure a resting heart rate of 55–60 beats/min, below 50 beats/min may be acceptable provided that heart block is avoided and there are no symptoms. It may not be possible to achieve low resting heart rates with newer drugs possessing intrinsic sympathomimetic activity (ISA) or added α-blocking properties. Reduction in exercise-induced tachycardia is an important determinant of the response to treatment, and one should aim to achieve an exercise heart rate of less than 100–110 beats/min during β-blockade therapy.

TABLE 1-2

PROPERTIES OF VARIOUS β-ADRENOCEPTOR ANTAGONIST AGENTS, NONSELECTIVE VERSUS CARDIOSELECTIVE AND VASODILATORY AGENTS

Generic name (Trade Names)	ISA‡	Plasma half-life (hr)	Lipid* solubility	First-pass effect	Loss by liver or kidney	Plasma protein binding %	Usual dose for angina	Usual doses as sole therapy for mild/moderate hypertension	IV dose (caution)
Noncardioselective									
Propranolol (Inderal®)	–	1–6	+++	++	Liver	90	120–140 mg/day; 3–4 divided doses but 80 mg 2× daily usually adequate. Start as for hypertension.	Start with 10–40 mg 2× daily to lessen side effects. Mean 160–320 mg/day, 1–2 doses; less with diuretic. Top dose 640–1000 mg/day	1–10 mg (0.1 mg/kg)
Oxprenolol† (Trasicor®)	++	2	++	++	Liver	80	As propranolol; Mean 160 mg/day.	160–800 mg/day; mean 260 mg/day, 444 mg, 2–3 divided doses.	1–12 mg†
Timolol (Blocadren®)	–	4–5	+	+	L,K	60	15–45 mg (in 3–4 divided doses)	20–60 mg/day = 160–480 mg propranolol, 2–3 doses/day.	0.4–1 mg†
Nadolol (Corgard®)	–	16–24	0	0	Kidney	20	80–240 mg 1× daily; mean 100 mg.	40–560 mg/day; mean 110 mg/day single dose.	–
Sotalol (Sotacor®)	–	15–17	0	0	Kidney	5	240–480 mg/day single dose.	80–320 mg/day; mean 190 mg.	10–20 mg†

Cardioselective									
Acebutolol (Sectral®)	++	8–12 (diacetolol)	0 (diacetolol)	++	L, K	15	200–400 mg 3 × daily 900 mg optimal.	400–1200 mg/day; can be given as a single dose.	12.5–50 mg†
Atenolol (Tenormin®)	–	6–9	0	0	Kidney	10	100 mg 1 × daily; 25 mg 2 × daily nearly as effective.	50–200 mg/day as single dose; usual dose 100 mg. Flat dose–response curve.	5–10 mg†
Metoprolol (Lopresso®, Betaloc®)	–	3	+	++	Liver	15	50–100 mg 3 × daily; mean total 200 mg.	50–400 mg/day, mean about 250 mg in 1 or 2 doses.	5–15 mg
Vasodilatory β-blockers									
Labetalol (Trandate®, Normodyne®)	–	3–4	+++	++	Liver	90	As for hypertension.	300–600 mg in 3 doses; top dose 2400 mg/day.	1–2 mg/kg
Pindolol (Visken®)	+++	4	+	+	L, K	55	2.5–7.5 mg 3 × daily	10–30 mg/day; mean 21 mg (some on diuretics); single dose.	–

* Octanol–water distribution coefficient (pH 7.4, 37°C) where 0 = <0.5; + = 0.5–2.0; ++ = 2–10; +++ = >10; see De Bono et al: Am Heart J 109:1212–1223, 1985. Data for plasma protein binding from same source. Loss = route of elimination of agent and pharmacologically active metabolites (Fig. 1-7). First-pass effect: ++ = high, + = moderate, 0 = low or none. † = not in USA; ISA = Intrinsic sympathomimetic activity. For other references, see Opie LH. Drugs and the Heart, Lancet, 1980, p 7.

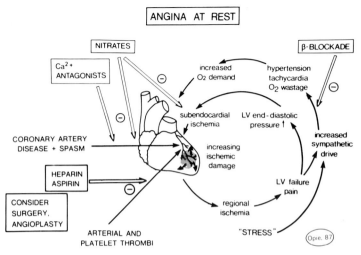

Fig. 1-3. Hypothetical mechanisms for angina at rest. The origin of this condition is partially related to coronary artery spasm in some patients. Once ischemia is established, vicious circle mechanisms may activate the sympathetic nervous system.

Combination Therapy

β-Blocking drugs are freely combined with nitrate vasodilators and calcium antagonists in the therapy of angina; they reduce the tachycardia resulting from nitrates and nifedipine. However, β-blockers should only be combined with verapamil and diltiazem with caution, as the combinations may occasionally produce extreme bradycardia or atrioventricular (AV) block.

Impaired LV function.   In patients with angina pectoris who have abnormal LV function, β-blockade may decrease the incidence of angina at the cost of lessening exercise tolerance; digitalis and diuretics can prevent this deterioration in exercise tolerance and reverse the cardiac enlargement induced by β-blockers.[20] Theoretically, β-blockers with either ISA or α-blocking properties depress myocardial function to a lesser extent and are preferred in such patients. Another alternative is the combination of nifedipine with a β-blocker.

β-Blockade withdrawal.   When β-blocking agents are suddenly withdrawn, angina may be exacerbated, sometimes resulting in myocardial infarction. Patients must be warned against abruptly stopping β-blocker therapy unless they are resting in bed when a sudden stop seems to be safe; added ISA (Fig. 1-1) as in pindolol may lessen withdrawal effects, but by the same token the resting heart rate is higher and there may be less protection against myocardial ischemia at rest. Treatment is by reintroduction of β-blockade.

Unstable Angina at Rest

In unstable angina (Fig. 1-3), it is important to distinguish between contributions to myocardial ischemia made by (1) coronary artery spasm that responds to calcium antagonists rather than β-blockade, (2) tachycardia and hypertension that respond to β-blockade, and (3) other mechanisms such as platelet aggregation and thrombosis that cannot be expected to respond well to either β-blockers or calcium antagonists, whereas specific antiplatelet agents (Chapter 8) may be more effective.

The clinical picture varies from threatened infarction when β-blockade benefits,[6] to short-lived attacks of chest pain (less than 15 minutes) when propranolol is less effective than verapamil.[7,18]

In patients with crescendo angina or prolonged ischemic chest pain poorly relieved by nitroglycerin and without evidence of Prinzmetal's angina, propranolol (initial dose 40 mg, increased to 80 mg 3× daily) is as effective as a calcium antagonist (diltiazem, initial dose 60 mg, followed by 120 mg also 3× daily).[49]

Prinzmetal's Variant Angina

β-Blockade is ineffective and may even be harmful, supposedly because of enhanced coronary spasm from unopposed α-receptor activity.[31] Such arguments favor calcium antagonists.

"Mixed" Angina, "Dynamic Stenosis," and Silent Ischemia

Much has been made of the possibility that coronary spasm contributes to the symptomatology of "mixed" angina, where in addition to ordinary effort angina, there may be anginal pain in response to cold or emotion or a varying exercise time before the onset of pain. The proposed mechanism may involve "dynamic stenosis" with a vasospastic element occurring at the site of organic stenosis. Despite cogent theoretical arguments, there appear to be few data proving that coronary spasm plays a role in "mixed" angina, and that therapy by calcium antagonism is better than β-blockade. Silent ischemic attacks, demonstrated by ST-deviations on the ambulatory ECG, are not necessarily evidence of coronary spasm, and appear to respond to β-blockade.[19]

ACUTE MYOCARDIAL INFARCTION

In acute myocardial infarction (AMI), very early IV β-blockade in patients without obvious clinical contraindications is now increasingly used despite occasional unpredictable hemodynamic effects. The risk of ventricular fibrillation (VF) may be lessened;[42,45] "infarct size" may be variably reduced by up to 30 percent.[20b,26,40] Theoretically, IV β-blockade is of most use in about the first 4 hours of the onset when VF might be most prevalent. For this use against VF, a nonselective agent like propranolol is probably best.[20b,30] The massive ISIS trial (the name of the river in Oxford, England) shows that about 150 patients need to be treated by early IV β-blockade (atenolol 5–10 mg) followed by oral therapy for one week to save one life.[27] Is this benefit really worth the effort and occasional risk? In the USA, metoprolol is the only β-blocker licensed for IV use in AMI; the package insert claims reduction of cardiovascular mortality without making it clear whether it is the early IV use or subsequent oral follow-up therapy that is beneficial.

Postinfarct Follow-up

In the postinfarct phase, β-blockade reduces the risk of sudden death and re-infarction. Timolol, propranolol, and metoprolol[43] are all effective, while β-blockers such as oxprenolol with ISA are ineffective.[52] (For selection of patients, see p 197.)

The only outstanding questions are: (1) whether low risk patients should be given β-blockade, which seems pointless because of their already excellent prognosis; (2) which β-blocker should be used—here it is safest to stick to those with documented efficacy and follow-up; (3) when to start—taking together the data on metoprolol and timolol, it seems reasonable to start as soon as the patient's condition allows but optimally once the patient has stablized at about 1–2 weeks; and (4) for how long should β-blockade be continued—in the absence of data to prove this point and bearing in mind the risk of β-blockade withdrawal in patients with angina, many clinicians are going to continue β-blockade administration "forever" once a seemingly successful result has been obtained. Yet unless adequate stratification of risk is undertaken postinfarct, many patients have to be treated for a long time before there is any benefit (an estimated 30 patient years of treatment for one extra year of life).[41] The high risk patients who should benefit most also have most contraindications to β-blockade.[25] Because of the possible benefit on mortality, β-blockers are usually preferred to calcium antagonists in postinfarct patients with angina or hypertension, although no good comparisons exist.

β-BLOCKERS FOR HYPERTENSION

Despite their widespread use, the exact mechanism whereby β-blockers lower blood pressure remains an open question. In general, the high doses

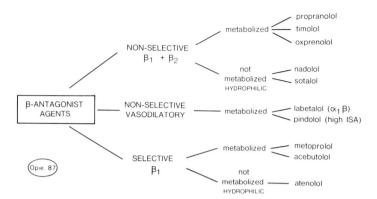

Fig. 1-4.   Classification of some common β-blocking agents. ISA = intrinsic sympathomimetic activity = partial agonist activity; such β-blocking agents not only inhibit β-adrenergic activity but also have limited sympathomimetic activity. Oxprenolol is not available in the USA. For details of lipid-solubility see Table 1-2.

previously used are now regarded as excessive, so that for propranolol 320 mg daily is usually the "top" dose. For initial therapy of hypertension, β-blockade is one of several strategies and is particularly suitable for younger patients with "increased adrenergic drive," nonsmoking men (see p 208), or for those patients with associated angina pectoris. Patients over 60 years, in whom the response rate may be as low as 20 percent, are better started on a mild diuretic or a mild vasodilator, while black patients are thought to respond better to a diuretic[11] or to the vasodilatory β-blocker, labetalol.[22]

Dosage.   Of younger patients with mild to moderate hypertension, 50–70 percent respond to "average" doses of β blockers,[10,11,12] but the optimal dose is hard to predict in the individual patient. It is best to start with a low dose to lessen the chances of initial fatigue, which is probably due in part to the fall in cardiac output. All patients should be closely observed in the early stages of treatment, both to assess side-effects and to gain the patient's confidence (hereby encouraging compliance). Though early uncontrolled observations suggested enhanced effects from higher doses, more recent studies with propranolol show little, if any, additional antihypertensive effect with doses above 80 mg/day, given either once or twice per day.[2,3,8] If the response to ordinary doses of β-blocker is inadequate, the preferred action is to add a diuretic and/or a vasodilator. Dose adjustment is more likely to be required with more lipid-soluble (lipophilic) agents, which have a high "first-pass" liver metabolism that may result in active metabolites (4-hydroxy-propranolol, diacetolol metabolite of acebutolol); the rate of formation will depend on liver blood flow and function. Hepatic metabolism of metoprolol and other lipid-soluble β-blockers also varies with genetic polymorphism[5] and interacting drugs such as verapamil.[38] Lipid-insoluble hydrophilic agents without hepatic metabolism include atenolol, sotalol, and nadolol (Fig. 1-4).

A pragmatic rule is that if a standard dose of a standard β-blocker does not work within a week, it is useless to try another.

Ideal β-Blocker for Hypertension

The ideal β-blocker for hypertension would be long-acting, cardioselective (Fig. 1-5), and usually effective in a standard dose; there would also be simple pharmacokinetics (no liver metabolism, little protein binding, no lipid-solubility, and no active metabolites). It would also possess vasodilatory β_2-ISA or α-blocking activity. Two compounds that go a long way to fulfil these requirements are atenolol (ideal pharmacokinetics; disadvantage: no ISA) and acebutolol (disadvantage: hepatic metabolism). Also widely used in the therapy of hypertension are metoprolol (cardioselective; disadvantages: no ISA, hepatic metabolism), nadolol or sotalol (long-acting, ideal pharmacokinetics; disadvantages: not cardioselective, no ISA), and labetalol (combined α-β-blocker; disadvantages: not cardioselective, no ISA, hepatic metabolism). Once a day therapy is satisfactory with atenolol, sotalol, nadolol and adequate doses of

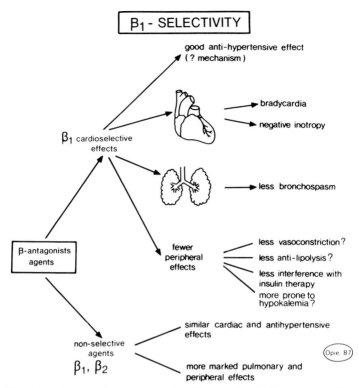

Fig. 1-5. β-antagonist agents may be either cardioselective or noncardiose-lective.

acebutolol, metoprolol, pindolol, propranolol, and oxprenolol, especially when the dose is high or when slow-release preparations (available for propranolol worldwide and for oxprenolol in Europe) are used. By contrast, in angina pectoris, long-acting compounds (atenolol) or ultralong-acting compounds (na-dolol, sotalol) have clear advantages; sometimes atenolol has to be used twice a day. When angina at rest is part of the picture, the higher heart rate and cardiac output of agents with ISA become undesirable.

Although propranolol is still the most widely used β-blocker, we can see no particular advantages for this drug with its high lipid solubility and high first-pass metabolism unless there is the coexistence of hypertension with some other condition in which experience with propranolol is greater than with other β-blockers (e.g. cardiomyopathy, migraine).

Side-Effects of β-Blockers

The three major mechanisms are through (1) central nervous penetration (dreams), (2) smooth muscle spasm (bronchospasm and cold extremities), and (3) exaggeration of the cardiac therapeutic actions (bradycardia, heart block, excess negative inotropic effect with heart failure). When patients are appropri-ately selected, double-blind studies show no differences between a cardio-selective agent such as *atenolol* and placebo.[9] This may be because atenolol does not penetrate the brain and should have lesser effects on bronchial and vascular smooth muscle than propranolol. When *propranolol* is given for hy-pertension, the rate of serious side-effects (bronchospasm, cold extremities, worsening of claudication) leading to withdrawal of therapy is about 10 per-cent.[9] The rate of withdrawal with atenolol is considerably lower (about 2 percent), but when it comes to dose-limiting side-effects then both agents can cause cold extremities, fatigue, dreams, worsening claudication, and broncho-spasm. The apparently lesser incidence of side-effects of 400 mg *acebutolol* compared with 100 mg atenolol[50] was not supported by strict statistical com-parisons; only acebutolol caused positive titers for antinuclear antibodies. Heart failure, although a theoretical hazard with β-blockade therapy, is in fact rare when the correct contraindications are observed (Table 1-1). Clearly if β-blockade is given to patients who are already severely ill, the risk of side-effects is increased.[4]

Occasionally β-blockade given alone produces a paradoxic hypertensive response, probably related to fluid retention in patients who start with low renin levels. During exercise, β-blockade reduces the total work possible by about 15 percent and increases the sense of fatigue. β-Blockers with high ISA (e.g. *pindolol*) or with added α-blockade (*labetalol*) cause less bradycardia and depression of cardiac output. Whether they cause fewer of the other side-effects such as cold extremities is still uncertain;[34] bronchospasm is reduced by labetalol.[24a] Pindolol, by maintaining sympathetic tone at night might create insomnia and dreams; propranolol acts likewise probably by central nervous system penetration.[15] Sometimes side-effects found with one β-blocker may be avoided by switching to another.

β-Blocker Co-Therapy with Other Drugs

Combinations of β-blockers with diuretics, vasodilators including hydralazine, methyldopa, calcium antagonists, angiotensin-converting enzyme (ACE) inhibitors, and α-blocking agents have all been successful in the therapy of hypertension. β-Blockade tends to counter the hypokalemic effect of some diuretics and the tachycardia induced by some vasodilators. **When monotherapy with a β-blocker begins to cause side-effects or is ineffective, there is much to be said for reducing the dose and adding a diuretic or a vasodilator.** Combinations of β-blockers with reserpine do not make sense (reserpine acts by catecholamine depletion), while the combination of β-blockade with clonidine is risky because the α-mediated rebound hypertension following sudden clonidine withdrawal may be exaggerated if the β-blocker is continued.

Diuretics plus β-blockers.   When combined with β-blockade, the dose of thiazide diuretics need be no more than 12.5 or at the most 25 mg daily.[35] Single-tablet combinations of β-blocker and diuretic are now being promoted for hypertension, but none should be used without a thorough knowledge of the properties and side-effects of both components. Particular problems arise when physicians are not aware that the combination contains a β-blocker (and therefore incorrectly give the combination to patients with asthma or early heart failure, for example) or when the dose of thiazide diuretic in the combination is high so that multiple doses lead to thiazide excess. Ideally, the total daily dose of β-blocker-thiazide combination should contain no more than 12.5 mg hydrochlorothiazide or 2.5 mg bendrofluazide or a similar low dose of another diuretic. Such low doses are not available as combination tablets with standard β-blocking doses. Double the ideal diuretic doses are provided in the USA by *Timolide®* (10 mg timolol, 25 mg hydrochlorothiazide) or *Corzide®* (80 mg nadolol, 5 mg bendrofluazide). Neither combination agent has a potassium-retaining component, provided in Europe by *Kalten®* with 50 mg atenolol, 25 mg hydrochlorothiazide and 2.5 mg amiloride.

β-Blocker-nifedipine (see p 44).   This combination is hemodynamically sound, with the powerful afterload reduction achieved by nifedipine offsetting the bradycardia and negative inotropic effects of β-blockade. There is an added hypotensive effect. Such combination therapy may be used both in mild to moderate hypertension not responding to monotherapy,[20a] and in severe or refractory hypertension when further combination with a diuretic is usual.[29a] In Europe, combination acebutolol-nifedipine tablets are available, and atenolol-nifedipine will shortly be introduced *(Tenif®,* atenolol 50 mg, slow nifedipine 20 mg).

Drug interactions.   Cimetidine reduces hepatic blood flow and therefore increases blood levels of propranolol (but not of agents such as atenolol, sotalol, and nadolol that are not metabolized in the liver). Verapamil may raise blood levels of metoprolol.[38] Nonsteroidal anti-inflammatory drugs (NSAIDs) such as indomethacin attenuate the antihypertensive effects of β-blockers and of thiazide diuretics.[51]

ARRHYTHMIAS

Both supraventricular and ventricular arrhythmias may respond to β-blocker therapy. The possible cardiodepressant effects of β-blockers argue against their use for arrhythmias when there are numerous alternative agents. In AMI, however, the desirable combination of a proven effect against VF and the possibility of "reduction of infarct size" has led to the increasing use of IV β-blockade although such use is still very far from general. A nonselective agent may be best (p 12). In the therapy of supraventricular tachycardias, verapamil (and diltiazem) are now the agents of first choice. β-Blockers are particularly effective in arrhythmias caused by increased circulating catecholamines (pheochromocytoma, anxiety, postoperative states, and some exercise-related arrhythmias) or by increased cardiac sensitivity to catecholamines (thyrotoxicosis), and in the arrhythmias of mitral valve prolapse. In the arrhythmias of digitalis intoxication, β-blockade is occasionally used, but coexisting AV block usually makes phenytoin or lidocaine a better choice. β-Blockers may stop the tachycardias of tricyclic antidepressant overdose.

In *chronic atrial fibrillation*, without LV failure, β-blockade can be used to reduce ventricular response rate. (See next section.)

IV dosage.   With the ECG and blood pressure monitored and with atropine at hand, β-blockers may be given slowly IV over 5–20 minutes (Table 1-2).

CARDIOMYOPATHIES, CONGENITAL HEART DISEASE, AND MITRAL STENOSIS

In *hypertrophic obstructive cardiomyopathy*, propranolol is standard therapy although increasingly challenged by verapamil. High dose propranolol (average 462 mg/day)[23] is thought to reduce ventricular arrhythmias. Lower dose β-blockade (mean: 280 mg propranolol or equivalent per day[36]) has been ineffective against the arrhythmias; amiodarone therapy may be required in patients at risk of sudden death.[37]

In *congestive cardiomyopathy*, low dose β-blockade may also be added very cautiously to conventional therapy especially when there is resting tachycardia; this indication remains highly controversial although increasingly supported by recent evidence.[21]

In *Fallot's tetralogy*, propranolol 2 mg/kg 2× daily is usually effective against the cyanotic spells, probably acting by inhibition of right ventricular contractility.

In *mitral stenosis* with sinus rhythm, β-blockade benefits by decreasing resting and exercise heart rates, thereby allowing longer diastolic filling and improved exercise tolerance.[32] In mitral stenosis with chronic atrial fibrillation, β-blockade may have to be added to digoxin to obtain sufficient ventricular slowing during exercise (see p 203).

OTHER INDICATIONS FOR β-BLOCKADE

Thyrotoxicosis

Together with antithyroid drugs or radioiodine, or as the sole agent before surgery,[13] β-blockade is now commonly used in thyrotoxicosis, although the hypermetabolic state is not decreased. β-Blockade controls tachycardia, palpitations, tremor, and nervousness and reduces the vascularity of the thyroid gland, thereby facilitating operation.[13] In *thyroid storm*, IV propranolol can be useful at a rate of 1 mg/min (to a total of 5 mg at a time); circulatory collapse is a risk, so that β-blockade should only be used in thyroid storm if LV function is normal as shown by conventional noninvasive tests. Because control of tachycardia is important, the choice of agent usually falls on those without ISA (see ISA, p 13). A cardioselective agent is advisable when there is bronchospasm.

Anxiety States

Although propranolol is most widely used in anxiety (and licensed for this purpose in several countries including the USA), probably all β-blockers are effective acting not centrally but by a reduction of peripheral manifestations of anxiety such as tremor.[28] Very low doses of either propranolol or oxprenolol can improve everyday skills impaired by anxiety. β-Blockade is usually thought to be the therapy of choice for hypertension related to stress or anxiety, but combination β-α-blockade might be more logical to combat excess adrenergic drive.

Glaucoma

The use of local timolol eye solution (Timoptic® in USA, Timoptol® in UK) is established for open-angle glaucoma; care needs to be exerted with occasional systemic side-effects such as sexual dysfunction,[24] bronchospasm, and cardiac depression. *Betaxolol* is a new cardioselective long-acting β-blocker, about to be introduced in the USA for glaucoma. (Oral betaxolol is used as an antihypertensive in Europe.)

Migraine

Propranolol (80–240 mg daily) reduces the incidence of migraine attacks in 60 percent of patients, as also do some other β-blockers without ISA,[44] which presumably inhibit the beneficial vasoconstriction. The anti-migraine effect is prophylactic, not for attacks once they have occurred. If there is no benefit within 4–6 weeks of top doses, propranolol should be tailed off and discontinued.

OVERDOSE OF β-BLOCKERS

Bradycardia may be countered by IV atropine 1–2 mg; if serious, temporary transvenous pacing may be required. When an infusion is required, glucagon (2.5–7.5 mg/hr) is the drug of choice because it stimulates formation of cyclic AMP by a route that bypasses the occupied β-receptor. Logically an infusion of amrinone (Chapter 6) should help cyclic AMP to accumulate. Alternatively, dobutamine is given in doses high enough to overcome the competitive β-blockade (15 μg/kg/min). In patients without ischemic heart disease, an infusion (up to 0.10 μg/kg/min) of isoproterenol may be used.

WHICH β-BLOCKER?

The major clinical division is into those β-blockers that are cardioselective (β_1-selective) and the noncardioselective agents (Fig. 1-5). New emphasis is on vasodilator β-blockers including those with ISA (Fig. 1-6) and added α-blockade. Membrane stabilizing activity (MSA) remains of little clinical importance. Pharmacokinetic properties are increasingly emphasized with advantages for long-acting lipid-insoluble compounds—nadolol, atenolol, and (not available in the USA) sotalol. (For trade names see Table 1-2.)

Cardioselectivity (β_1-selectivity)

The noncardioselective β-blockers antagonize catecholamine effects at both cardiac β_1-receptors and at noncardiac β_2-receptors. Cardioselective agents (atenolol, metoprolol, acebutolol) are therefore preferable in patients with chronic lung disease or asthma or chronic smoking, peripheral vascular disease, and insulin-requiring diabetes mellitus. Cardioselectivity varies between agents. As judged by bronchospasm in asthmatics (fall in forced expiratory volume), atenolol is somewhat more cardiospecific than metoprolol and both are more so than acebutolol.[1] Cardioselectivity declines or is lost at high doses. **No β-blocker is completely safe in the presence of asthma; low dose cardioselective agents can be used with care in patients with bronchospasm or chronic lung disease or chronic smoking.** In angina and hypertension, cardioselective agents are just as effective as noncardioselective agents. In AMI and hypokalemia, nonselective blockers should theoretically be better antiarrhythmics than β_1-selective blockers.[30]

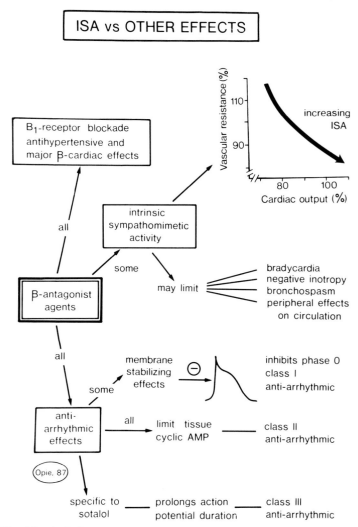

Fig. 1-6. Intrinsic sympathomimetic activity (ISA) and antiarrhythmic effects of some β-blockers.

Vasodilatory β-Blockers

Intrinsic Sympathomimetic Activity (ISA or Partial Agonist Activity)

Pindolol is the β-blocker with most ISA and nonselective β-blocking quali-ties (Fig. 1-6). *Acebutolol* has less ISA but is cardioselective. The effect of a β-blocker with ISA (Fig. 1-6) on resting heart rate depends upon the level of sympathetic stimulation at rest. If the resting sympathetic tone is high, a β-blocker with ISA reduces the resting heart rate. If the sympathetic activity is low, the heart rate either does not decrease or may increase. Compared to drugs without ISA, β-blockers with ISA lower resting heart rate and cardiac output to a lesser extent. With a high degree of ISA, such as xamoterol (investi-gational), the agent becomes more of an agonist than an antagonist with dominant inotropic qualities. When there is bronchospasm, a β-blocker with high ISA, such as pindolol, may diminish β-blockade-induced spasm, although cardioselectivity is more desirable because ISA may lessen the bronchodilator effects of β_2-stimulants such as albuterol in USA (Proventil®), salbutamol in UK (Ventolin®). ISA, like β-blockade, may be selective for β_1-receptors or be nonse-lective. β_1-selective ISA, as in the new agent xamoterol (not in the USA), im-pairs the hypotensive effect of β-blockade[33b] while maintaining a positive ino-tropic effect, so that xamoterol is mostly used in patients with modest degrees of heart failure (see p 104). ISA introduces a quality of potential β-receptor stimulation that is probably useful in patients with hypertension (provided that the ISA is β_2-stimulant), but not in patients with ischemic heart disease when a slow heart rate might be best. In elderly patients, where fatigue might be caused by limitation of cardiac output, a higher heart rate with ISA may improve the symptomatic response.

The potential disadvantage of ISA is the stimulation of the central nervous system at night, when sympathetic tone is low, with sleep impairment and fewer erections.[33a]

α-Blocking Activity

Labetalol is a combined α- and β-blocking agent that causes less bronchospasm and vasoconstriction than propranolol and lowers the blood pressure more rapidly; but these advantages are bought at the cost of two potential side-effects—postural hypotension with high doses and occasional retrograde ejaculation (α-blockade relaxes the bladder neck sphincter and is used in the therapy of prostatism). Besides α-blockade, labetalol may possess significant ISA.[47a] Labetalol is a more powerful β-blocker than α-blocker (β:α ratio 3:1 after oral and 7:1 after IV dosage) so that a high dose may be required for adequate α-blockade. Nevertheless, a standard dose of labetalol (200 mg 2 × daily) was as effective as atenolol (100 mg daily) in controlling angina in patients with coexisting hypertension.[29] For angina without hypertension, labetalol is not well documented. For black hypertensives or patients with airways obstruction, labetalol seems better than propranolol.[22,24a] IV labetalol is also effective for severe hypertension (Table 11-5) and is well-tested in pregnancy hypertension (IV or oral). The acute benefit in hypertension is explained by the vasodilator properties (see p 141).

Combined Vasodilatory β-Blocking Molecules

Bucindolol, a developmental drug, has a hydralazine-like moiety built into the molecule.

Optical isomers.   There are two optical isomers of propranolol—only the l-form is β-blocking while both possess MSA. Thus the ratio of β-blockade to MSA can be increased by penbutolol which has only the l-isomer; it is widely used in Germany. Whether this structural change really results in any properties of clinical significance remains to be shown.

Membrane stabilizing activity.   MSA, as in propranolol, is important experimentally because in high concentrations certain β-blockers have a quinidine-like, membrane-stabilizing effect on the action potential. Such activity is not relevant to clinical management of arrhythmias. There is no evidence that MSA is responsible for the negative hemodynamic effects of β-blocking agents. For example, propranolol (with MSA) and nadolol and timolol (without MSA) equally depress myocardial performance.

Renal Blood Flow

β-Blockers tend to lessen renal blood flow because they depress cardiac output. Ultimate excretion of β-blockers is usually by the kidneys, so in renal failure the dose may have to be lowered; but with pindolol the plasma half-life is unaltered in renal failure. There is no evidence (contrary to claims) that some β-blockers such as nadolol are better at maintaining glomerular filtration rates (GFR) in patients with renal impairment (for review, see reference 16, Table 2).

Antirenin Properties

All β-blockers reduce circulating renin levels. High ISA (as in pindolol) reduces this effect. Thus, in general, the more the heart rate falls with a β-blocker, the more the renin falls. The antihypertensive action of β-blockers is not directly related to the antirenin effect.

Pharmacokinetic Properties

The plasma half-life (Table 1-2) of propranolol is only 3 hours, but continued administration saturates the hepatic process that removes propranolol

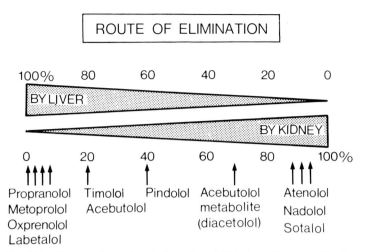

Fig. 1-7. Comparative routes of elimination of β-blockers. Those most hydrophilic and least lipid-soluble are excreted unchanged by the kidneys. Those most lipophilic and least water-soluble are largely metabolized by the liver. Note that the metabolite of acebutolol, diacetolol, is largely excreted by the kidney, in contrast to the parent compound. (Modified from Meier J: β-Adrenoceptor blocking agents: Pharmacokinetic differences and their clinical implications illustrated on pindolol. Cardiology 64 [suppl 1]:1–13, 1979; by permission of S. Karger AG, Basel. Data points for acebutolol and sotalol changed on basis of Smith et al: Br J Clin Pharm 16:253–258, 1983; and Antilla et al: Arch Pharm Toxicol 39:118–126, 1976.)

from the circulation; the active metabolite 4–hydroxypropranolol is formed, and the effective half-life then becomes longer. The biological half-life of propranolol and metoprolol (and all other β-blockers) exceeds the plasma half-life considerably, so that *2× daily dosage is effective even in angina pectoris.* Clearly, the higher the dose of any β-blocker, the longer the biologic effects. Long-acting compounds such as nadolol, atenolol, and slow-release oxprenolol (Slow Trasicor®, not in the USA) or slow-release propranolol (Inderal LA®) should theoretically be best for hypertension and ordinary angina, whereas shorter-acting drugs are preferable in unstable angina and threatened infarction when hemodynamic changes may call for withdrawal of β-blockade.

Brain penetration by certain compounds such as *propranolol* may be connected with vivid dreams[15] and subtle degrees of mental impairment.[47] Whether the beneficial anxiolytic effects of propranolol result from brain penetration is doubtful.[28] **Eventually even the lipid-insoluble β-blockers penetrate into the cerebrospinal fluid (CSF),**[14] which may explain why even atenolol produces some impairment of very fast mental reactions despite its lipid-insolubility.[46] Nonetheless atenolol produces far fewer central side-effects than propranolol.[21a]

Protein binding of β-blockers is variable (Table 1-2); propranolol, pindolol, labetalol, and oxprenolol are bound much more to plasma proteins than are the others. Hypoproteinemia calls for lower doses of the highly bound compounds.

First-pass liver metabolism is found especially with the highly lipid-soluble compounds such as propranolol, labetalol, and oxprenolol; acebutolol, metoprolol, and timolol have only modest lipid-solubility yet with hepatic clearance; first-pass metabolism varies greatly between patients and alters the dose required. In liver disease or low-output states the dose should be decreased. First-pass metabolism produces active metabolites with, in the case of propranolol, properties different from those of the parent compound. Acebutolol produces large amounts of diacetolol, also cardioselective with ISA, but with a longer half-life and chiefly excreted by the kidneys (Fig. 1-7).[14]

Ideal kinetics. Lipid-insoluble hydrophilic compounds (*atenolol, sotalol, nadolol*) are excreted only by the kidneys (Fig. 1-7) and have low brain penetration. In patients with renal or liver disease, the simpler pharmacokinetic patterns of lipid-insoluble agents make dosage easier. As a group, these agents have low protein binding (Table 1-2). The diacetolol metabolite of acebutolol may fall into this category (Table 1-2).

New β-Blockers

Of the large number of β-blockers in development, the ideal agent for hypertension or angina might have (1) advantageous pharmacokinetics (lipid-insolubility); (2) cardioselectivity; (3) long duration of action; and (4) vasodilatory properties.

Betaxolol.   This agent is a new long-acting lipid-soluble cardioselective β-blocker (oral dose 10–40 mg once daily) now available in Europe and undergoing trials for angina and for hypertension elsewhere.[15a] For its use in glaucoma, see p 12.

Esmolol.   Recently introduced in the USA by American Critical Care, esmolol (Brevebloc®) is an ultrashort-acting cardioselective β-blocker, rapidly converted to inactive metabolites by blood esterases. The dose range is 50–400 μg/kg/min intravenously,[24b] and full recovery from β-blockade occurs within 30 minutes in patients with a normal cardiovascular system. The indications of esmolol are situations where "on-off" control of β-blockade is desired, as in supraventricular tachycardia[17] or perioperative tachycardias or perioperative hypertension. Exploratory uses are in unstable angina and AMI, when the hemodynamic effects of β-blockade may be uncertain.

CONCLUSIONS

β-Blockade is very effective treatment, alone or combined with other drugs, in 70–80 percent of patients with classic angina or 50–70 percent of those with mild to moderate hypertension; elderly or black hypertensives respond less well. Propranolol (Inderal®) is likely to remain the gold standard because it is still so widely used and licensed for so many different indications, including angina, hypertension, arrhythmias, migraine, anxiety states, and postinfarct follow-up. However, propranolol is not β_1-selective. Being lipid-soluble, propranolol has a high brain penetration and undergoes extensive hepatic first-pass metabolism. Propranolol also has a short half-life so that it must be given 2× daily (4× daily, still sometimes used, is bad practice because it leads to poor patient compliance). **Other compounds are increasingly used because of specific attractive properties:** cardioselectivity (atenolol, metoprolol, acebutolol); lipid-insolubility and no hepatic metabolism (atenolol, nadolol, sotalol); long action (nadolol > sotalol > atenolol); ISA to help avoid myocardial depression (pindolol, acebutolol); added α-blockade to achieve more arterial dilation (labetalol); and superior antiarrhythmic properties (sotalol—not in the USA). Every clinician should become thoroughly familiar with only a limited number of β-blocking agents, one of which must be cardioselective. Where side-effects are encountered, they can sometimes be avoided by a switch to another β-blocker. Generally, if one agent in adequate dose will not work, nor will another; nor should one β-blocker be added to another in the hope of improved therapeutic response. As concluded in previous editions of this book, in clinical practice the differences between existing β-blockers are slight and hardly justify the vast commercial pressures applied in competitive promotion.

REFERENCES

References from Previous Edition

For details see previous edition of Opie et al, Drugs for the Heart, American Edition. Orlando, FL, Grune & Stratton, 1984, pp 1–22.

1.   Decalmer PBS, Chatterjee SS, Cruickshank JM, et al: Br Heart J 40:184–189, 1978
2.   Douglas-Jones AP, Baber NS, Lee A: Eur J Clin Pharmacol 14:163–166, 1978

3. Galloway DB, Glover SC, Hendry WG, et al: Br Med J 2:140–142, 1976
4. Greenblatt DJ, Koch-Weser J: Am Heart J 86:478–484, 1973
5. Lennard MS, Silas JH, Freestone S, et al: New Engl J Med 307:1558–1560, 1982
6. Norris RM, Clarke ED, Sammel NL, et al: Lancet ii:907–909, 1978
7. Parodi O, Simonetti I, L'Abbate A, et al: Am J Cardiol 50:923–928, 1982
8. Serlin MJ, Orme MLE, Baber NS, et al: Clin Pharmacol Ther 27:586–592, 1980
9. Simpson WT: Postgrad Med J 53 (suppl 3):162–167, 1977
10. Veterans Administration Cooperative Study Group on Antihypertensive Agents: JAMA 237:2303–2310, 1977
11. Veterans Administration Cooperative Study Group on Antihypertensive Agents: JAMA 248:1996–2003, 1982
12. Wilcox RG, Hampton JR: Br Heart J 46:498–502, 1981
13. Zonszein J, Santangelo RP, Mackin JF, et al: Am J Med 66:411–416, 1979

New References

14. Abernethy DR, Arendt RM, Greenblatt DJ: Pharmacologic properties of acebutolol: Relationship of hydrophilicity to central nervous system penetration. Am Heart J 109: 1120–1125, 1985.
15. Betts TA, Alford C: β-Blocking drugs and sleep. A controlled trial. Drugs 25 (suppl 2): 268–272, 1983
15a. Beresford R, Heel RC: Betaxolol. Drugs 31:6–28, 1986
16. Brater DC, Anderson S, Kaplan NM, et al: Beta-adrenergic blockade alone does not decrease renal perfusion in black hypertensives. J Hypertens 2:43–48, 1984
17. Byrd RC, Sung RJ, Marks J, et al: Safety and efficacy of esmolol (ASL-8052: an ultrashort-acting beta-adrenergic blocking agent) for control of ventricular rate in supraventricular tachycardias. J Am Coll Cardiol 3:394–399, 1984
18. Capucci A, Bassein L, Bracchetti D, et al: Propranolol v. verapamil in the treatment of unstable angina. A double-blind cross-over study. Eur Heart J 4:148–154, 1983
19. Chierchia S, Smith G, Morgan M, et al: Role of heart rate in pathophysiology of chronic stable angina. Lancet ii:1353–1357, 1984
20. Crawford MH, LeWinter MM, O'Rourke RA, et al: Combined propranolol and digoxin therapy in angina pectoris. Ann Intern Med 83:449–455, 1975
20a. Daniels AR, Opie LH: Atenolol plus nifedipine for mild to moderate systemic hypertension after fixed doses of either agent alone. Am J Cardiol 57:965–970, 1986
20b. Editorial: Intravenous β-blockade during acute myocardial infarction. Lancet ii :79–80, 1986
21. Engelmeier RS, O'Connell JB, Walsh R, et al: Improvement in symptoms and exercise tolerance by metoprolol in patients with dilated cardiomyopathy: A double-blind, randomized, placebo-controlled trial. Circulation 72:536–546, 1985
21a. Engler RL, Conant J, Maisel A, et al: Lipid solubility determines the relative CNS effects of beta-blocking agents. J Am Coll Cardiol 7:25A, 1986
22. Flamenbaum W, Weber MA, McMahon FG, et al: Monotherapy with labetalol compared with propranolol. Differential effects by race. J Clin Hypertens 1:56–69, 1985
23. Frank MJ, Abdulla AM, Canedo MI, et al: Long-term medical management of hypertrophic obstructive cardiomyopathy. Am J Cardiol 42:993–1001, 1978
24. Fraunfelder FT, Meyer SM: Sexual dysfunction secondary to topical ophthalmic timolol. JAMA 253:3092–3093, 1985
24a. George RB, Light RW, Hudson LD, et al: Comparison of the effects of labetalol and hydrochlorothiazide on the ventilatory function of the hypertensive patient with asthma and propranolol sensitivity. Chest 88:815–818, 1985
24b. Gorczynski RJ, Quon CY, Krasula RW, Matier WL: Esmolol, in Scriabine A (ed): New Drugs Annual: Cardiovascular Drugs, Vol 3. New York, Raven Press, 1985, pp 99–119
25. Hansteen V, Moinichen E, Lorentsen E, et al: One year's treatment with propranolol after myocardial infarction: Preliminary report of Norwegian multicentre trial. Br Med J 284:155–160, 1982
26. International Collaborative Study Group: Reduction of infarct size with the early use of timolol in acute myocardial infarction. New Engl J Med 310:9–15, 1984
27. ISIS-1 Group: Randomized trial of intravenous atenolol among 16027 cases of suspected acute myocardial infarction. Lancet ii:57–65, 1986
28. James I, Savage I: Beneficial effect of nadolol on anxiety-induced disturbances of performance in musicians: A comparison with diazepam and placebo. Am Heart J 108:1150–1155, 1984
29. Jee LD, Opie LH: Double-blind trial comparing labetalol with atenolol in the treatment of systemic hypertension with angina pectoris. Am J Cardiol 56:551–554, 1985
29a. Jennings AA, Jee LD, Smith JA, et al: Acute effect of nifedipine on blood pressure and left ventricular ejection fraction in severely hypertensive outpatients. Predictive effects of acute therapy and prolonged efficacy when added to existing therapy. Am Heart J 111:557–563, 1986
30. Johansson BW, Dziamski R: Malignant arrhythmias in acute myocardial infarction.

Relationship to serum potassium and effect of selective and non-selective β-blockade. Drugs 28 (suppl 1):77–85, 1984

31. Kern MJ, Ganz P, Horowitz JD, et al: Potentiation of coronary vasoconstriction by beta-adrenergic blockade in patients with coronary artery disease. Circulation 67:1178–1185, 1983

32. Klein HO, Sareli P, Schamroth C, et al: Effects of atenolol on exercise capacity in patients with mitral stenosis with sinus rhythm. Am J Cardiol 56:598–601, 1985

33. Kostis JB, Lacy CR, Krieger SD, et al: Atenolol, nadolol and pindolol in angina pectoris on effort: Effect of pharmacokinetics. Am Heart J 108:1131–1136, 1984

33a. Kostis JB, Rosen RC: Beta-blocker effects on central nervous system. A controlled comparative study. J Am Coll Cardiol 7:25A, 1986

33b. Leonetti G, Sampieri L, Cuspidi C, et al: Does β_1-selective agonistic activity interfere with the antihypertensive efficacy of β_1-selective blocking agents? J Hypertens 3 (suppl 3):S243–S245, 1985

34. Louis WJ, McNeil JJ: Beta-adrenoceptor blocking drugs: The relevance of intrinsic sympathomimetic activity. Br J Clin Pharmacol 13 (suppl):317–320, 1982

35. MacGregor GA, Banks RA, Markandu ND, et al: Lack of effect of beta-blocker on flat dose response to thiazide in hypertension: Efficacy of low dose thiazide combined with beta-blocker. Br Med J 286:1535–1538, 1983

36. McKenna WJ, Chetty S, Oakley CM, et al: Arrhythmia in hypertrophic cardiomyopathy: Exercise and 48 hour ambulatory electrocardiographic assessment with and without beta-adrenergic blocking therapy. Am J Cardiol 45:1–5, 1980

37. McKenna WJ, Harris L, Rowland E, et al: Amiodarone for long-term management of patients with hypertrophic cardiomyopathy. Am J Cardiol 54:802–810, 1984

38. McLean AJ, Knight R, Harrison PM, et al: Clearance-based oral drug interaction between verapamil and metoprolol and comparison with atenolol. Am J Cardiol 55:1628–1629, 1985

39. Meier J: β-Adrenoceptor blocking agents: Pharmacokinetic differences and their clinical implications illustrated on pindolol. Cardiology 64 (suppl 1):1–13, 1979

40. MIAMI Trial Research Group: Metoprolol in acute myocardial infarction (MIAMI). A randomized placebo-controlled international study. Eur Heart J 6:199–226, 1985

41. Mitchell JRA: "But will it help my patients with myocardial infarction." The implications of recent trials for everyday country folk. Br Med J 285:1140–1148, 1982

42. Norris RM, Barnaby PF, Brown MA, et al: Prevention of ventricular fibrillation during acute myocardial infarction by intravenous propranolol. Lancet ii:883–886, 1984

43. Olsson G, Rehnqvist N, Sjogren A, et al: Long-term treatment with metoprolol after myocardial infarction: Effect on 3 year mortality and morbidity. J Am Coll Cardiol 5:1428–1437, 1985

44. Ryan RE: Comparative study of nadolol and propranolol in prophylactic treatment of migraine. Am Heart J 108:1156–1159, 1984

45. Ryden L, Ariniego R, Arnman K, et al: A double-blind trial of metoprolol in acute myocardial infarction. Effects on ventricular tachyarrhythmias. New Engl J Med 308:614–618, 1983

46. Salem SS, McDevitt DG: Central effects of beta-adrenoceptor antagonists. Clin Pharmacol Ther 33:52–57, 1983

47. Solomon S, Hotchkiss E, Saravay SM, et al: Impairment of memory function by antihypertensive medication. Arch Gen Psychiatry 40:1109–1112, 1983

47a. Tadepalli AS, Novak PJ: Intrinsic sympathomimetic activity of labetalol. J Cardiovasc Pharmacol 8:44–50, 1986

48. Thadani U, Davidson C, Singleton W, et al: Comparison of five beta-adrenoceptor antagonists with different ancillary properties during sustained twice daily therapy in angina pectoris. Am J Med 68:243–250, 1980

49. Theroux P, Taeymans Y, Morissette D, et al: A randomized study comparing propranolol and diltiazem in the treatment of unstable angina. J Am Coll Cardiol 5:717–722, 1985

50. Turner AS, Brocklehurst JC: Once-daily acebutolol and atenolol in essential hypertension: Double-blind crossover comparison. Am Heart J 109:1178–1183, 1985

51. Webster J: Interactions of NSAIDs with diuretics and β-blockers. Mechanisms and clinical implications. Drugs 30:32–41, 1985

52. Yusuf S, Peto R, Lewis JA, et al: β-Blockade during and after myocardial infarction: An overview of the randomized trials. Prog Cardiovasc Dis 27:335–371, 1985

Reviews

Editorial: Choice of a β-blocker. Med Lett 28:20–22, 1986

Prichard BNC, Tomlinson B: The additional properties of β-adrenoceptor blocking drugs. J Cardiovasc Pharmacol 8 (Suppl 4): S1–S15, 1986

U. Thadani
L. H. Opie

2

Nitrates

MECHANISM OF ACTION

In 1933 Sir Thomas Lewis held that the effect of amyl nitrite was probably due mainly to its powerful dilatation of the coronary vessels, rather than to its effect in lowering the blood pressure, as originally suggested by Lauder Brunton in Scotland in 1867. Emphasis swung back to the peripheral effect of nitrates when Gorlin, Brachfeld, and coworkers[16] found that overall coronary blood flow was unchanged by nitroglycerin. This conflict has been resolved by realizing that both coronary and peripheral effects are important.

Two current problems are: first, whether the numerous new nitrate preparations are more effective than those already in established use; and second, whether nitrate tolerance is a real clinical problem.

Vasodilatory Effects, Coronary and Peripheral

Three new observations now emphasize the effects of nitrates on the coronary arteries. First, in animal preparations nitrates can cause vasodilation* in the ischemic zone. Second, coronary artery spasm is an additional major factor in precipitating chest pain, even in the presence of coronary artery disease,[23] and nitrates are very effective against vasospastic angina and angina at rest.[10] Third, "dynamic stenosis" emphasizes that coronary artery spasm and organic stenosis can occur at the same site; the dynamic component responds to vasodilators such as nitrates[38] and calcium antagonists.

A distinction must be made between antianginal and vasodilator properties. Nitrates (1) redistribute blood flow along collateral channels and from epicardial to endocardial regions and (2) relieve coronary spasm and "dynamic stenosis" especially at epicardial sites.[38] Thus nitrates are "effective" vasodilators for angina; but dipyridamole and many other vasodilators are not, and may increase angina by diverting blood from the ischemic area—a "coronary steal" effect.

The peripheral hemodynamic effects of nitrates cannot, however, be ignored, because nitrates reduce the afterload and especially the preload of the heart (Fig. 2-1). Hence, nitrates are now being used not only for angina pectoris but also to unload the heart in left ventricular (LV) failure and in selected cases of myocardial infarction.[32]

---

*Terminology: Vasodilation vs vasodilatation. Because "vasodilators" and not "vasodilatators" is correct, "vasodilation" makes more sense although both forms are correct according to the Oxford English dictionary.

Drugs for the Heart, Second Expanded Edition
Copyright © 1987 by Grune & Stratton, Inc.

ISBN 0-8089-1840-0
All rights reserved.

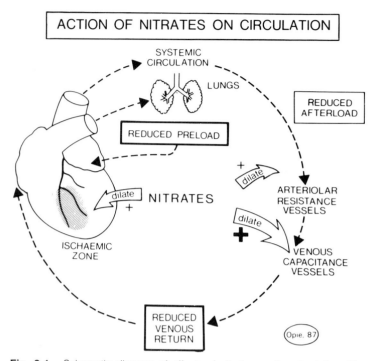

Fig. 2-1.   Schematic diagram of effects of nitrates on the circulation. The major effect is on the venous capacitance vessels.

Vascular Receptors

The cellular mechanism of these vascular effects may be as follows. An intact vascular endothelium is required for the vasodilatory effects of some other agents (thus serotonin physiologically vasodilates but constricts when the endothelium is damaged). Nitrates vasodilate whether or not the endothelium is intact. The postulated "nitrate receptor" is therefore likely to be situated on the myocyte rather than on the endothelium. Nitrates, after binding to the receptor, form the NO group which is thought to stimulate guanylate cyclase to produce cyclic GMP (Fig. 2-2). The cyclic nucleotide thus formed causes vasodilation either by inhibition of calcium ion entry or by interfering with actin-myosin interaction or by promoting calcium exit. Sulfhydryl (SH) groups are required for the stimulation of guanylate cyclase. Vascular tolerance occurs when the SH groups are oxidized by excess exposure to nitrates, which can occur within 10 minutes and is remedied by the SH donor n-acetylcysteine;[87] some similar principles may apply to man.[52] Why nitrates are better as venous than arteriolar dilators is not clear. Nitroglycerin powerfully dilates when injected into an artery, an effect that is probably limited in man by reflex vasoconstriction in response to preload reduction.[54]

Oxygen Demand

Effects of nitrates on the oxygen demand are even more important than effects on the oxygen supply unless coronary spasm is dominant. Nitrates increase the venous capacitance, causing pooling of blood in the peripheral veins and thereby a reduction in venous return and in ventricular volume, to lessen the stress on the myocardial wall and to reduce the oxygen demand. Furthermore, a modest fall in arterial pressure also reduces the oxygen demand, although offset by a reflex increase in heart rate. The latter can be attenuated by concurrent β-blockade. The beneficial effect of nitrates in congestive heart failure (CHF) depends on venodilation.

PHARMACOKINETICS

Nitroglycerin is absorbed from skin and oral mucosa, and less readily from the gut.

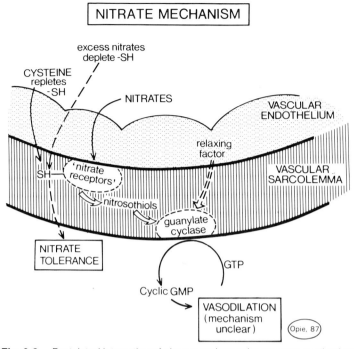

Fig. 2-2. Postulated interaction of nitrates and vascular receptor to stimulate guanylate cyclase to produce vasodilatory cyclic GMP. For this sequence, an intact vascular endothelium is not required so that nitrates can dilate even diseased coronary arteries. SH = sulfhydryl.

Sublingual nitroglycerin. Bioavailability is incomplete but clinical effects start within a minute or two and last up to an hour (Table 2-1); peak blood levels occur at 2 minutes and the half-life is 7 minutes.

Nitroglycerin ointment. Nitroglycerin ointment is slow in its onset of action. The effects persist for 4–6 hours, the amount of nitroglycerin absorbed being dependent upon the surface area covered by the ointment.

Nitroglycerin patches. Nitroglycerin patches containing nitroglycerin in a reservoir or matrix form give plasma levels that are fairly constant between 2–24 hours or longer. Although the nitroglycerin content of the patches is variable (Table 2-1), the amount of nitroglycerin delivered over 24 hours is dependent upon the surface area covered by the patch rather than the content of nitroglycerin.[59] The total nitroglycerin delivered over a 24-hour period is 0.5 mg/cm² from Transderm Nitro® and Nitrodur® patches and 0.625 mg/cm² from Nitrodisc® patches. Recent studies have failed to show 24-hour efficacy of the patches.

Isosorbide dinitrate. Isosorbide dinitrate is absorbed from the oral mucosa and gut, with slower onset and longer action; after liver metabolism, ultimate excretion of active mononitrate metabolites is by the kidney with a half-life of about 10 hours. Significant accumulation of intact isosorbide dinitrate occurs in plasma after 4× daily dosing at 30 mg, 60 mg and 120 mg for 1 week.[14] The elimination half-life is about 30 minutes after a sublingual dose, and 1.5–4 hours after oral dosing.[14] Metabolites of isosorbide dinitrate, i.e. 2– and 5–mononitrates, may also contribute to its action.[4,14]

Mononitrates. Mononitrates are active after absorption without liver metabolism and are of variable half-life, mostly long.[37] Isosorbide-5–mononitrate is nearly fully bioavailable after oral administration; it reaches peak plasma values between half to 2 hours before being excreted by the kidney partially unchanged and partially as an inactive glucuronide metabolite, with an elimination half-life of 4–6 hours. Its clinical efficacy correlates with its plasma concentration, being about 8 hours for 20 mg dose when the dosage is 20–40 mg 3× daily.[62]

TABLE 2-1

NITRATE PREPARATIONS: DOSES, PREPARATIONS, AND DURATION OF EFFECTS

Compound	Route	Preparation and dose	Duration of effects and comments	References
Amyl nitrite	Inhalation for diagnosis	2–5 mg	10 sec—10 min	
Nitroglycerin (trinitrin, TNT, glyceryl trinitrate)	(a) Sublingual	0.3–1.5 mg as needed Tablets: usually 0.3, 0.5, or 0.6 mg	1½ min–1 hr; peak blood levels at 2 min (½- time of 7½ min)	18
	(b) Spray	0.4 mg/metered dose, as needed	Effects apparent within 5 min, duration of effects not known	70
	(c) Percutaneous	2% ointment 15×15 cm or 12.5–40 mg	3–4 hr	2, 17, 39, 53
	(d) Transdermal patches			
	i) Nitrodur®	2%; 5 mg/cm²; 5–20 cm² 26–104 mg	Initial reports up to 24 hr; not confirmed	45, 55, 56, 67,
	ii) Transderm-Nitro®	5 mg/24 hr (10 cm² up to 10–25 mg/24 hr; 2.5 mg/24 hr to decrease dose gradually after effect achieved	Initial reports up to 24 hr; not confirmed	71, 74, 78, 83
	iii) Nitrodisc®	5 mg/24 hr released from each 8 cm² patch	Initial reports up to 24 hr; not confirmed	
	(e) Oral: sustained release	2.6 mg, 1–2 tablets 3× daily	8–12 hr	27, 40
	(f) Intravenous	0.6–12.0 mg/hr when urgent 0.1 mg bolus (care, lower dose for new sets) Tridil® 0.5 mg/ml Nitrostat® 0.8 mg/ml Nitrol® IV 0.8 mg/ml	During infusion and 30 min postinfusion high K^+ may cause VF	3, 47a, 58, 60, 72, 88

	Route / form	Dose	Effect / comments	Ref.
Isosorbide dinitrate (= sorbide nitrate)	(a) Sublingual	5–15 mg	Onset 5–10 min, effect up to 60 min	50
	(b) Oral*	5–80 mg 4–6 hourly (top dose 480 mg daily)	Exercise time raised for 2–8 hr (see text for tolerance)	9, 21, 22, 28, 29
	(c) Chewable	5 mg as single dose	Exercise time raised for 2 min–2½ hr	18
	(d) Oral; sustained release*	40 mg once or 2 × daily	2–6 hr free from angina	6
	(e) Intravenous	1.25–5.0 mg/hr (care: absorbed onto tubing)	Effective for repetitive attacks of angina at rest	10
	(f) Ointment	100 mg/24 hr	Not effective during continuous therapy	71
Isosorbide-5-mononitrate (not in USA)	Oral	10–40 mg 2–4 × day	6–10 hr	79, 81
	Sustained release	40–100 mg 1 × daily	Claimed 24 hr efficacy not proven	82, 84
Pentaerythritol tetranitrate	(a) Sublingual	10 mg as needed	45 min; classified as "possibly effective" in USA	19
Erythrityl tetranitrate	(a) Sublingual	5–10 mg as needed	10–45 min	19
	(b) Oral	10–30 mg 3 × daily, chew before swallowing	Effects begin after 20–30 min Not intended for acute attacks	

* Duration of hemodynamic effects has been most closely studied, but there is good correlation between such effects and antianginal action.

VF = ventricular fibrillation

NITRATES FOR ACUTE EFFORT ANGINA

Sublingual nitroglycerin is very well established in the therapy (Table 2-1) and diagnosis of angina of effort, yet may be ineffective—frequently because the patient has not received proper instruction. When angina starts, the patient should rest in the sitting position (standing promotes syncope, lying enhances venous return and heart work) and take sublingual nitroglycerin (0.3–0.5 mg) every 3 minutes until the pain goes or a maximum of 4–5 tablets have been taken.

Nitroglycerin spray (Nitrolingual Spray®) has recently become available and is an alternative to sublingual nitroglycerin. Each spray is absorbed over a wide mucosal surface and releases 0.4 mg of nitroglycerin/metered dose and the vial contains 200 doses. The effects are similar to those of sublingual nitroglycerin.[70]

Buccal nitroglycerin (Suscard Buccal® in UK, not in USA) is available in tablet form 1–5 mg and when placed against the gum above the upper incisor teeth, exerts immediate effects within a few minutes that persist for 4–5 hours. It has to be taken 3× daily. Its rapid onset and disappearance of action may be why tolerance seems not to develop.[69]

Isosorbide dinitrate may be given *sublingually* (5 mg) to abort an anginal attack and then exerts antianginal effects for about 1 hour. As the dinitrate requires hepatic conversion to the mononitrate, the onset of antianginal action must be slower than with nitroglycerin. After *oral* ingestion, hemodynamic and antianginal effects persist for several hours.[28] Single doses of isosorbide dinitrate confer longer protection against angina than can single doses of sublingual nitroglycerin (Table 2-1).

Side-effects and failure of nitrate therapy. (For side-effects, see Table 2-2.)   Causes of failure are: increasing severity of angina or development of nitrate-resistant myocardial ischemia; loss of potency of tablets; incorrect route of administration (some sublingual preparations should not be taken orally, and vice versa); arterial hypoxemia, especially in chronic lung disease (caused by increased venous admixture); and noncompliance, usually because of headaches. Dry mucous membranes impair oral absorption. Nitrates are more effective if taken before the expected onset of anginal pain. When nitrates are less effective than expected owing to tachycardia, combination with β-blockade should give better results. A wrong diagnosis may be made, because nitrates sometimes relieve the pain of esophageal spasm and renal or biliary colic. During prophylactic therapy with long-acting nitrates (next section), tolerance is a frequent cause of apparent failure.

LONG-ACTING NITRATES FOR ANGINA PROPHYLAXIS

The "nitrate controversy" relates to the long-held opinion that the so-called long-acting nitrates have no truly long-lasting effects. For the patient requiring protection for several hours, a single dose of long-acting nitrates, whether taken sublingually or orally, has obvious advantages.[15] There are long-lasting hemodynamic effects lasting for hours both in CHF[12] and in coronary heart disease without failure.[30] Single doses of long-acting nitrates can confer longer protection against angina than can single doses of sublingual nitroglycerin (Table 2-1). **What is unsure is whether long-acting nitrates are continuously effective if regularly taken over a prolonged period.**

Isosorbide dinitrate is frequently used in the prophylaxis of angina. An important question is whether regular therapy with isosorbide dinitrate gives long-lasting protection against angina. Improvement in exercise tolerance for up to 3 hours during acute and for up to 5 hours during sustained therapy with isosorbide dinitrate has been reported.[9] In a critical placebo-controlled study, exercise duration improved significantly for 6–8 hours after single oral doses of 15–120 mg isosorbide dinitrate, but for only 2 hours when the same doses were given repetitively 4× daily.[29] The development of partial tolerance to the antianginal effects during sustained therapy occurred, despite higher plasma isosorbide dinitrate concentrations during sustained therapy than those of acute therapy.[29] Conversely, high doses of isosorbide dinitrate are reported to

TABLE 2-2

PRECAUTIONS AND SIDE-EFFECTS IN USE OF NITRATES

Precautions

Nitrate tablets should be kept in airtight containers and stored in cold. Some nitrates are inflammable (especially the spray).

Serious Side-Effects

Syncope and hypotension from reduction of preload and afterload; alcohol may enhance. Treat by recumbency.

Tachycardia frequent, but unexplained bradycardia occasionally arises in acute myocardial infarction. Hypotension may cause cerebral ischemia. Prolonged high dosage can cause methemoglobinemia; treat by intravenous methylene blue.

Other Side-Effects

Headaches frequently limit dose. Facial flushing. Sublingual nitrates may cause halitosis.

Contraindications

In angina caused by *hypertrophic obstructive cardiomyopathy*, nitrates may exaggerate outflow obstruction and are contraindicated except for diagnosis. *Cardiac tamponade* or constrictive pericarditis; the already compromised diastolic filling may be aggravated by reduced venous return.

Relative Contraindications

Acute inferior myocardial infarction with right ventricular involvement; fall in filling pressure may lead to hemodynamic and clinical deterioration. In *cor pulmonale* and arterial hypoxemia, nitrates decrease arterial O_2 tension by venous admixture. Although *glaucoma* is usually held to be a contraindication, there is no objective evidence to show any increase in intraocular pressure (possible exception: amyl nitrite).[33] In *mitral stenosis*, nitrates may reduce the preload excessively.

Tolerance

Shown experimentally and clinically. Continuous therapy and high-dose frequent therapy leads to tolerance that low-dose interval therapy may avoid. Cross-tolerance likely.

Withdrawal Symptoms

Established in munition workers when withdrawal may precipitate symptoms and sudden death. Some evidence for a similar clinical syndrome. Therefore, only gradually discontinue long-term nitrate therapy.

reduce anginal frequency by more than 50 percent over many months of therapy.[77] That study was not placebo-controlled in a double-blind manner. Yet placebo alone is nearly as effective,[85] so that the frequency of angina is not, by itself, a sufficiently firm end-point. The duration of antianginal effects of long-term therapy with isosorbide dinitrate tablets thus remain highly controversial.

Transdermal isosorbide dinitrate, only recently being studied, is effective in angina for 8 hours when given acutely, whereas tolerance develops during sustained therapy.[71]

Transdermal nitroglycerin patches come in various sizes. For example, patches 5–30 cm^2 in size contain 2–5 mg/cm^2 nitroglycerin in different vehicles to permit the timed release of nitroglycerin over a 24-hour period. Despite initial claims of 24-hour efficacy,[22,31,49] many studies[45,55,68,74,78,83] with the exception of only two[75,76] have all failed to show prolonged improvement. The criteria used to show tolerance were the failure to maintain improvement in exercise tolerance or a decreased effect on exercise-induced ST-segment depression 24 hours after single or repeated application of patches of 5–45 cm^2. Thus nitroglycerin patches do not provide 24 hour prophylaxis against exertional angina. In unstable angina they may be more effective (for use in angina at rest, see p 26). *A new use for nitrate patches* is on the forearms of patients receiving prolonged IV infusion to keep the drip open.[91]

Nitroglycerin paste may be used for nocturnal angina or angina at rest. For convenience, it is applied to the skin of the chest. Usually oral isosorbide dinitrate is the long-acting agent of choice but the paste may be better in acute myocardial infarction (AMI) because it can be wiped off in the event of an adverse reaction.

Mononitrates (not yet available in the USA; Elantan®, Monit®, Mono-Cedocard® in UK) are logical successors to isosorbide dinitrate, because the latter becomes active by hepatic conversion to mononitrates. Thus the potentially variable effect of liver metabolism can be avoided and mononitrates have a high bioavailability. Dosage and effects of mononitrates are similar to those of isosorbide dinitrates; nitrate tolerance is likewise a potential problem. There have only been a few clinical reports comparing the mononitrate with the dinitrate preparations as far as effects on angina pectoris are concerned. The mean incidence of attacks and use of nitroglycerin during the mononitrate therapy was lower than during medication with slow-release dinitrate or with placebo.[65] What is particularly difficult to know is whether optimal doses of both preparations were used.

Nicorandil is a nicotinamide mononitrate, with hemodynamic effects similar to those of isosorbide dinitrate, currently under investigation.[40a]

Mononitrate tolerance.   In a placebo-controlled study, 50 and 100 mg of slow-release preparation of isosorbide-5-mononitrate increased exercise duration at 4 hours but not at 20 or 24 hours despite high plasma concentrations,[84] suggesting the rapid attenuation of antianginal effects. Furthermore, even with the ordinary formulation, tolerance develops when larger doses of isosorbide-5-mononitrate such as 50 mg $3\times$ or $4\times$ daily are used.[79] It may be possible to avoid such tolerance by giving lower doses such as 20 mg $2\times$ or $3\times$ daily.[79]

Causes of failure.   During therapy with long-acting preparations, two of the chief causes of failure are (1) **the development of tolerance,** treated by gradually decreasing the dose till there is a nitrate-free interval (see section on tolerance); (2) **worsening of the disease process,** treated by combination therapy (see p 29) while excluding aggravating factors such as hypertension, atrial fibrillation or anemia, and considering surgical intervention.

NITRATES FOR ANGINA AT REST

In angina at rest and unstable angina, nitrates (both short-acting and long-acting) are widely used but there is surprisingly little objective evidence of their long-term efficacy on morbidity or mortality.

IV nitroglycerin is very effective in the management of patients with unstable angina. The initial starting dose, usually 5–10 μg/min, that can be titrated up to 200 μg/min or higher depending upon the clinical course and aiming at a fall of mean blood pressure of 10 percent, the infusion being maintained for up to 36 hours.[60] IV therapy, given up to 5 days, reduced the number of episodes of rest angina, the requirement for sublingual nitroglycerin, and the dose of morphine needed in over 90 percent of patients with angina at rest not responding to standard nitrate therapy, whether or not they were also receiving propranolol.[58] In some patients the dose has to be increased to control anginal episodes during maintenance therapy. IV therapy allows more rapid titration to an effective dose and permits rapid reversal of hemodynamic effects if an adverse reaction develops. IV nitroglycerin is also used for relief of coronary spasm occurring during angiography; some IV preparations contain enough K^+ to cause risk of ventricular fibrillation (VF).[72,88]

IV isosorbide dinitrate, infused in patients with repetitive episodes of angina at rest at a rate of 1.25–5.0 mg/hr, relieves pain and reduces the incidence of ischemic episodes as judged by spontaneous ST-deviations[10] with few side-effects. Why **the IV route is so much more effective than the oral route,** is not well understood. However, the blood levels are almost $10\times$ higher for equivalent doses given IV than when given orally,[80] stressing the poor bioavailability of oral isosorbide dinitrate, due to extensive presystemic metabolism.

Nitrate patches are frequently used in angina at rest despite evidence that tolerance to the antianginal effect develops within 24 hours. There are no good data to justify a prolonged antianginal efficacy. A change over from IV nitroglycerin to patches can be made without any problems;[60] about 20–25 mg/24 hr was the equivalent of about 120 mg/24 hr of IV nitroglycerin, using a reduction of arterial pressure by 10 percent as end-point.

Nitroglycerin ointment, likewise frequently used, is subject to the same reservations.

In *Prinzmetal's angina at rest*, caused by coronary artery spasm, nitroglycerin is given in acute attacks and long-acting nitrates for prophylaxis.

Isosorbide dinitrate (mean titrated daily dose, 75 mg) was about as effective as nifedipine (mean titrated daily dose, 65 mg) in a double-blind trial over 5 weeks.[51] Combination of nitrates with one of the calcium antagonists (verapamil, nifedipine, or diltiazem) is usual.

ACUTE MYOCARDIAL INFARCTION

In AMI, nitrates are effective in carefully monitored patients who have LV failure and pulmonary congestion.[47a] A nitroglycerin infusion at an initial dose of 5–10 μg/min is titrated upwards under careful hemodynamic monitoring. This form of therapy should not be used indiscriminately.[25,34] A fall in cardiac output with clinical deterioration may occur especially in patients with acute inferior myocardial infarction with right ventricular involvement who are highly dependent on the preload. Therefore IV nitroglycerin should be reserved for those who have postinfarct angina and/or LV failure.

Mortality in Acute Infarction

When pooling the data from several studies (a procedure not statistically immaculate), it seems that nitrates may reduce mortality in the early phases of AMI.[92]

CONGESTIVE HEART FAILURE

Both short- and long-acting nitrates are used in the therapy of acute and chronic heart failure. Their dilating effects are more pronounced on veins than on arterioles, so they are best suited to patients with raised pulmonary wedge pressure and clinical features of pulmonary congestion.

In *acute pulmonary edema*, from various causes including AMI, nitroglycerin can be strikingly effective. There is, however, some risk of precipitious falls in blood pressure and of tachycardia or bradycardia. Sublingual nitroglycerin in repeated doses of 0.8–2.4 mg every 5–10 minutes can relieve coarse rales and dyspnea within 15–20 minutes with a fall of LV filling pressure and a rise in cardiac output.[8] Isosorbide dinitrate has a similar effect.[7] IV nitroglycerin, however, is usually a better method to administer nitroglycerin as the dose can be rapidly adjusted upwards or downwards depending upon the clinical and hemodynamic response. One study compared IV isosorbide dinitrate with IV furosemide and the hemodynamic consequences of the nitrate seemed preferable.[66] Little has been reported on the combination of nitrates with conventional therapy in acute pulmonary edema.

In *severe CHF*, nitrates may be used as the sole vasodilator agent (as in mitral stenosis[43]), or added to converting enzyme inhibitors, hydralazine, or nifedipine. Excess reduction of the preload may lead to syncope or hypotension. IV nitroglycerin has also been combined with dopamine.[61] Oral isosorbide dinitrate, 20–80 mg 4 × daily, can be added to digitalis and diuretics[44] and to hydralazine in chronic oral therapy of heart failure[24,44a] with beneficial hemodynamic and symptomatic effects. So too has nitroglycerin paste been used.

Tolerance may develop. Isosorbide dinitrate (orally 40 mg 4 × daily), given to 16 patients with severe CHF, increased the maximal exercise duration when compared with placebo.[13] The dinitrate was effective over a 2-month period in one study[48] and a dose of 40 mg 4 × daily was better than placebo, during 3 months treatment in another study.[21] In another study, however, hemodynamic tolerance developed and was restored by discontinuation of therapy for 36 hours.[5] (For isosorbide plus hydralazine, see p 28.)

Nitrate patches have also given variable results varying from only transient benefit[46,56,67] to sustained effects over 24 hours.[73] The fact that the ideal dose could be at least 60 mg/24 hr[56] suggests at least partial tolerance.

POST-BYPASS HYPERTENSION; HYPERTENSION WITH LV FAILURE

IV nitroglycerin controls hypertension and reduces myocardial ischemia following coronary artery bypass surgery; the doses required are variable, up to 1 mg/min or higher may be required.[57] Similar protocols are sometimes followed for the therapy of severe essential hypertension especially when complicated by LV failure with pulmonary congestion.

NITRATE TOLERANCE

"In contradistinction to the conclusions of my previous reviews of this subject, I now feel that sufficient clinical investigational data exists to support the concept that nitrate tolerance is relevant in some patients" states Abrams.[36] Many apparently conflicting studies can be resolved by taking into account the exact dosage schedule—thus effort tests in the morning may show an apparent absence of nitrate tolerance, yet the tolerance that had been achieved during the previous day could have worn off during the night.

Effort angina.   Recent studies by Thadani et al[29] and Parker and others[71] show that repetitive dosage of isosorbide dinitrate or mononitrates[81] leads to a decreased effect on effort tolerance. Even worse, the efficacy of 24-hour release patches may wear off completely after about 12 hours, despite what should have been (not measured) sustained blood nitrate levels over 24 hours.[74] The relatively modest benefit achieved with sustained release nitroglycerin (6.5 mg 3× daily) over 2 weeks of therapy[40] could be the result of partial tolerance. On the other hand, tolerance can seemingly be avoided by interval-dosing,[41,47,79] which may explain why some nitrate efficacy seems to be kept during chronic sustained oral therapy (see-saw blood levels) in contrast to loss of efficacy with the nitrate patches (sustained blood levels). Even a short nitrate-free interval of a few hours could theoretically restore sensitivity. **While this controversy continues, it is reasonable to (1) give isosorbide dinitrate or mononitrates with a dose-free interval at night (or during the day if angina is chiefly nocturnal); (2) avoid an excessively high dose. Thus two doses of isosorbide dinitrate or mononitrate of about 20 mg each during the day (morning and midday) could be the "average" dose designed to avoid tolerance during the therapy of effort angina.**

Angina at rest.   IV nitroglycerin or isosorbide is frequently given for 24–36 hours and the clinical impression is that benefit is sustained, although in some patients higher and higher doses are needed to control anginal attacks. The plasma concentrations of an IV infusion are extremely high,[80] over 100× those reached during sublingual administration of nitroglycerin.[89] Thus far there are no studies on possible tolerance during unstable angina. Although it is frequent custom to change from IV nitrates to nitrate patches[60] or to high-dose sustained oral release preparations or to nitroglycerin ointment every 4–6 hours, first principles would suggest that efficacy is likely to be better maintained with high-dose oral isosorbide dinitrate given 4× daily with a 10 hour interval-free period at night (or during the day). As yet, no firm recommendations can be made.

Congestive heart failure.   The maintained benefit of oral isosorbide dinitrate 40 mg 4× daily,[21,48] also in combination with hydralazine,[44a] does not prove that there was no tolerance; as Cohn[44] points out, a test dose after 3 months was given 16 hours after the last dose so that hemodynamic effects could, theoretically, have been restored. Further, efficacy of 24-hour release nitroglycerin patches may wear off completely by 4 hours in patients with chronic heart failure.[67] Thus also in the therapy of chronic CHF, nitrate tolerance should be considered if the response seems to wane or if sustained release preparations of isosorbide or nitroglycerin are used.[56a]

Nitrate tolerance may attenuate the therapeutic effects, especially in the case of long-acting nitrates. A nitrate-free interval should be built into the dose regime whenever possible. Yet there are such individual and wide dose-response spectra that each patient merits specific evaluation of the optimal dose.

Nitrate Cross-Tolerance

Long and short-acting nitrates are frequently combined.[35] However, the issue of tolerance with repetitive doses of long-acting nitrates remains a problem in patients already receiving isosorbide dinitrate. In patients already receiving isosorbide dinitrate, addition of sublingual nitroglycerin gives a further small (10 percent) therapeutic effect without nitrate cross-tolerance in one study.[20] Hypotensive effects of sublingual nitroglycerin or sublingual isosorbide dinitrate are, however, rapidly attenuated during chronic therapy with oral isosorbide dinitrate.[5,30] Logically, tolerance to long-acting nitrates should cause cross-tolerance to short-acting nitrates, as shown for the capacitance vessels of the forearm.[63]

COMBINATION THERAPY FOR ANGINA

β-Blockade and Nitrates

β-Blockade is often combined with nitrates in the therapy of angina (Table 2-3). Both β-blockers and nitrates decrease the oxygen demand and nitrates increase the oxygen supply; β-blockade cancels the tachycardiac effect of nitrates. β-Blockade tends to increase heart size, nitrates to decrease it. Anginal patients on β-blockers are better able to withstand pacing-stress when nitroglycerin is added,[26] and patients already receiving β-blockade respond no less well than others to nitroglycerin.[11] The combination of isosorbide dinitrate (mean daily dose, 90 mg) and β-blockade (propranolol mean dose 120 mg/day) is more effective than β-blockade by itself,[64] although less effective than the combination propranolol-nifedipine.

Calcium Antagonists and Nitrates

In the therapy of angina of effort or rest, verapamil, nifedipine or diltiazem can be combined with nitrates (see Chapter 3 for calcium antagonists). In a double-blind trial in 47 patients with effort angina, verapamil 80 mg 3× daily decreased the use of nitroglycerin tablets by 25 percent and prolonged the exercise time by 20 percent.[1]

Nifedipine, when added to propranolol and titrated to the maximum tolerated dose (mean 77 mg/day) and then given for 3 weeks, was more effective in effort angina than isosorbide dinitrate likewise titrated and given.[64]

Nitrates, β-Blockers, and Calcium Antagonists

Such combined antianginal therapy, frequently deemed to be "maximal," may be less effective than only two of the components, possibly because triple therapy predisposes to excess hypotension.[86] High-dose diltiazem, when added to maximum tolerated doses of propranolol and isosorbide dinitrate, improved persistent effort angina.[42] However, the high daily dose of dinitrates used (mean 137 mg daily) suggests that nitrate tolerance had occurred. There is also added benefit of nifedipine after nitrates and β-blockers.[90] Individual

TABLE 2-3

PROPOSED STEP-CARE FOR ANGINA OF EFFORT

1. General therapy: History and physical examination to exclude valvular disease, anaemia, hypertension, thromboembolic disease, and heart failure. Check risk factors for coronary artery disease (smoking, hypertension, blood lipids, diabetes).

2. Nitrates, short/long-acting given *intermittently* as needed to control pain.

3. *Intermittent* short/long-acting nitrates plus β-adrenergic blocker
                                      or
    Intermittent short/long-acting nitrates plus calcium antagonist.

4. *Intermittent* short/long-acting nitrates plus calcium antagonists plus β-blocker (triple therapy).

5. Failure to respond to medical therapy and/or left main stem lesion requires bypass surgery.

6. In selected patients PTCA* may be attempted at any stage.

As an alternative to steps 3–4, replace intermittent long-acting nitrates by *prophylactic long-acting nitrates* taken regularly while trying to avoid nitrate tolerance (low dose, 2× daily), in which case, intermittent short-acting nitrates are still used as needed.

* PTCA = percutaneous transluminal angioplasty

variations between patients mean that some will tolerate one type of combination therapy better than another, so that triple therapy should not be automatic when dual therapy fails.

NEW ANTIANGINAL AGENTS

Molsydomine (2 mg 3× daily) acts by release of vasodilatory metabolites formed during first-pass liver metabolism. *Nicorandil*, a nicotinamide nitrate, acts chiefly by dilation of the large coronary arteries. Both these agents are still investigational.

SUMMARY

Nitrates act by venodilation and relief of coronary spasm to treat anginal attacks; their unloading effect also benefits patients with "backward" CHF and high LV filling pressures. New nitrate preparations are not a substantial advance over the old, especially not the nitrate patches that seem to predispose to tolerance by sustained blood nitrate levels. Mononitrates, not yet available in the USA, are an advance over dinitrates because they eliminate variable hepatic metabolism upon which the action of the dinitrates depend. Yet with all nitrate preparations the fundamental problem of potential tolerance remains. During the treatment of effort angina by isosorbide dinitrate, early evidence suggests that 2× daily low doses (20–30 mg) may be best to avoid tolerance. During the treatment of unstable angina at rest and CHF, much higher doses may be required to exert a sustained therapeutic effect.

REFERENCES

References from Previous Edition

For details see previous edition of Opie et al, Drugs for the Heart, American Edition. Orlando, FL, Grune & Stratton, 1984, pp 23–37.

1. Andreasen F, Boye E, Christoffersen P, et al: Eur J Cardiol 2:443–452, 1975
2. Armstrong PW, Armstrong JA, Marks GS: Am J Cardiol 46:670–678, 1980a
3. Armstrong PW, Armstrong JA, Marks GS: Circulation 62:160–166, 1980b
4. Assinder DE, Chasseaud LF, Taylor T: J Pharm Sci 66:775–778, 1979
5. Blasini R, Froer KL, Blumel G, et al: Herz 7:250–258, 1982
6. Brunner D, Meshulam N, Zeriekar F: Chest 66:282–287, 1974
7. Bussmann W-D, Lhner J, Kaltenbach M: Am J Cardiol 39:91–96, 1977
8. Bussmann W-D, Schupp D: Am J Cardiol 41:931–936, 1978
9. Dahany DT, Burwell DT, Aronow WS, et al: Circulation 55:381–387, 1977
10. Distante A, Maseri A, Severi S, et al: Am J Cardiol 44:533–539, 1979
11. Fox KM, Dyett JF, Portal RW, et al: Eur J Cardiol 5:507–515, 1977
12. Franciosa JA, Mikulic E, Cohn JN, et al: Circulation 50:1020–1024, 1974
13. Franciosa JA, Nordstrom LA, Cohn JN: JAMA 240:443–446, 1978
14. Fung HL, McNiff EF, Ruggirello D, et al: Br J Clin Pharmacol 11:579–590, 1981
15. Glancy DL, Richter MA, Ellis EV, et al: Am J Med 62:39–46, 1977
16. Gorlin R, Brachfeld N, MacLeod C, et al: Circulation 19:705–718, 1959
17. Hardarson T, Henning H, O'Rourke RA: Am J Cardiol 40:90–98, 1977
18. Kattus AA, Alvaro AB, Zohman LR, et al: Chest 75:17–23, 1979
19. Klaus AP, Zaret BL, Pitt BL, et al: Circulation 48:519–525, 1973
20. Lee G, Mason DT, DeMaria AN: Am J Cardiol 41:82–87, 1978
21. Leier CV, Huss B, Margorien D, et al: Circulation 67:817–822, 1983
22. Livesley B, Catley PF, Campbell RC, et al: Br Med J 1:375–378, 1973
23. Maseri A, L'Abbate A, Pesola A, et al: Lancet i:713–717, 1977
24. Massie B, Chatterjee K, Werner J, et al: Am J Cardiol 40:794–801, 1977
25. Miller RR, Awan NA, DeMaria AN, et al: Am J Cardiol 40:504–508, 1977
26. Schang SJ Jr, Pepine CJ: Br Heart J 40:1221–1228, 1978
27. Strumza P, Riggaud M, Mechmeche R, et al: Am J Cardiol 43:272–277, 1979
28. Thadani U, Fung HL, Darke AC, et al: Circulation 62:491–502, 1980
29. Thadani U, Fung HL, Darke AC, et al: Am J Cardiol 49:411–419, 1982
30. Thadani U, Manyari D, Parker JO, et al: Circulation 61:526–535, 1980
31. Thompson RH: Angiology 34:23–31, 1983
32. Warren SE, Francis GS: Nitroglycerin and nitrate esters. Am J Med 65:53–62, 1978

33. Whitworth CG, Grant WM: Arch Opthalmol 7:492–497, 1964
34. Williams DO, Amsterdam EA, Mason DT: Circulation 51:421–427, 1975
35. Zelis R, Mason DT: JAMA 234:166–170, 1975

New References

36. Abrams J: Nitrate tolerance in angina pectoris, in Cohn JN, Rittinghausen R (eds): Mononitrates. Berlin, Springer-Verlag, 1985, pp 154–170
37. Abshagen U: Pharmacokinetics of ISDN, sustained release ISDN and IS-5-MN, in Cohn JN, Rittinghausen R (eds): Mononitrates. Berlin, Springer-Verlag, 1985, pp 53–66
38. Badger RS, Brown BG, Gallery CA, et al: Coronary artery dilation and hemodynamic responses after isosorbide dinitrate therapy in patients with coronary artery disease. Am J Cardiol 56:390–395, 1985
39. Bennett D, Davies A, Davis A: Sustained antianginal action of glyceryl trinitrate cream. Br J Clin Pharmacol 15:173–180, 1983
40. Berkenboom GM, Sobolski JC, Degre SG: Oral sustained-release nitroglycerin in chronic stable angina: A multicenter, double-blind, randomized crossover trial. Am J Cardiol 53:15–17, 1984
40a. Belz GG, Mathews JH, Beck A, et al: Hemodynamic effects of nicorandil, isosorbide dinitrate and dihydralazine in healthy volunteers. J Cardiovasc Pharmacol 7:1107–1112, 1985
41. Blasini R, Reiniger G, Brugmann U: Tolerance to the anti-ischemic effect of isosorbide dinitrate during continuous but not during intermittent oral therapy, in Cohn JN, Rittinghausen R (eds): Mononitrates. Berlin, Springer-Verlag, 1985, pp 124–129
42. Boden WE, Bough EW, Reichman MJ, et al: Beneficial effects of high-dose diltiazem in patients with persistent effort angina on β-blockers and nitrates: a randomized, double-blind, placebo-controlled cross-over study. Circulation 71:1197–1205, 1985
43. Bornheimer JF, Kim JS, Sambasivan V, et al: Effects of nitroglycerin on supine and upright exercise in mitral stenosis. Am Heart J 104:1288–1293, 1982
44. Cohn JN: Nitrate therapy of congestive heart failure, in Cohn JN, Rittinghausen R (eds): Mononitrates. Berlin, Springer-Verlag, 1985, pp 299–305
44a. Cohn JN, Archibald DG, Phil M, et al: Effect of vasodilator therapy on mortality in chronic congestive heart failure. New Engl J Med 314:1547–1552, 1986
45. Crean PA, Ribeiro P, Crea F, et al: Failure of transdermal nitroglycerin to improve chronic stable angina: A randomized, placebo-controlled double-blind, double crossover trial. Am Heart J 108:1494–1500, 1984
46. Elkayam U, Roth A, Henriquez B, et al: Hemodynamic and hormonal effects of high-dose transdermal nitroglycerin in patients with chronic congestive heart failure. Am J Cardiol 56:555–559, 1985
47. Flaherty JT: Hemodynamic attenuation and the nitrate-free interval: alternative dosing strategies for transdermal nitroglycerin. Am J Cardiol 56:321–326, 1985
47a. Flaherty JT, Becker LC, Bulkley BH, et al: A randomized prospective trial of intravenous nitroglycerin in patients with acute myocardial infarction. Circulation 68:576–588, 1983
48. Franciosa JA, Cohn JN: Sustained hemodynamic effects without tolerance during long-term isosorbide dinitrate treatment of chronic left ventricular failure. Am J Cardiol 45:648–654, 1980
49. Georgopolous AJ, Markis A, Georgiadis H: Therapeutic efficacy of a new transdermal system containing nitroglycerin in patients with angina pectoris. Eur J Clin Pharmacol 22:481–485, 1982
50. Goldstein RE, Rosing DR, Redwood DR, et al: Clinical and circulatory effects of isosorbide dinitrate—comparison with nitroglycerin. Circulation 43:629–635, 1971
51. Hill JA, Feldman RL, Pepine CJ, et al: Randomized double-blind comparison of nifedipine and isosorbide dinitrate in patients with coronary arterial spasm. Am J Cardiol 49:431–438, 1982
52. Horowitz JD, Antman EM, Lovell BH, et al: Potentiation of the cardiovascular effects of nitroglycerin by N-acetylcysteine. Circulation 68:1247–1253, 1983
53. Hubner PJB, Jones PRM, Galler IAR: Assessment of dermal glyceryl trinitrate and isosorbide dinitrate for patients with angina pectoris. Br Med J 290:514–516, 1985
54. Imaizumi T, Takeshita A, Ashihara T, et al: The effects of sublingually administered nitroglycerin on forearm vascular resistance in patients with heart failure and in normal subjects. Circulation 72:747–752, 1985
55. James MA, Walker PR, Papouchado M, et al: Efficacy of transdermal glyceryl trinitrate in the treatment of chronic stable angina pectoris. Br Heart J 53:631–635, 1985
56. Jordan RA, Seth L, Henry DA, et al: Dose requirements and hemodynamic effects of transdermal nitroglycerin compared with placebo in patients with congestive heart failure. Circulation 71:980–986, 1985
56a. Jordan RA, Seth L, Casebolt P, et al: Rapidly developing tolerance to transdermal nitroglycerin in congestive heart failure. Ann Intern Med 104:295–298, 1986
57. Kaplan JA, Dunbar RW, Jones EL: Nitroglycerin infusion during coronary artery surgery. Anesthesiology 45:14–21, 1976

58. Kaplan K, Davidson R, Parker M, et al: Intravenous nitroglycerin for the treatment of angina at rest unresponsive to standard nitrate therapy. Am J Cardiol 51:694–698, 1983

59. Karim A: Transdermal absorption of nitroglycerin from microseal drug delivery (MDD) system. Angiology 34:11–22, 1983

60. Lin S-G, Flaherty JT: Crossover from intravenous to transdermal nitroglycerin therapy in unstable angina pectoris. Am J Cardiol 56:742–748, 1985

61. Loeb HS, Ostrenga JP, Gaul W, et al: Beneficial effects of dopamine combined with intravenous nitroglycerin on hemodynamics in patients with severe left ventricular failure. Circulation 68:813–820, 1983

62. Maclean D, Feely J: New drugs. Calcium antagonists, nitrates and new anti-anginal drugs. Br Med J 286:1127–1130, 1983

63. Manyari DE, Smith ER, Spragg J: Isosorbide dinitrate and glyceryl trinitrate: Demonstration of cross-tolerance in the capacitance vessels. Am J Cardiol 55:927–931, 1985

64. Morse JR, Nesto RW: Double-blind crossover comparison of the antianginal effects of nifedipine and isosorbide dinitrate in patients with exertional angina receiving propranolol. J Am Coll Cardiol 6:1395–1401, 1985

65. Muller G, Hacker W, Schneider B: Intra-individual comparison of the action of equal doses of isosorbide-5-mononitrate, slow-release isosorbide dinitrate and placebo in patients with coronary heart disease. Klin Wochenschr 61:409–416, 1983

66. Nelson GIC, Silke B, Ahuja RC, et al: Haemodynamic advantages of isosorbide dinitrate over frusemide in acute heart failure following myocardial infarction. Lancet i:730–733, 1983

67. Packer M, Medina N, Yushak M, et al: Hemodynamic factors limiting the response to transdermal nitroglycerin in chronic congestive heart failure. Am J Cardiol 57:260–267, 1986

68. Parker JO, Fung HL: Transdermal nitroglycerin in angina pectoris. Am J Cardiol 54:471–476, 1984

69. Parker JO, Vankoughnett KA, Farrell B: Comparison of buccal nitroglycerin and oral isosorbide dinitrate for nitrate tolerance in stable angina pectoris. Am J Cardiol 56:724–728, 1985

70. Parker JO, Vankoughnett KA, Farrell B: Nitroglycerin lingual spray. Clinical efficacy and dose response relations. Am J Cardiol 57:1–5, 1986

71. Parker JO, Vankoughnett KA, Fung HL: Transdermal isosorbide dinitrate in angina pectoris: Effect of acute and sustained therapy. Am J Cardiol 54:8–13, 1984

72. Quigley PJ, Maurer BJ: Ventricular fibrillation during coronary angiography: Association with potassium-containing glyceryl trinitrate. Am J Cardiol 56:191, 1985

73. Rajfer SI, Demma FJ, Goldberg LI: Sustained beneficial hemodynamic responses to large doses of transdermal nitroglycerin in congestive heart failure and comparison with intravenous nitroglycerin. Am J Cardiol 54:120–125, 1984

74. Reichek N, Priest C, Zimrin D, et al: Anti-anginal effects of nitroglycerin patches. Am J Cardiol 54:1–7, 1984

75. Scardi S, Pivotti F, Fonda F, et al: Effect of a new transdermal therapeutic system containing nitroglycerin on exercise capacity in patients with angina pectoris. Am Heart J 110:546–551, 1985

76. Schneider W, Michel O, Kaltenbach M, et al: Antiangiose Wirkung von transdermal appliziertem Nitroglycerin in Abhangigkeit von der Pflastergosse. Dtsch Med Wochenschr 110:87–90, 1985

77. Schneider WH, Bussmann WD, Stahl B, et al: Dose response relationship of antianginal activity of isosorbide dinitrate. Am J Cardiol 53:700–705, 1984

78. Sullivan M, Savvides M, Abouantoun S, et al: Failure of transdermal nitroglycerin to improve exercise capacity in patients with angina pectoris. J Am Coll Cardiol 5:1220–1223, 1985

79. Tauchert M, Jansen W, Osterspey A, et al: Dose dependence of tolerance during treatment with mononitrates. Z Kardiol 72 (suppl 3):218–228, 1983

80. Taylor T, Chasseaud LF: Pharmacokinetics of isosorbide dinitrate in human subjects, in Lichtlen PR, Engel H-J, Schrey A, et al (eds): Nitrates. III. Cardiovascular effects. Berlin, Springer-Verlag, 1981, pp 40–46

81. Thadani U: Nitrates for angina. A critical review of therapeutic efficacy and tolerance. Hertz 9:123–136, 1984

82. Thadani U: Antianginal and anti-ischemic efficacy of conventional and slow release formulation of isosorbide-5-mononitrate in angina pectoris. A review. Z Kardiol 74 (suppl 4):19–22, 1985

83. Thadani U, Brady DC, Klutts SJ, et al: Dose titration and duration of effects of transdermal nitroglycerin patches in angina pectoris. Circulation 72 (suppl III):III-431, 1985a

84. Thadani U, Hamilton S, Teague S, et al: Slow release isosorbide-5-mononitrate for the treatment of angina pectoris: Duration of effects, in Cohn JN, Rittinghausen R (eds): Mononitrates. Berlin, Springer-Verlag, 1985b, pp 188–189

85. Thadani U, Shapiro W, DiBianco R: Effect of long-term placebo therapy on angina

frequency and exercise tolerance in patients with stable angina pectoris. Circulation 70 (suppl II):I-44, 1984

86. Tolins M, Weir K, Chesler E, et al: 'Maximal' drug therapy is not necessarily optimal in chronic angina pectoris. J Am Coll Cardiol 3:1051–1057, 1984

87. Torresi J, Horowitz JD, Dusting GJ: Prevention and reversal of tolerance to nitroglycerin with N-acetylcysteine. J Cardiovasc Pharmacol 7:777–783, 1985

88. Webb SC, Canepa-Anson R, Rickards AF, et al: High potassium concentration in a parenteral preparation of glyceryl trinitrate. Need for caution if given by intracoronary injection. Br Heart J 50:395–396, 1983

89. Wei JY, Reid PR: Relation of time course of plasma nitroglycerin levels to echocardiographic, arterial pressure and heart rate changes after sublingual administration of nitroglycerin. Am J Cardiol 48:778–782, 1981

90. White HD, Polak J, Wynne J, et al: Addition of nifedipine to maximal nitrate and beta-adrenoceptor blocker therapy in coronary artery disease. Am J Cardiol 55:1303–1307, 1985

91. Wright A, Hecker JF, Lewis GBH: Use of transdermal glyceryl trinitrate to reduce failure of intravenous infusion due to phlebitis and extravasation. Lancet ii:1148–1150, 1985

92. Yusuf S, Collins R: IV nitroglycerin (NG) and nitroprusside (NP) therapy in acute myocardial infarction reduces mortality: Evidence from randomized controlled trials (RCTS). Circulation 72 (suppl III):III-224, 1985

Reviews

Abrams J: Transdermal nitroglycerin and nitrate tolerance. Ann Intern Med 104:424–426; 1986

Cowan JC: Nitrate tolerance. Int J Cardiol 12:1–19, 1986

Thadani U: Nitrates for angina. A critical review of therapeutic efficacy and tolerance. Hertz 9:123–136, 1984

L. H. Opie
B. N. Singh

3

Calcium Channel Antagonists (Slow Channel Blockers)

The single most important property of calcium antagonists (= *calcium entry blockers* = *slow channel blockers*) is to selectively inhibit, the slow inward calcium current in those tissues where there is a slowly rising calcium-dependent upstroke to the action potential not fired by a fast sodium signal. Such tissues are vascular smooth muscle and nodal tissue (sinus and atrioventricular [AV] nodes). Only at higher concentrations do the potentially inhibitory effects on the calcium channel in the myocardium become apparent, with a negative inotropic effect (Table 3-1). Why different calcium antagonists have different effects on nodal and vascular tissues is unknown; however, they are structurally different. Verapamil is a papaverine derivative, nifedipine a dihydropyridine, and diltiazem a benzothiazepine. Verapamil and diltiazem interact with similar but different binding sites, and both depress nodal tissue as well as vascular tissue. Dihydropyridines such as nifedipine bind to a different site and have little clinical effect on nodal tissue.

Clinically, each of the "first generation" calcium antagonists, verapamil, nifedipine and diltiazem, has a slightly different spectrum of clinical activity (Fig. 3-1, Table 3-2). Their common denominator is their ability to block the calcium channel, which results in their vasodilatory effect. They are virtually exchangeable when used for coronary artery spasm; all may be used for mild to moderate hypertension. All three benefit angina of effort, acting through a mixture of mechanisms: all may increase coronary blood flow; diltiazem has a negative chronotropic effect and mildly reduces the afterload; verapamil has a mild negative inotropic effect and decreases the afterload; while the major effect of nifedipine is to reduce the afterload.

Cellular mechanism: β-Blockade versus calcium antagonists. Both calcium antagonists and β-blockade have a negative inotropic effect, whereas only calcium antagonists relax vascular and other smooth muscle (Fig. 3-2). Calcium antagonists "block" the entry of calcium through the calcium channel in both smooth muscle and myocardium, so that less calcium is available to the contractile apparatus in both tissues. The result is vasodilation and a negative inotropic effect; the latter is usually modest and overridden, especially in the case of nifedipine, by peripheral vasodilation.

β-Blockade has contrasting effects on smooth muscle and on the myocardium. Whereas it tends to promote smooth muscle contraction, β-blockade impairs myocardial contraction (negative inotropic effect). In explaining this difference, a fundamental difference lies in the regulation of the contractile mechanism by calcium ions in these two tissues. In the myocardium, calcium ions interact with troponin C to allow actin-myosin interaction; β-stimulation enhances the entry of calcium ions via the slow channel, and also the rate of uptake in the sarcoplasmic

Drugs for the Heart, Second Expanded Edition
Copyright © 1987 by Grune & Stratton, Inc.

ISBN 0-8089-1840-0

TABLE 3-1
RELATIVE EFFECTS OF CALCIUM CHANNEL BLOCKERS IN EXPERIMENTAL
PREPARATIONS COMPARED WITH THERAPEUTIC LEVELS IN MAN

	Verapamil	Nifedipine	Diltiazem
Therapeutic level in man ng/ml molecular weight molar value protein binding molar value, corrected for protein binding	80–400 455 $2-8 \times 10^{-7}M$ about 90% $2-8 \times 10^{-8}M$	25–100 346 $0.5-2 \times 10^{-7}M$ about 95% $0.3-1 \times 10^{-8}M$	50–300 415 $1-7 \times 10^{-7}M$ about 85% $1-5 \times 10^{-8}M$
Isolated coronary artery contraction 50 percent inhibition	$10^{-7}M$	$10^{-8}M$	$10^{-7}M$
Myocardial depression 40% depression of contractile force	$5 \times 10^{-6}M$	$5 \times 10^{-7}M$	$5 \times 10^{-4}M$†
Fast sodium current depression	$10^{-4}M$	no effect	$10^{-4}M$
Alpha-blockade, K_i (myocardium)	$5 \times 10^{-7}M$	$4 \times 10^{-6}M$	$7 \times 10^{-6}M$
Slowing of heart rate by 20%	$10^{-6}M$	$10^{-5}M$	$10^{-8}M$
Relative effect on AV node versus contractile force	6.5 : 1	1 : 1	20 : 1
Inhibition of enzyme release from infarcting myocardium	$2 \times 10^{-7}M$	$10^{-7}M$	$10^{-7}M$
Inhibition of ventricular automaticity (ventricular fibrillation threshold in coronary ligated rat heart)	$10^{-7}M$	$10^{-6}M$	$5 \times 10^{-6}M$

† Caution: The failing myocardium is probably more sensitive to the negative inotropic effect of diltiazem[76] and other agents too. (For references, see previous edition.)

reticulum so that calcium ions rise and fall more rapidly; hence both contraction and relaxation are speeded up as cyclic AMP forms under β-stimulation. Furthermore, the peak force of contraction is enhanced. β-Blockade opposes all these effects.

In smooth muscle (Fig. 3-2), calcium ions regulate the contractile mechanism by interaction with calmodulin to form calcium-calmodulin which then stimulates myosin light chain kinase (MLCK) to phosphorylate the myosin light chains to allow actin-myosin interaction. Cyclic AMP inhibits the light chain kinase. β-Blockade, by inhibiting the effect of cyclic AMP, removes the inhibition on light chain kinase activity, and therefore promotes contraction in smooth muscle.

In addition, in the case of arterial smooth muscle, a further mechanism is that β-blockade may permit unopposed α-induced vasoconstriction.

VERAPAMIL

Introduced in Europe in 1963, verapamil (Isoptin®, Calan®) remains the prototype of calcium antagonists, and the one that has been most extensively studied experimentally and clinically. Although originally used as an antianginal and antihypertensive agent, these properties were soon overshadowed by a dramatic effect in supraventricular arrhythmias[79] so that only recently has the wide therapeutic potential of verapamil again come to be appreciated (Fig. 3-3). The use of this agent, especially in angina, is now increasing. Its use for mild to moderate hypertension is pending approval in the USA. Its role in obstructive cardiomyopathy and Raynaud's phenomenon is reasonably well defined, while its use in pulmonary hypertension is less encouraging.

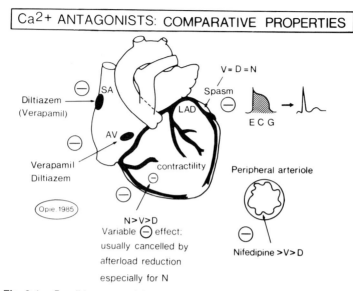

Fig. 3-1.   Possible comparable potency of the three major calcium antagonist drugs. V = verapamil; D = diltiazem; N = nifedipine. These potencies are based on a consideration of literature reports, but may not accurately reflect any particular experimental or clinical situation and must therefore be regarded as provisional. (From Opie LH: Calcium ions, drug action and the heart with special reference to calcium antagonist drugs. Pharmacol Ther 25:271–295, 1984, by permission of Pergamon Press Ltd.)

Pharmacologic Properties

Electrophysiologically, verapamil inhibits the action potential of the upper and middle nodal regions (Fig. 3-1) where the slow inward Ca^{2+}-mediated current is the major cause of depolarization. Verapamil thus inhibits one limb of the re-entry circuit, which is believed to underlie most paroxysmal supraventricular tachycardias (PSVTs). Increased AV block and the increase in effective refractory period of the AV node explain the reduction of ventricular rate in atrial flutter and fibrillation. On electrophysiologic grounds, one might expect verapamil not to be very effective in ventricular arrhythmias except in certain uncommon forms.

Hemodynamically, verapamil combines arteriolar dilation with a direct

TABLE 3-2

CALCIUM ANTAGONISTS: COMPARATIVE INDICATIONS

Condition	Verapamil	Nifedipine	Diltiazem
Coronary artery spasm (Prinzmetal's)	+ +	+ +	+ +
Chronic stable angina of effort	+ +	+/+ +[‡]	+ +
Angina with hypertension	+ +	+ +	+ +
Angina with heart failure	+/−	+ +	+
Angina at rest	+ +	+ +	+ +
Unstable angina (threatened infarction)	+ +	+/−	+ +
Unstable angina already treated by β-blockade	+	+ +	+
Combination with β-blockade	+	+ +	+
Supraventricular tachycardia,[*] acute IV use	+ +	−	+
Supraventricular tachycardia,[†] oral prophylaxis	+ +	−	+ +
Chronic atrial fibrillation or flutter[*] (± digitalis)	+ +	−	+ +
Severe hypertension[†]	+	+ +	+
Hypertension (2nd or 3rd line therapy)[*]	+	+ +	+
Hypertension, monotherapy[*]	+	+	+
Raynaud's phenomenon[†]	+ +	+ +	+ +
Hypertrophic cardiomyopathy[†]	+ +	+	+

[*] only verapamil approved in USA
[†] not approved in USA
[‡] careful titration needed

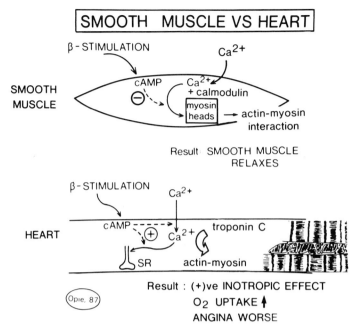

Fig. 3-2. Proposed comparative effects of β-blockers (BB) and calcium antagonists (Ca²⁺ antag) on smooth muscle and myocardium. The opposing effects on vascular smooth muscle are of critical therapeutic importance. SR = sarcoplasmic reticulum. (For further details, see reference 70, Figs 17-5 and 18-3.)

negative inotropic effect. The cardiac output and left ventricular (LV) ejection fraction do not increase as expected following peripheral vasodilation,[2] which may be an expression of the negative inotropic effect. Peripheral vasodilation generally overcomes the direct depressant effect of verapamil on the sinus node so that the heart rate is unchanged or variably altered.

Pharmacokinetics. The hemodynamic effects (hypotension) of IV verapamil are short-lived, with a peak at 5 minutes and loss of activity by 10–12 minutes, but the peak effect on the AV node occurs at 10–15 minutes and lasts up to 6 hours, suggesting preferential binding by nodal tissues. Oral verapamil takes 2 hours to act and peaks at 3 hours. Therapeutic blood levels (80–400 ng/ml) are seldom measured.[39] The elimination half-life is usually 3–7 hours, but increases significantly during chronic administration and in patients with liver or advanced renal insufficiency. Despite nearly complete absorption of oral doses, bioavailability is only 10–20 percent (high first-pass liver metabolism). The usual oral daily dose is 12–40× the standard IV dose (10 mg). Ultimate excretion of the parent compound as well as the active hepatic metabolite norverapamil is 75 percent by the kidneys and 25 percent by the gastrointestinal (GI) tract. Verapamil is 87–93 percent protein-bound, but no interaction with coumadin has been reported. When both verapamil and digoxin are given together, there is an important interaction in which digoxin levels rise, probably due to a reduction in the renal clearance of digoxin.[7]

Norverapamil is a hepatic metabolite of verapamil which appears rapidly in the plasma after oral administration of verapamil, and in concentrations similar to those of the parent compound; like verapamil, norverapamil undergoes delayed clearance during chronic dosing.

Dose. The usual *oral dose* is 80–120 mg 3× daily; large differences of pharmacokinetics between individuals mean that dose titration is required. Lower or higher doses may therefore be needed; the highest reported daily dose is 960 mg[95] but such levels are rarely tolerated. During chronic oral dosing, the formation of norverapamil metabolites and altered rates of hepatic metabolism may mean that a lower total daily dose of verapamil is preferable;[81] for example, if verapamil has been titrated upwards to a dose of 160 mg 3× daily during chronic dosing, the "correct" dose would be 160 mg 2× daily.

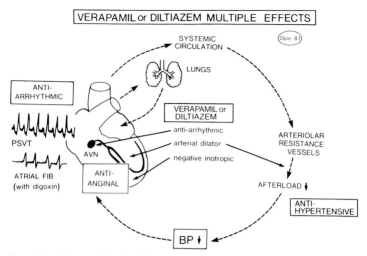

Fig. 3-3. Verapamil and diltiazem have a broad spectrum of therapeutic effects. PSVT = paroxysmal supraventricular tachycardia.

Lower doses are also required in elderly patients or those with advanced renal or hepatic disease.[83] Several *slow-release preparations* are now available in Europe. The usual dose is 1–2 capsules daily (160–320 mg).

IV verapamil should be used only in monitored patients. When used for uncontrolled atrial fibrillation combined with myocardial disease, verapamil is infused at a very low dose (0.0001 mg/kg/min) and titrated against the ventricular response, especially if the patient has already received β-blockade or when digitalis toxicity is suspected. In the absence of these relative contraindications, verapamil may safely be given at a higher rate (0.005 mg/kg/min, increasing) or as an IV bolus of 5 mg (0.075 mg/kg) followed by double the dose if needed.[86] For supraventricular tachycardias when there is risk of hypotension (prior β-blockade, myocardial disease, disopyramide therapy), pretreatment with calcium gluconate (90 mg, see reference 91) should be tried before a bolus or an infusion (1 mg/min for 10 minutes). When there is no myocardial depression, a bolus of 5–10 mg (0.1–0.15 mg/kg) can be given over 1 minute and repeated 10 minutes later if needed; the infusion rate after a successful bolus is 0.005 mg/kg/min for about 30–60 minutes, decreasing thereafter (for another regime, see reference 77).

Minor side-effects. Relatively minor side-effects are those of vasodilation—headaches and dizziness, with occasional palpitations and hypotension.[84] The side-effect causing most trouble, especially in elderly patients, is constipation found in the majority of patients given high-dose verapamil.[74,84] Other side-effects may include pain in the gums, facial pains, and epigastric pains.[43]

Severe side-effects. When incorrectly given as a bolus to patients with pre-existing AV inhibition caused by disease or by β-adrenergic blockade, IV verapamil can be fatal. When correctly used, verapamil seldom causes serious cardiac depression. In the average patient with angina pectoris, verapamil therapy is probably as safe as or safer than β-adrenergic blockade.[84] Two extreme reactions reported for β-blockade—fatal bronchospasm and gangrene—have thus far not been found with verapamil, nor can be expected. The side-effects of verapamil itself are somewhat less than those of nifedipine when both are used in doses equally potent for chronic stable angina.[28]

Myocardial depressant effects. A striking negative inotropic effect is seen with verapamil and other calcium antagonists in isolated preparations. These are seldom encountered with normal therapeutic concentrations[12] and intact autonomic nervous reflexes. IV verapamil may cause very serious

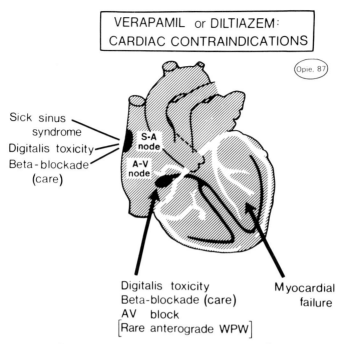

VERAPAMIL or DILTIAZEM:
CARDIAC CONTRAINDICATIONS

(Opie, 87)

Sick sinus
syndrome
Digitalis toxicity
Beta-blockade
(care)

S-A
node

A-V
node

Digitalis toxicity
Beta-blockade (care)
AV block
[Rare anterograde WPW]

Myocardial
failure

Fig. 3-4. Contraindications to verapamil and diltiazem. For use of verapamil and diltiazem in patients already receiving β-blockers, see text.

cardiodepression in hypodynamic hearts;[2] on the other hand, when given to patients with coronary artery disease without heart failure or conduction block, IV verapamil improves LV performance, because of afterload reduction.[3] In supraventricular arrhythmias, the hemodynamic benefits of restoration of sinus rhythm may outweigh any negative inotropic effect.[18]

Contraindications to verapamil (Fig. 3-4). Sick sinus syndrome, pre-existing AV nodal disease, excess therapy with β-adrenergic blockade or digitalis or quinidine or disopyramide, or myocardial depression are all still contra-indications that especially apply in the IV therapy of supraventricular tachycardias.[69,82] In the rarer type of Wolff-Parkinson-White (WPW) syndrome with anterograde (= antegrade) conduction through the bypass tract, the risk is that the impulses of atrial fibrillation can be too rapidly conducted to the ventricles with fear of ventricular fibrillation (VF). Nonetheless, verapamil can safely be used in the vast majority of patients with supraventricular tachycardias and narrow QRS complexes. (For use in digitalis toxicity, see p 41.)

Therapy of verapamil toxicity effects. There are few clinical reports on manage-ment of verapamil toxicity. Calcium gluconate helps in heart failure and when excess hypotension is induced by verapamil; 1–2 g IV may be tried. Calcium therapy, however, is not effective against excess AV block.[4] Alternatively, atropine (1 mg IV) can shorten prolonged AV conduction. β-Agonists (especially isopro-terenol) should also be effective.

Verapamil for Chronic Stable Angina, Unstable Angina and Prinzmetal's Variant Angina

In *chronic stable effort angina*, verapamil acts by a combination of after-load reduction and a mild negative inotropic effect; there may also be an increase in the blood supply.[18] The heart rate usually stays the same as in controls. Thus verapamil can logically be combined with β-blockade (for pre-cautions, see p 41). In several recent studies, verapamil has been as effective as propranolol for effort angina, or more so, and there is less risk of serious side-effects. A daily dose of about verapamil 360 mg is the approximate equivalent of propranolol 300 mg daily[10] or metoprolol 200 mg twice daily[23] or nifedipine 60 mg daily.[28]

In *unstable angina at rest* oral verapamil gives symptomatic and electro-cardiographic short-term benefit (dose 480 mg daily, divided).[13,14] Is there sustained benefit? In 22 patients followed for 1 year, verapamil (320–480 mg daily) continued to relieve anginal pain, but the high incidence of death and myocardial infarction seemed unaltered.[80] In some patients, pain-relief is not maintained for unknown reasons.[66]

In *variant angina* (Prinzmetal's syndrome), verapamil (average daily dose 450 mg in 3–4 divided doses) and nifedipine (average daily dose 70 mg in 3–4 divided doses) were equally effective with fewer dose-limiting side-effects with verapamil.[20] Combinations of verapamil or nifedipine with oral isosorbide dini-trate are more effective than isosorbide alone in reducing anginal frequency and ischemic ECG changes in variant angina.[94]

In *acute myocardial infarction* (AMI), verapamil, when given early enough, may reduce enzymatically measured infarct size in man. A large trial failed to show any benefit of acute followed by *postinfarct* long-term verapamil therapy;[27] however, the design was imperfect and more studies are needed to settle the issue.

Verapamil for Supraventricular Arrhythmias

In *PSVT*, an IV bolus of 5–10 mg restores sinus rhythm in 75 percent or more of cases.[101] Thereafter, oral prophylactic therapy against recurrent PSVT may be either by verapamil[65] or by verapamil-propranolol.[96] Verapamil by itself is about as effective as digoxin or propranolol.[94]

In rapid *atrial fibrillation*, whether or not previously treated with digitalis, IV verapamil reduces the ventricular rate with "regularization" in some and con-version to sinus rhythm in a few, especially in those of recent onset. But the blood pressure may drop,[5] so that a slow infusion or oral treatment (taking only 2 hours to act) is preferred to bolus infusion unless reduction of ventricular rate is urgent, for example, in AMI when there are no facilities for cardioversion.

In *atrial flutter*, the block is increased; occasionally sinus rhythm is restored (especially in acute infarction), or atrial fibrillation ensues.[101]

In the *WPW syndrome*, verapamil usually has no effects on the accessory pathway, but depresses the AV node and inhibits the reciprocating re-entry tachycardias at the site of the AV node. Verapamil does not work and may be dangerous when there is anterograde (antegrade) conduction down the anom-alous bundle with atrial flutter or fibrillation (Fig. 3-4, Chapter 4). Like digoxin, verapamil may accelerate the ventricular response and is contraindicated.[45]

Verapamil for Hypertension

All three calcium antagonists can be effective in systemic hypertension (p 49). Verapamil is pending approval for mild to moderate hypertension in the USA.

Verapamil for hypertrophic cardiomyopathy. In hypertrophic cardiomyopathies, the role of verapamil has been best evaluated of all the calcium antagonists. It improves symp-toms, reduces the outflow tract gradient, and improves exercise tolerance by 20–25 percent, at least when administered acutely.[15] Diastolic function is also improved by vera-pamil.[47] However, verapamil should not be given to patients with resting outflow tract obstruction,[92] when disopyramide (see p 65) may be better. At present there is no evi-dence of an effect against ventricular arrhythmias associated with the disease. A large number of patients on the drug develop significant side-effects with long-term verapamil, including sino-atrial and AV nodal dysfunction, and occasionally severe heart failure.[15] It is not known whether calcium antagonists produce a regression in the ventricular hypertro-phy so characteristic of hypertrophic cardiomyopathy. Although strict comparisons with β-blockade are lacking,[56] verapamil may offer better symptomatic improvement and fewer side-effects than with β-blockade, possibly because of improved diastolic mechanics.[47]

Verapamil for ventricular tachycardia (VT). "For most patients with recurrent, sustained VT, verapamil is not effective and frequently deleterious."[24] However, some patients with exercise-induced VT presumably due to triggered automaticity may respond well[95] as well as young patients with the following combination: idiopathic VT with right bundle branch block and left axis deviation.

Verapamil and β-Blockers: Interactions and Combination Therapy

Special care is required when verapamil is acutely added by IV injection in the presence of pre-existing β-adrenergic blockade.[90] Also in patients with angina pectoris already receiving propranolol or metoprolol, IV[57] or oral vera-pamil[72] can reduce contractility[72] and increase heart size[53] and cause symptomatic sinus bradycardia.[93] There may be a hepatic pharmacokinetic interaction.[46] Depending on the dose, the combination may be well tolerated[53] or not.[48] In practice, clinicians can safely combine verapamil and β-blockade in the therapy of angina pectoris provided that due care is taken; the combination improves myocardial function during exercise more than does either agent alone.[52] Verapamil-β-blocker is a combination that should work well for hypertension, although heart rate, AV conduction, and LV function may be adversely affected.[62a] Similarly, with care, the combination verapamil-propranolol is used for the chronic prevention of supraventricular tachycardia.[96]

In comparison, the combination of nifedipine-β-blockade is generally well tolerated.[71] The combination diltiazem-β-blockade may cause concern if bradycardia or hypotension develops.[48]

Other Drug Interactions with Verapamil

Digoxin.   Verapamil can interact with digitalis to increase blood digoxin levels.[61] In digitalis toxicity, rapid IV verapamil is *absolutely contraindicated* because it can lethally exaggerate AV block. There is no reason why, in the absence of digitalis toxicity or AV block, oral verapamil and digitalis compounds should not be combined (checking the digoxin level) because digitalis does not inhibit the slow inward calcium current. Experimentally, verapamil has proved effective against ventricular arrhythmias due to digitalis, but in practice IV verapamil should only be given with great caution to patients with digitalis poisoning.

Prazosin.   Verapamil has also been used combined with prazosin in hypertension, with added and possibly synergistic effects;[33] the latter may be explained by pharmacokinetic interactions.[73]

Quinidine.   Verapamil may adversely interact with quinidine, presumably due to the combined effect on peripheral alpha-receptors causing hypotension,[64] or by increasing quinidine levels (see p 60).

Disopyramide.   The combined negative inotropic potential of verapamil and disopyramide is considerable so that the combination can only be given with care.

New Derivatives of Verapamil

Gallopamil (D_{600}) is closely related in structure to verapamil with similar clinical effects. *Anapamil* is long-acting and also under clinical investigation. *Tiapamil* is a combined sodium-calcium blocking agent (p 49).

NIFEDIPINE

The newer dihydropyridine calcium antagonists, of which nifedipine (Procardia®; Adalat®) is the prototype, inhibit the calcium channel at a different site from verapamil and diltiazem. Nifedipine was first introduced in Europe (Adalat®) and is now widely used in the USA. **Dihydropyridines are, in general, powerful arteriolar vasodilators with relatively scant effects on the AV node in clinical doses and their direct negative inotropic effect is usually outweighed by arteriolar unloading effects in clinical practice** (Fig. 3-5).

Nifedipine, the most widely used dihydropyridine, is a powerful arterial vasodilator, very successful in severe hypertension, Prinzmetal's variant angina, and other syndromes produced by arterial vasoconstriction. Nifedipine's action on isolated coronary smooth muscle is 10 or 12× more powerful than that of verapamil, although in clinical practice nifedipine is only marginally better for coronary spasm.[58] The arterial unloading qualities of nifedipine have also been used in the management of all grades of hypertension, acute pulmonary edema, and angina of effort. In congestive heart failure (CHF), arterial vasodilation usually offsets a mild direct negative inotropic effect.

Lacking a clinically significant effect against the AV node, nifedipine is

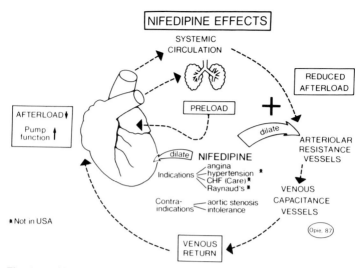

Fig. 3-5. Nifedipine acts chiefly as a powerful arteriolar dilator. CHF = congestive heart failure.

ineffective against supraventricular arrhythmias, and in combination with β-blocking agents is theoretically less hazardous than verapamil or diltiazem.

Pharmacologic Properties

Pharmacokinetics. Nifedipine (capsule form) is almost fully absorbed after an oral dose, reaching peak blood values within 20–45 minutes; it remains detectable for up to 6 hours. The hypotensive effect starts within 20 minutes of an oral dose and within 5 minutes of a sublingual dose; duration of action is 8–12 hours in some studies with an effect of only 4–6 hours in other studies.

Dose. Nifedipine capsules: the usual dose for *angina* is 10–20 mg (1–2 capsules) 3× daily, going up to 20 mg 4× daily.[35] In effort angina, dose-titration is advisable to avoid precipitation of pain by nifedipine in some patients. In *severe hypertension*, 10 mg sublingually usually brings down the pressure within 20–60 minutes. In mild to moderate hypertension, the required dose as monotherapy may be up to 20 mg 3× daily. In *elderly patients*, the fear of abrupt peripheral vasodilation with cerebral underperfusion suggests that the initial dose should be 5 mg (available in capsule form in many countries, otherwise cut a 10 mg capsule in half).

Nifedipine tablets (Adalat Retard® 20 mg) cause blood levels to fall and rise more slowly. As an approximation, the dose of nifedipine tablets may be about twice as high as that of nifedipine capsules. *IV nifedipine* (available in Europe) is seldom used because of light sensitivity.

Contraindications. These are few (Table 3-3): aortic stenosis (exaggeration of pressure gradient across the valve), obstructive hypertrophic cardiomyopathy and severe myocardial depression (added negative inotropic effect). Relative contraindications are subjective intolerance to nifedipine, previous adverse reactions, and pre-existing tachycardia.

Minor side-effects. Overall the drug is very safe when the above contraindications are observed. There may be unpleasant subjective reactions in some subjects such as peripheral vasodilation with flushing, dizziness, headaches, and palpitations. Sometimes angina may be precipitated about 30 minutes after the dose.[50] In the therapy of Prinzmetal's angina, significant side-effects occurred in 37 percent of patients but in only 5 percent were they severe enough to require discontinuation.[1] Subjectively the bilateral ankle edema of nifedipine is distressing but not serious and not due to cardiac failure; the edema can usually be left alone but, if required, therapy is by conventional diuretics or captopril. Nifedipine itself has a mild diuretic effect. Although the incidence of subjective vasodilatory side-effects may be higher with nifedipine than with verapamil, it should be emphasized that all such effects are rather trivial and subjective.

TABLE 3-3
COMPARATIVE CONTRAINDICATIONS OF β-ADRENERGIC BLOCKING AGENTS, VERAPAMIL, NIFEDIPINE AND DILTIAZEM

Contraindications	β-Blockade	Verapamil	Nifedipine	Diltiazem
Absolute:				
Sinus bradycardia	+ +	0/ +	0	0/ +
Sick sinus syndrome	+ +	+	0	+
AV conduction defects	+	+ +	0	+ +
Digitalis toxicity with AV block*	+	+ +	0	+ +
Asthma	+ + +	0	0	0
Bronchospasm	+ +	0	0	0
Heart failure	+ +	+	0	+
Hypotension	+	+	+ +	+
Coronary artery spasm	+	0	0	0
Raynaud's and active peripheral vascular disease	+	0	0	0
Severe mental depression	+	0	0	0
Severe aortic stenosis	+	+	+ +	+
Obstructive cardiomyopathy	0	0/ +	+ +	0/ +
Relative:				
Adverse blood lipid profile	Care	0	0	0
Digitalis without toxicity	Care	Care	0	Care
β-blockade	0	Care	Hypotension	Care
Verapamil therapy	Care	0	Hypotension	Avoid
Quinidine therapy	Care	Care/avoid†	Care‡	Care
Disopyramide therapy	Care	Care/avoid†	0	Care

* Contraindication to rapid intravenous administration.
† However, the combination can be effective in antiarrhythmic therapy.
‡ Nifedipine depresses blood quinidine levels with rebound upon nifedipine-withdrawal.

Severe side-effects.   Occasionally in very ill patients, the direct negative inotropic effect is a problem. Side-effects compatible with the effects of excess hypotension and organ underperfusion have rarely occurred: myocardial ischemia and even infarction; retinal and cerebral ischemia[75] and renal failure.[29]

Nifedipine for Ischemic Syndromes

In *chronic stable angina*, extensive studies show that nifedipine is consistently better than placebo. In a double-blind study on ambulatory patients where ST-segment shifts were monitored, propranolol (380 mg daily) was more effective than nifedipine 60 mg daily while the combination was possibly most effective.[11] Likewise, nifedipine with metoprolol[90a] or atenolol[37a] is more effective in effort angina than either agent alone, while the β-blocker was marginally superior as monotherapy. Nifedipine causes a modest reflex increase in heart rate which may be dose-dependent to limit the antianginal effect; furthermore, the absence of any significant direct negative inotropic effect may also be a disadvantage in the therapy of angina of effort. **Combination with β-blockade is therefore logical therapy, giving better antianginal efficacy than nifedipine or β-blockade alone**[6,11,37,93] or propranolol-isosorbide dinitrate (see p 29). When combined with nitrates, hypotension or syncope from excess peripheral vasodilation may become troublesome, even though nifedipine plus nitrates may give added vasodilator effects at the site of "dynamic stenosis."[9]

In *Prinzmetal's angina* (vasospastic angina), nifedipine 40–80 mg in 4 divided daily doses gives consistent relief,[1,35,87] and is more effective combined with isosorbide dinitrate.[94]

In *unstable angina at rest,* the closer the angina is to Prinzmetal's variety, the better is the effect of nifedipine.[19] In the *standard* type of unstable angina at rest (Fig. 1-3), nifedipine by itself can usually achieve freedom from pain, yet better results are obtained by the combination β-blocker-nifedipine-nitrates.[42a,67] The best studied β-blocker is propranolol and the usual dose of nifedipine is 60–80 mg daily, taking care to avoid hypotension. The problem with these two trials is that neither was able to randomize both agents (propranolol and nifedipine) so that the true efficacy of nifedipine remains unknown. *After the acute phase of unstable angina* is over, follow-up therapy with nifedipine, diltiazem or verapamil is usually successful although additional therapy may often be needed.[74]

In *threatened and very early myocardial infarction*, routine therapy with oral nifedipine for 14 days apparently increased mortality.[67] Perhaps careful patient selection (angina combined with hypertension or heart failure) and avoidance of hypotension might have given different results.

After the onset of AMI sublingual nifedipine has been given as an unloading agent; almost all the hemodynamic benefit results from the first dose of 10 mg[41] and routine prolonged therapy cannot be advised.[67]

> **Other uses of nifedipine** (not approved in the USA).   In *hypertrophic cardiomyopathy* nifedipine may have two opposing effects: peripheral vasodilation could exaggerate resting outflow tract obstruction (which is a contraindication), whereas benefit presumably results from enhanced diastolic relaxation. The combination of nifedipine and propranolol reduces peak systolic and end-diastolic pressures, the peripheral resistance, and the outflow gradient.[8]
>
> In *CHF*, nifedipine is somewhat less effective an arterial vasodilator than is hydralazine,[32] although neither agent increases glomerular filtration rates (GFR).[32] Other reports stress the possible benefits of nifedipine therapy.[60,63] IV nitroprusside is also better than oral nifedipine.[36]
>
> In *acute pulmonary edema* caused by hypertension, nifedipine 10 mg sublingually is effective.[34,44]
>
> In *chronic hypertensive heart failure* nifedipine (20 mg 4× daily) seems better than verapamil (160 mg 3× daily) in reducing symptoms and pulmonary wedge pressure.[44]
>
> In *Raynaud's phenomenon*, nifedipine is usually effective and much better than prazosin.[55]
>
> In *progressive systemic sclerosis* nifedipine improves myocardial perfusion defects.

Nifedipine for Hypertension

In *systemic hypertension* (use not approved in the USA), nifedipine is increasingly seen (together with other calcium antagonists) as third-line therapy (after diuretics and β-blockade). Some centers are using nifedipine as second-line therapy (in combination with β-blockade) and occasionally nifedipine is used as monotherapy. In combination with methyldopa and (probably) β-blockers, nifedipine capsules have a prolonged action up to 8–12 hours in mild to moderate hypertension. However, slow-release tablets are better for 2× daily dosage.

For *severe hypertension* (DBP > 120 mmHg), nifedipine 10 mg sublingually, which can be repeated once after 30–60 minutes, is increasingly used. The efficacy of nifedipine is apparently maintained during subsequent chronic therapy without development of tolerance when combined with other agents.[51] In true *hypertensive crises*, however, it is not yet clear that such rapid reduction of blood pressure is safe or desirable (see p 211).

> In *systolic hypertension of the elderly*, nifedipine 10 mg may also be given but fear of abrupt peripheral vasodilation with possible cerebral ischemia suggests that the initial dose should be 5 mg.
>
> In *primary pulmonary hypertension*, nifedipine seems better than hydralazine,[38] yet must be used with care.

Rebound after Cessation of Nifedipine Therapy

In patients with vasospastic angina, abrupt cessation of nifedipine therapy may markedly increase the frequency and duration of attacks.[62] Nifedipine (40–80 mg/day), isosorbide dinitrate (30 mg 4× daily) or verapamil (80–120 mg 4× daily) all reduced the rebound phenomenon. In another placebo-controlled double-blind study, abrupt withdrawal of nifedipine also increased the attack rate in vasospastic angina, but not to pretreatment levels.[16] In patients with previous unstable angina, who become stable on therapy, nifedipine may be withdrawn unless pain at rest persists.[42]

Combination therapy including β-blockade

In patients with reasonable LV function, nifedipine may be freely combined with β-blockade (Fig. 3-6), provided that excess hypotension is guarded against. In the therapy of angina pectoris, nifedipine-propranolol seems better

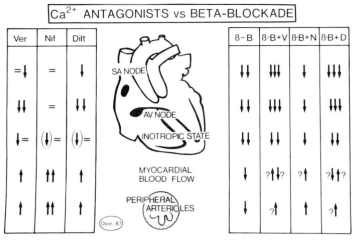

Fig. 3-6.   Proposed hemodynamic effects of calcium antagonists, singly or in combination with β-blockade. Note that some of these effects are based on animal data and extrapolation to man needs to be made with caution.
Ver = verapamil; Nif = nifedipine; Dilt = diltiazem; BB = β-blockade.

than propranolol-isosorbide dinitrate (p 29). In the therapy of angina caused by spasm, nifedipine may be combined with nitrates. In the therapy of hypertension, nifedipine may be combined with β-blockade (see p 10), diuretics, methyldopa, or captopril. Combination with prazosin occasionally leads to adverse interactions so a test dose is required.

Nifedipine—Summary

Nifedipine is a widely used and powerful arterial vasodilator with few serious side-effects and now part of the accepted therapy of all types of angina and hypertension. Nifedipine is especially useful in patients with contraindications to β-blockade such as bronchospasm, LV failure or active peripheral vascular disease. Contraindications to nifedipine are few, and combination with β-blockade is usually simple.

DILTIAZEM

Diltiazem (Cardizem® in USA; Tildiem® in UK; Herbesser® or Tilazem® elsewhere), initially developed in Japan, is now available worldwide. Initially thought to bind at the same cellular site as verapamil, modern opinion suggests that there are different sites for each of the three major calcium antagonists (nifedipine, diltiazem and verapamil). Clinically, **diltiazem is used for the same spectrum of disease as verapamil** (Fig. 3-3)—angina pectoris, hypertension and when AV nodal inhibition is required. Of these indications, only angina is approved in the USA. Diltiazem may have a more powerful inhibitory effect on the sinus node than verapamil, so part of its antianginal effect results from a modest bradycardia. Diltiazem seems to have a very **low side-effect profile,** but whether this would also be so in the higher doses sometimes needed for a full therapeutic effect (360 mg/day) is not yet certain. Like all the other first generation calcium antagonists, diltiazem must be given several times a day for optimal therapy.

Pharmacologic Properties

Pharmacokinetics.   Following oral administration, over 90 percent is absorbed, but bioavailability is about 45 percent (first-pass hepatic metabolism). The onset of action is within 15–30 minutes (oral) with a peak at 1–2 hours. The elimination half-life is 4–7 hours; hence dosage every 8 hours is required for sustained therapeutic effect. The therapeutic plasma concentration range is 50–300 ng/ml. Protein binding is 80–86 percent. Diltiazem is acetylated in the liver to deacyldiltiazem (40 percent of the activity of the parent compound), which accumulates with chronic therapy. Unlike verapamil and nifedipine, only 35 percent of diltiazem is excreted by the kidneys (65 percent by the GI tract).

Dose.   For all varieties of angina, the dose of diltiazem is 120–360 mg, usually in 4 daily doses. Strict 6-hour dosing may be needed for severe angina. Yet a single 120 mg dose improves exercise tolerance for 8 hours and 3× daily dosing may be effective even in unstable or variant angina.[26] Slow-release diltiazem-SR permits 2× daily doses. For hypertension and prophylaxis of supraventricular tachycardia, doses are similar. IV diltiazem, not yet available in the USA and United Kingdom, is given like verapamil with a dose of 0.15–0.25 mg/kg over 2 minutes with ECG and blood pressure control.

Side-effects.   Normally side-effects are few. With high-dose diltiazem (360 mg daily) one series reported no side-effects in the treatment of angina,[48] whereas leg edema, abdominal discomfort, and constipation limited the dose when added to digoxin for atrial fibrillation (Chapter 11, reference 83a). Side-effects of IV diltiazem should resemble those of IV verapamil (p 38).

Contraindications.   These resemble those of verapamil (Fig. 3-4, Table 3-3)—pre-existing marked depression of the sinus or AV node. Myocardial depression may be less of a contraindication.

Drug interactions and combinations.   Like verapamil, diltiazem may increase the blood digoxin level. *Diltiazem plus long-acting nitrates* may lead to excess hypotension.[25]

Combination with β-blockade.   *Diltiazem plus propranolol* (Fig. 3-6) may be used for angina; the combination may cause excess bradycardia or hypotension;[48] however, the combination may be better tolerated from the subjective point of view than propranolol-nifedipine.[53] When propranolol is ineffective in patients with coronary artery spasm, then the combination of diltiazem-propranolol becomes effective although without any advantage over diltiazem alone.[89]

Diltiazem for Ischemic Syndromes

In *chronic stable effort angina*, the combination of vasodilatory and a mild bradycardiac effect seems very desirable. The efficacy of diltiazem in chronic angina is at least as good as propranolol and in some studies the combination was no more effective than diltiazem itself, presumably because of the bradycardia already induced by diltiazem.[48] The doses required vary from 120–360 mg daily in 3 divided doses. The drug is generally safe with no effect on the PR or QRS intervals, and subjective side-effects are unusual.

In *Prinzmetal's variant angina*, diltiazem 240–360 mg/day reduces the number of episodes of pain. At doses of 240 mg daily 30 percent of patients become pain-free with the frequency of angina reduced in the remaining majority.[17]

In *unstable angina at rest*, the properties of diltiazem should be ideal—vasodilation and bradycardia, with only a relatively slight negative inotropic effect. In comparison with β-blockade (propranolol), diltiazem is at least as good[88] or possibly even better.[22,89] Different results probably reflect different population groups with varying degree of coronary spasm as cause of angina at rest.

In *AMI, without Q waves,* diltiazem 360 mg daily helps to prevent early re-infarction, starting 24–72 hours after the onset.[78]

Diltiazem as a peripheral vasodilator.   In *systemic hypertension*, diltiazem has been used against mild to moderate hypertension, where it is as good as hydrochlorothiazide[49] and compares well with nifedipine.[59] In *Raynaud's phenomenon*, diltiazem seems about as effective as nifedipine although there are no strict comparisons.[54,55]

Antiarrhythmic Properties of Diltiazem

The electrophysiological properties of diltiazem closely resemble those of verapamil. The main effect is a depressant one on the AV node; the functional and effective refractory periods are prolonged by diltiazem. Diltiazem is likely to be used for the elective as well as prophylactic control (90 mg 3× daily[97]) of most supraventricular tachyarrhythmias (use not approved in the

USA). A particularly useful therapy for termination of PSVT is single oral dose diltiazem (120 mg) and propranolol (160 mg) which usually works within 20–40 minutes.[98] Diltiazem is unlikely to be effective in ventricular arrhythmias except in those complicating coronary artery spasm. In chronic atrial fibrillation, diltiazem (optimal dose 240 mg daily) added to digoxin improves control of ventricular rate (see p 198).

Hypertrophic cardiomyopathy. In *hypertrophic cardiomyopathy*, diltiazem is not well studied, but apparently more successful than low doses of propranolol (up to 120 mg daily) in improving diastolic function.[85]

Diltiazem—Summary

Diltiazem is a widely used calcium antagonist with a relatively low side-effect profile. In the USA its use is confined to anginal syndromes, but elsewhere it is also used for systemic hypertension, supraventricular arrhythmias and Raynaud's phenomenon.

NEW AGENTS UNDER EVALUATION

New Dihydropyridines (Table 3-4)

Nitrendipine (Baypress®) is a long-acting agent likely to be available in the USA in the near future; it is already used in Europe for hypertension. From the point of efficacy and pharmacokinetics, nitrendipine probably resembles slow-release nifedipine tablets. *Nimodipine* appears to benefit acute ischemic strokes[40] and cerebral arterial spasm as found in subarachnoid hemorrhage.[21] Of the other agents, *nicardipine* and *felodipine* are among the new calcium antagonists (Table 3-4) undergoing widespread clinical testing. Felodipine may be of particular benefit in CHF secondary to coronary artery disease.[89a]

Mixed Agents

Sodium-Calcium Channel Blockers. Combined sodium-calcium channel blockers could be very effective antiarrhythmics as well as having antianginal properties. *Bepridil*, still available in Europe, has been withdrawn from the USA market reportedly because of QT-prolongation. *Tiapamil* has therapeutic potential in angina, hypertension, AMI[30] and supraventricular arrhythmias. Although a promising compound, its commercial development has been stopped.

Flunarizine. This agent, also under evaluation, appears to have a predominant cerebral vasodilator effect and belongs to a different category of agent from verapamil, nifedipine, or diltiazem. Rather, it resembles *cinnarizine* in some ways. When used for vertigo, its benefit may result from nonspecific antihistaminic properties.

TABLE 3-4

SOME NEW CALCIUM ANTAGONISTS

	Possible Dose	Proposed Indications
Dihydropyridines *		
Nicardipine	5–30 mg 3× daily	Hypertension, angina, congestive heart failure.
Felodipine	5–10 mg 2–3× daily	Hypertension, angina, congestive heart failure.
Nitrendipine	10–20 mg 1–2× daily	Hypertension, (angina).
Nimodipine	0.35 mg/kg 4 hourly	Cerebral spasm, subarachnoid hemorrhage, early stroke.
Nisoldipine	10–20 mg 2–3× daily	Hypertension, angina.
Verapamil-like *		
Tiapamil (mixed sodium blocker)	500 mg 3× daily	Similar to verapamil, but slows sinus rate.
Other mixed agents *		
Bepridil (mixed sodium blocker)	200–400 mg 1 × daily	Angina, arrhythmias (problem: QT prolonged)
Flunarizine (mixed antihistaminic)	5–10 mg 1 × daily	Migraine, vertigo, transient ischemic attacks.

* None of above approved in the USA; nicardipine approved in Europe.

TABLE 3-5

CALCIUM ANTAGONISTS: INDICATIONS AND DOSAGE

Agent	Indications	Dose
Verapamil (Isoptin®, Calan®)	Paroxysmal supraventricular tachycardia (PSVT) narrow QRS complexes	1. IV bolus 5–10 mg repeated after 10 min, then 0.005 mg/kg/min if needed 2. IV infusion 1 mg/min to total of 10 mg 3. If myocardial disease, pretreat with calcium gluconate 90 mg (see p 38) before infusion
	Atrial flutter/fibrillation (control of ventricular rate)	IV infusion, if needed, work up from 0.0001 mg/kg/min, titrating against heart rate; or 80–120 mg 3 × daily increasing to 80–120 mg 4 × daily, beware of digitalis toxicity
	"Prophylaxis" of PSVT*	Orally 80–120 mg 3× daily
	Angina of effort, angina at rest	Orally 80–120 mg 3 × daily increasing to 80–120 mg 4× daily
	Prinzmetal's angina and hypertrophic cardiomyopathy*	(rarely higher doses). Later reduced dose to 2× daily
Nifedipine (Procardia®, Adalat®)	Angina of effort	Orally 30–80 mg/day in 3 or 4 doses
	Angina at rest and Prinzmetal's angina	Orally 10 mg 3× daily up to 20 mg every 4 hr
	Hypertension*	Orally 10 mg 2–4× daily
	Acute left ventricular failure (pulmonary edema) in the setting of acute ischemia*	10 mg sublingually 6-hourly
Diltiazem (Cardizem®, Tildiem®, Herbesser®, Tilazem®)	PSVT with narrow QRS complexes*	IV 0.15–0.25 mg/kg given over 2 min (infusion regimen not established)
	Atrial flutter/fibrillation (control of ventricular rate)*	IV 0.15–0.25 mg/kg given over 2 min
	Angina of effort and angina at rest including Prinzmetal.	Oral 30–90 mg 3× daily increasing to 4 × daily as indicated
	"Prophylaxis" of PSVT*	
	Hypertrophic cardiomyopathy*	Indication not well established

* Not FDA approved at present.
PSVT = paroxysmal supraventricular tachycardia
IV = intravenous

CALCIUM ANTAGONISTS FOR HYPERTENSION

All three calcium antagonists have hypotensive actions in addition to their effects against supraventricular arrhythmias (verapamil and diltiazem) and against coronary spasm (verapamil, diltiazem, and nifedipine); the mechanism is by arteriolar dilatation. Although verapamil is the calcium antagonist likely first to be approved for hypertension in the USA, **all three agents are increasingly used.** Nifedipine rather than verapamil is generally chosen against severe or apparently refractory hypertension, or when a calcium antagonist is used as a third-line agent (vasodilator after diuretic-β-blockade combination). In mild to moderate hypertension, verapamil (360–480 mg daily) is the equivalent of nifedipine (40–120 mg daily; nifedipine tablets 2× daily) with similar side-effects.[43] In Europe, nifedipine is now being used more and more as a standard vasodilator in the therapy of systemic hypertension. In Japan, diltiazem is standard. All three agents may be used either as monotherapy or in combination with diuretics or angiotensin-converting enzyme (ACE) inhibitors. Only nifedipine has been well studied in combination with β-blockers in the therapy of hypertension.[26a,51] Caution is required when combining α-blockers such as prazosin with calcium antagonists for fear of excess hypotension.[45a,50a]

RATIONAL CHOICE OF CALCIUM ANTAGONISTS

The striking clinical differences between verapamil and diltiazem on the one hand and nifedipine on the other hand (Table 3-5) suggest that there might be more than one type of binding site on the calcium channel for such drugs to act on.[99-103] Alternatively, the calcium channels in different tissues may differ in sensitivity to various antagonists with the channels of the AV node being most sensitive to verapamil and diltiazem, those of the sinus node to diltiazem, and the channels of smooth muscle responding to all three agents. The predominant action on the AV node is the explanation for the striking efficacy of IV verapamil and diltiazem in the acute therapy of paroxysmal supraventricular tachycardia. As coronary artery vasodilators, all three agents are first-line therapy for vasospastic or Prinzmetal's angina; by analogy they can also be used in mixed angina (partially Prinzmetal's and partially chronic stable angina of effort).

When combination of a calcium antagonist with β-blockade is desired, the additive effects of verapamil or diltiazem on the AV node occasionally result in heart block or excess sinus bradycardia, so that the preferred combination is nifedipine-β-blockade.

Verapamil

The agent verapamil has the widest range of approved indications including angina pectoris, supraventricular tachycardias and hypertension; compared with propranolol in the therapy of effort angina, it is at least as effective, has less risk of serious side-effects, and fewer contraindications. In vasospastic angina, verapamil is preferable to propranolol. Verapamil is now one of a number of early options in the therapy of hypertension.

Nifedipine

In vasospastic angina, nifedipine works consistently. In chronic stable angina, nifedipine is more effective than placebo yet appears to be somewhat less effective than the other agents, possibly because of the reflex tachycardia. An advantage of nifedipine, however, is that it may be combined with β-blockade with less monitoring than in the case of verapamil or diltiazem, and with better benefit than isosorbide dinitrate combined with β-blockade. Nifedipine is also selected for angina combined with CHF or conduction problems or hypertension and for a powerful and rapid hypotensive effect.

Diltiazem

The major advantages of diltiazem are the relatively few subjective side-effects and the modest negative inotropic effect. Diltiazem, with its properties of peripheral vasodilation and a mild negative inotropic effect, is increasingly seen as having hemodynamic advantages in the therapy of angina pectoris. In the USA, diltiazem is not approved for supraventricular tachycardias nor for hypertension, although widely used elsewhere for these indications.

Comparison with β-Blockers

Calcium antagonists are being used increasingly in preference to β-blockade early on in the therapy of anginal syndromes because of their efficacy against a wide variety of ischemic syndromes including coronary spasm, the fewer contraindications, and the absence of bronchial side-effects. Like β-blockers, calcium antagonists are now used earlier and earlier in the therapy of hypertension.

SUMMARY

Each agent has its own advantages and the choice will be partially dictated by the experience of the clinician with a particular agent and the anticipated side-effects. As a group, they are being used sooner and sooner in the therapy of anginal syndromes and of hypertension; other uses include Raynaud's syndrome and (in the case of verapamil and diltiazem) supraventricular tachycardias and obstructive cardiomyopathies.

REFERENCES

References from Previous Edition

For details see previous edition of Opie et al Drugs for the Heart, American Edition. Orlando, FL, Grune & Stratton, 1984, pp 39–64.

1. Antman E, Muller J, Goldberg S, et al: New Engl J Med 302:1269–1273, 1980
2. Chew CYC, Hecht HS, Collett JT, et al: Am J Cardiol 47:917–922, 1981
3. Ferlinz J, Easthope JL, Aronow WS: Circulation 59:313–319, 1979
4. Hariman RJ, Mangiardi LM, McAllister RG, et al. Circulation 59:797–804, 1979
5. Heng MK, Singh BN, Roche AHG, et al: Am Heart J 90:487–498, 1975
6. Kenmure ACF, Scruton JH: Br J Clin Prac 33:49–51, 1979
7. Klein HO, Kaplinsky L: Am J Cardiol 50:894–902, 1982
8. Landmark K, Sire S, Thaulow E, et al: Br Heart J 48:19–26, 1982
9. Lichtlen PR, Engel H-J, Rafflenbeul W: In Opie LH (ed): Calcium Antagonists and Cardiovascular Disease. New York, Raven Press, 1984, pp 221–236
10. Livesley B, Catley PF, Campbell RC, et al: Br Med J 1:375–378, 1973
11. Lynch P, Dargie H, Krikler S, et al: Br Med J 2:184–187, 1980
12. Mangiardi LM, Hariman RJ, McAllister RG, et al: Circulation 57:366–372, 1977
13. Mehta J, Pepine CJ, Day M, et al: Am J Med 71:977–982, 1981
14. Parodi O, Maseri A, Simometti I: Br Heart J 41:167–174, 1979
15. Rosing DR, Kent KM, Maron BJ, et al: Circulation 60:1208–1213, 1979
16. Schick EC, Heupler FA, Kerin NZ, et al: Am Heart J 104:690–697, 1982
17. Schroeder JS, Feldman RL, Giles TD, et al: Am J Med 72:227–232, 1982
18. Singh BN, Roche AHG: Am Heart J 94:593–599, 1977
19. Stone PH, Muller JE, Turi ZG, et al: Am Heart J 106:644–652, 1983
20. Winniford MD, Johnson SM, Mauritson DR, et al: Am J Cardiol 50:913–918, 1982

New References

21. Allen GS, Ahn HS, Preziosi TJ, et al: Cerebral arterial spasm—a controlled trial of nimodipine in patients with subarachnoid hemorrhage. New Engl J Med 308:619–624, 1983
22. Andre-Fouet X, Usdin JP, Gayet C, et al: Comparison of short-term efficacy of diltiazem and propranolol in unstable angina at rest. A randomized trial in 70 patients. Eur Heart J 4:691–698, 1983
23. Arnman K, Ryden L: Comparison of metoprolol and verapamil in the treatment of angina pectoris. Am J Cardiol 49:821–827, 1982
24. Belhassen B, Horowitz LN: Use of intravenous verapamil for ventricular tachycardia. Am J Cardiol 54:1131–1133, 1984
25. Bruce RA, Hossack KF, Kusumi F, et al: Excessive reduction in peripheral resistance during exercise and risk of orthostatic symptoms with sustained-release nitroglycerin and diltiazem treatment of angina. Am Heart J 109:1020–1026, 1985
26. Chaitman BR, Wagniart P, Pasternac A, et al: Improved exercise tolerance after propranolol, diltiazem or nifedipine in angina pectoris: Comparison at 1, 3 and 8 hours and correlation with plasma drug concentration. Am J Cardiol 53:1–9, 1984
26a. Daniels AR, Opie LH: Atenolol plus nifedipine for mild to moderate systemic hypertension after fixed doses of either agent alone. Am J Cardiol 57:965–970, 1986

27. Danish Study Group on verapamil in myocardial infarction: Verapamil in acute myocardial infarction. Eur Heart J 5:516–528, 1984

28. Dawson JR, Whitaker NHG, Sutton GC: Calcium antagonist drugs in chronic stable angina. Comparison of verapamil and nifedipine. Br Heart J 46:508–512, 1981

29. Diamond JR, Cheung JY, Fang LST: Nifedipine-induced renal dysfunction. Alterations in renal hemodynamics. Am J Med 77:905–909, 1984

30. Eichler HG, Mabin T, Commerford PJ, et al: Tiapamil, a new calcium antagonist: Hemodynamic effects in patients with acute myocardial infarction. Circulation 71:779–786, 1985

31. Elkayam U, Weber L, Campese VM, et al: Renal hemodynamic effects of vasodilation with nifedipine and hydralazine in patients with heart failure. J Am Coll Cardiol 4:1261–1267, 1984

32. Elkayam U, Weber L, McKay CR, et al: Differences in hemodynamic response to vasodilation due to calcium channel antagonism with nifedipine and direct-acting agonism with hydralazine in chronic refractory congestive heart failure. Am J Cardiol 54:126–131, 1984

33. Elliott HL, Pasanisi F, Meredith PA, et al: Acute hypotensive response to nifedipine added to prazosin. Br Med J 288:238, 1984

34. Ellrodt AG, Ault MJ, Riedinger MS, et al: Efficacy and safety of sublingual nifedipine in hypertensive emergencies. Am J Med 79 (suppl 4A):19–25, 1985

35. Endo M, Kanda I, Hosoda S, et al: Prinzmetal's variant form of angina pectoris. Re-evaluation of mechanisms. Circulation 52:33–37, 1975

36. Fifer MA, Colucci WS, Lorell BH, et al: Inotropic, vascular and neuroendocrine effects of nifedipine in heart failure: Comparison with nitroprusside. J Am Coll Cardiol 5:731–737, 1985

37. Findlay IN, Dargie HJ: The effects of nifedipine, atenolol and that combination on left ventricular function. Postgrad Med J 59 (suppl 2):70–73, 1983

37a. Findlay IN, MacLeod K, Ford M, et al: Treatment of angina pectoris with nifedipine and atenolol: Efficacy and effect on cardiac function. Br Heart J 55:240–245, 1986

38. Fisher JF, Borer JS, Moses JW, et al: Hemodynamic effects of nifedipine versus hydralazine in primary pulmonary hypertension. Am J Cardiol 54:646–650, 1984

39. Frishman W, Kirsten E, Klein M, et al: Clinical relevance of verapamil plasma levels in stable angina pectoris. Am J Cardiol 50:1180–1184, 1982

40. Gelmers HJ: The effects of nimodipine on the clinical course of patients with acute ischemic stroke. Acta Neurol Scand 69:232–239, 1984

41. Gordon GD, Mabin TA, Isaacs S, et al: Hemodynamic effects of sublingual nifedipine in acute myocardial infarction. Am J Cardiol 53:1228–1232, 1984

42. Gottlieb SO, Ouyang P, Achuff SC, et al: Acute nifedipine withdrawal: Consequences of preoperative and late cessation of therapy in patients with prior unstable angina. J Am Coll Cardiol 4:382–388, 1984

42a. Gottlieb SO, Weisfeldt M, Ouyang P, et al: Effect of addition of propranolol to therapy with nifedipine for unstable angina pectoris. Circulation 73:331–337, 1986

43. Gould BA, Hornung RS, Mann S, et al: Slow channel inhibitors verapamil and nifedipine in the management of hypertension. J Cardiovasc Pharmacol 4:S369–S373, 1982

44. Guazzi MD, Cipolla C, Bella PD, et al: Disparate unloading efficacy of the calcium channel blockers, verapamil and nifedipine, on the failing hypertensive left ventricle. Am Heart J 108:116–123, 1984

45. Gulamhusein S, Ko P, Carruthers SG, et al: Acceleration of the ventricular response during atrial fibrillation in the Wolff-Parkinson-White syndrome after verapamil. Circulation 65:348–354, 1982

45a. Halperin AK, Cubeddu LX: The role of calcium channel blockers in the treatment of hypertension. Am Heart J 111:363–382, 1986

46. Hamann SR, Kaltenborn KE, Vore M, et al: Cardiovascular and pharmacokinetic consequences of combined administration of verapamil and propranolol in dogs. Am J Cardiol 56:147–156, 1985

47. Hess O, Grimm J, Krayenbuehl HP: Diastolic function in hypertrophic cardiomyopathy: Effects of propranolol and verapamil on diastolic stiffness. Eur Heart J 4 (suppl F):47–56, 1983

48. Hung J, Lamb IH, Connolly SJ, et al: The effect of diltiazem and propranolol, alone and in combination, on exercise performance and left ventricular function in patients with stable effort angina: a double-blind, randomized, and placebo controlled study. Circulation 68:560–567, 1983

49. Inouye IK, Massie BM, Benowitz N, et al: Antihypertensive therapy with diltiazem and comparison with hydrochlorothiazide. Am J Cardiol 53:1588–1592, 1984

50. Jariwalla AG, Anderson EG: Production of ischaemic cardiac pain by nifedipine. Br Med J i:1181–1182, 1978

50a. Jee LD, Opie LH: Acute hypotensive response to nifedipine added to prazosin in treatment of hypertension. Br Med J 287:1514, 1983

51. Jennings AA, Jee LD, Smith JA, et al: Acute effect of nifedipine on blood pressure and left ventricular ejection fraction in severely hypertensive outpatients. Predictive effects of acute therapy and prolonged efficacy when added to existing therapy. Am Heart J 111:557–563, 1986

52. Johnston DL, Gebhardt VA, Donald A, et al: Comparative effects of propranolol and

verapamil alone and in combination on left ventricular function and volumes in patients with chronic exertional angina: A double-blind, placebo-controlled, randomized, crossover study with radionuclide ventriculography. Circulation 68:1280–1289, 1983

53. Johnston DL, Lesoway R, Humen DP, et al: Clinical and hemodynamic evaluation of propranolol in combination with verapamil, nifedipine and diltiazem in exertional angina pectoris: A placebo-controlled, double-blind, randomized, crossover study. Am J Cardiol 55:680–687, 1985

54. Kahan A, Amor B, Menkes CJ: A randomized double-blind trial of diltiazem in the treatment of Raynaud's phenomenon. Ann Rheum Dis 44:30–33, 1985

55. Kahan A, Foult JM, Weber S, et al: Nifedipine and alpha$_1$-adrenergic blockade in Raynaud's phenomenon. Eur Heart J 6:702–705, 1985

56. Kaltenbach M, Hopf R: Treatment of hypertrophic cardiomyopathy: Relation to pathological mechanisms. J Mol Cell Cardiol 17 (suppl 2):59–68, 1985

57. Kieval J, Kirsten EB, Kessler KM, et al: The effects of intravenous verapamil on hemodynamic status of patients with coronary artery disease receiving propranolol. Circulation 65:653–659, 1982

58. Kimura E, Kishida H: Treatment of variant angina with drugs: A survey of 11 cardiology institutes in Japan. Circulation 63:844–848, 1981

59. Klein W, Brandt D, Vrecko K, et al: Role of calcium antagonists in the treatment of essential hypertension. Circ Res 52(suppl 1):174–181, 1983

60. Klugmann S, Salvi A, Camerini F: Haemodynamic effects of nifedipine in heart failure. Br Heart J 43:440–446, 1980

61. Lessem J, Bellinetto A: Interaction between digoxin and calcium antagonist. Am J Cardiol 49(abs):1025, 1982

62. Lette J, Gagnon RM, Lemire JG, et al: Rebound of vasospastic angina after cessation of long-term treatment with nifedipine. Can Med Assoc J 130:1169–1171, 1984

62a. McInnes GT, Findlay IN, Murray G, et al: Cardiovascular responses to verapamil and propranolol in hypertensive patients. J Hypertens 3 (suppl 3):S219–S221, 1985

63. Magorien RD, Leier CV, Kolibash AJ, et al: Beneficial effects of nifedipine on rest and exercise myocardial energetics in patients with congestive heart failure. Circulation 70:884–890, 1984

64. Maisel AS, Motulsky HJ, Insel PA: Hypotension after quinidine plus verapamil. Possible additive competition at alpha-adrenergic receptors. New Engl J Med 312:167–171, 1985

65. Mauritson DR, Winniford MD, Walker WS, et al: Oral verapamil for paroxysmal supraventricular tachycardia. A long-term, double-blind randomized trial. Ann Int Med 96:409–412, 1982

66. Mauritson DR, Johnson SM, Winniford MD, et al: Verapamil for unstable angina at rest: A short-term randomized, double-blind study. Am Heart J 106:652–658, 1983

67. Muller JE, Morrison J, Stone PH, et al: Nifedipine therapy for patients with threatened and acute myocardial infarction. A randomized double-blind placebo-controlled comparison. Circulation 69:740–747, 1984

68. Muller JE, Turi ZG, Pearle DL, et al: Nifedipine and conventional therapy for unstable angina pectoris. A randomized, double-blind comparison. Circulation 69:728–739, 1984

69. Opie LH: Drugs and the Heart. London, Lancet, 1980, pp 27–38

70. Opie LH: The Heart: Physiology, Metabolism, Pharmacology and Therapy. London, Grune & Stratton, 1984

71. Opie LH: Calcium ions, drug action and the heart with special reference to calcium antagonist drugs. Pharmacol Ther 25:271–295, 1984

72. Packer M, Meller J, Medina N, et al: Hemodynamic consequences of combined beta-adrenergic and slow calcium channel blockade in man. Circulation 65:660–668, 1982

73. Pasanisi F, Elliott HL, Meredith PA, et al: Combined alpha-adrenoceptor antagonism and calcium channel blockade in normal subjects. Clin Pharmacol Ther 36:716–723, 1984

74. Pepine CJ, Feldman RL, Hill JA, et al: Clinical outcome after treatment of rest angina with calcium blockers: Comparative experience during the initial year of therapy with diltiazem, nifedipine and verapamil. Am Heart J 106:1341–1347, 1983

75. Pitlik S, Manor RS, Lipshitz I, et al: Transient retinal ischaemia induced by nifedipine. Br Med J 287:1845–1846, 1983

76. Porter CB, Walsh RA, Badke FR, et al: Differential effects of diltiazem and nitroprusside on left ventricular function in experimental chronic volume overload. Circulation 68:685–692, 1983

77. Reiter MJ, Shand DG, Aanonsen LM, et al: Pharmacokinetics of verapamil: Experience with a sustained intravenous infusion regimen. Am J Cardiol 50:716–721, 1982

78. Roberts R, Gibson RS, Boden WE, et al: Prophylactic therapy with diltiazim prevents re-infarction (abstract). J Am Coll Cardiol 7:68A, 1986

79. Schamroth L, Krikler DM, Garrett C: Immediate effects of intravenous verapamil in cardiac arrhythmias. Br Med J 1:660–662, 1972

80. Scheidt S, Frishman WF, Packer M, et al: Long-term effectiveness of verapamil in stable and unstable angina pectoris. One-year follow-up of patients treated in placebo-controlled double-blind randomized clinical trials. Am J Cardiol 50:1185–1190, 1982

81. Schwartz JB, Keefe DL, Kirsten E, et al: Prolongation of verapamil elimination kinetics during chronic oral administration. Am Heart J 104:198–203, 1982

82. Singh BN, Opie LH: Drugs for the heart. III. Calcium antagonists. Orlando, Grune and Stratton, 1984, pp 39–64

83. Storstein L, Larsen A, Midtbo K, et al: Pharmacokinetics of calcium blockers in patients with renal insufficiency and in geriatric patients. Acta Med Scand (suppl 681):25–30, 1983

84. Subramanian VB: Calcium antagonists in chronic stable angina pectoris. Amsterdam, Excerpta Medica, 1983, pp 97–116, 217–229

85. Suwa M, Hirota Y, Kawamura K: Improvement in left ventricular diastolic function during intravenous and oral diltiazem therapy in patients with hypertrophic cardiomyopathy: An echocardiographic study. Am J Cardiol 54:1047–1053, 1984

86. Talano JV, Tommaso C: Slow channel calcium antagonists in the treatment of supraventricular tachycardia. Prog Cardiovasc Dis 25:141–156, 1982

87. Theroux P, Waters DD, Affaki GS, et al: Provocative testing with ergonovine to evaluate the efficacy of treatment with calcium antagonists in variant angina. Circulation 60:504–510, 1979

88. Theroux P, Taeymans Y, Morissette D, et al: A randomized study comparing propranolol and diltiazem in the treatment of unstable angina. J Am Coll Cardiol 5:717–722, 1985

89. Tilmant PY, Lablanche JM, Thieuleux FA, et al: Detrimental effect of propranolol in patients with coronary arterial spasm countered by combination with diltiazem. Am J Cardiol 52:230–233, 1983

89a. Tweddel AC, Hutton I: Felodipine in ventricular dysfunction. Eur Heart J 7:54–60, 1986

90. Urthaler F, James TN: Experimental studies on the pathogenesis of asystole after verapamil in the dog. Am J Cardiol 44:651–656, 1979

90a. Uusitalo A, Arstila M, Bae AE, et al: Metoprolol, nifedipine, and the combination in stable effort angina pectoris. Am J Cardiol 57:733–737, 1986

91. Weiss AT, Lewis BS, Halon DA, et al: The use of calcium with verapamil in the management of supraventricular tachyarrhythmias. Int J Cardiol 4:275–280, 1983

92. Wigle ED, Sasson Z, Henderson MA, et al: Hypertrophic cardiomyopathy. The importance of the site and the extent of hypertrophy. A review. Prog Cardiovasc Dis 28:1–83, 1985

93. Winniford MD, Fulton KL, Corbett JR, et al: Propranolol-verapamil versus propranolol-nifedipine in severe angina pectoris of effort: a randomized, double-blind, crossover study. Am J Cardiol 55:281–285, 1985

94. Winniford MD, Gabliani G, Johnson SM, et al: Concomitant calcium antagonist plus isosorbide dinitrate therapy for markedly active variant angina. Am Heart J 108:1269–1273, 1984

95. Woelfel A, Foster JR, McAllister RG, et al: Efficacy of verapamil in exercise-induced ventricular tachycardia. Am J Cardiol 56:292–297, 1985

96. Yee R, Gulamhusein SS, Klein GJ: Combined verapamil and propranolol for supraventricular tachycardia. Am J Cardiol 53:757–763, 1984

97. Yeh S-J, Kou H-C, Lin F-C, et al: Effects of oral diltiazem in paroxysmal supraventricular tachycardia. Am J Cardiol 52:271–278, 1983

98. Yeh S-J, Lin F-C, Chou Y-Y, et al: Termination of paroxysmal supraventricular tachycardia with a single oral dose of diltiazem and propranolol. Circulation 71:104–109, 1985

Review Articles

99. Chaffman M, Brogden RN: Diltiazem: A review of its pharmacological properties and therapeutic efficacy. Drugs 29:387–454, 1985

100. Opie LH: Calcium ions, drug action and the heart—with special reference to calcium antagonist drugs. Pharmacol Therap 25:271–295, 1984

101. Singh B, Ellrodt G, Peter CT: Verapamil: A review of its pharmacological properties and therapeutic use. Drugs 15:169–197, 1978

102. Sorkin EM, Clissold SP, Brogden RN: Nifedipine. A review of its pharmacodynamic and pharmacokinetic properties and therapeutic efficacy in ischemic heart disease, hypertension and related cardiovascular diseases. Drugs 30:182–274, 1985

103. Sorkin EM: Verapamil. Its safety and efficacy in angina pectoris and hypertension. Drugs, in press, 1986

B. N. Singh, L. H. Opie
D. C. Harrison, F. I. Marcus

4

Antiarrhythmic Agents

Singh and Vaughan Williams[36,37] have categorized antiarrhythmic compounds by their effects on (1) the fast sodium current, (2) the sympathetic activity of the heart, (3) the repolarization currents, and (4) the slow inward calcium current (Table 4-1). Antiarrhythmics that fall into Class I antagonize the fast sodium channel (Fig. 4-1), which is responsible for the rapid phase of depolarization (phase 0) in conduction and myocardial fibers. Class II agents are β-antagonists, which are antiarrhythmic probably by limiting formation of the arrhythmogenic second messenger, cyclic AMP. The best studied Class III agent is amiodarone, which prolongs the action potential duration, while having a variety of other pharmacological effects. The Class IV agents verapamil and diltiazem owe their antiarrhythmic effects to inhibition of the slow calcium current, particularly in the atrioventricular (AV) node. Common to most antiarrhythmics is their lengthening of the effective refractory period (Fig. 4-1), not always evident in normal heart tissue stimulated at physiologic frequencies.

CLASS IA: QUINIDINE AND SIMILAR COMPOUNDS

Class IA agents (quinidine, disopyramide, procainamide) lengthen the effective refractory period by two mechanisms in the usual therapeutic concentrations. First, they inhibit the fast sodium current and the upstroke of the action potential, thereby delaying the return of excitability ("pure" Class I effect; very much rate-dependent); second, they prolong the action potential duration and thereby have a mild Class III effect. In addition, as a group, these agents interact with muscarinic receptors (vagolytic effect). Such compounds can have a pro-arrhythmic effect by prolonging the QT-interval in certain predisposed patients (see QT-prolongation). Despite newly reported side-effects, quinidine still has a place.[178]

Quinidine

Electrophysiology. Quinidine (Fig. 4-2) is the prototype of Class I agents; it inhibits the fast sodium channel or slow phase 0 of the action potential while leaving the resting membrane potential unaltered. Quinidine also prolongs the action potential duration by inhibition of the outward potassium current.[69] In addition, it slows phase 4 depolarization in automatic Purkinje fibers. It inhibits conduction along the fast limb of AV nodal or bypass Wolff-Parkinson-White (WPW) syndrome re-entrant arrhythmias (Fig. 4-3). Quinidine has a wide spectrum of activity against re-entrant as well as ectopic atrial and ventricular tachyarrhythmias.

Drugs for the Heart, Second Expanded Edition
Copyright © 1987 by Grune & Stratton, Inc.

ISBN 0-8089-1840-0
All rights reserved.

TABLE 4-1

CLASSIFICATION OF ANTIARRHYTHMIC AGENTS BY EFFECTS ON
INTRACELLULAR ACTION POTENTIAL

I.	Membrane stabilizing agents (fast sodium channel blockers)	A.	Quinidine and quinidine-like agents (Na^+ blockade; repolarization delayed with widening of action potential): quinidine, procainamide, disopyramide (amiodarone).
		B.	Lidocaine and lidocaine-like agents (Na blockade; repolarization accelerated; action potential abbreviated): lidocaine, phenytoin, mexiletine, tocainide, ethmozine*
		C.	Na^+ blockers with marked inhibition of His-Purkinje tissue and QRS prolongation: flecainide, encainide, propafenone, lorcainide, cibenzoline, indecainide.
II.	β-Blocking agents		Propranolol and all other β-blockers.
III.	Agents widening action potential duration as major effect (repolarization inhibitors)		Amiodarone, bretylium, sotalol, d-sotalol, N-acetyl-procainamide (amiodarone: mixed I and III; sotalol: mixed II and III).
IV.	Calcium antagonist agents (inhibit slow calcium channel in AV node)		Verapamil, diltiazem (Mixed Na^+-Ca^{2+} blockers: bepridil, tiapamil).

Modified from Singh BN, Vaughan Williams M: A fourth class of antidysrhythmic action. Effect of verapamil on ouabain toxicity, on atrial and ventricular potentials and on other features of cardiac function. Cardiovasc Res 6:109–119, 1972; and from Singh BN, Hauswirth O: Comparative mechanisms of action of antiarrhythmic drugs. Am Heart J 87:367–382, 1974. See also Campbell TJ: Cardiovasc Res 17:344–352, 1983.

* = some Class IC properties

Receptor Effects. Quinidine inhibits peripheral and myocardial α-adrenergic receptors[124] so that there is risk of hypotension with IV administration. By inhibiting muscarinic receptors, quinidine has an anticholinergic effect (vagolytic) which may cause tachycardia.[117]

Pharmacokinetics and therapeutic levels. Quinidine is metabolized primarily by hydroxylation in the liver and a small amount is excreted by the kidneys; mean

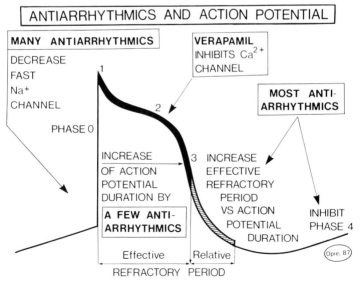

Fig. 4-1. Class I agents decrease phase zero of the rapid depolarization of the action potential (rapid sodium channel). β-Blocking agents (Class II) have no specific effects on intracellular action potential. Class III agents increase the duration of the action potential. The Class IV agents, verapamil and diltiazem, inhibit the inward calcium channel. Most antiarrhythmic agents have nonspecific effects on phase 4 depolarization and increase the effective refractory period.

bioavailability is about 75 percent but varies greatly with up to 3–fold differences between individuals.[172] Many studies on quinidine kinetics have used a protein precipitate extraction method followed by fluorometric assay, which also measures the antiarrhythmic metabolites such as hydroxyquinidine and oxoquinidone. A double-extraction method is more specific. Modern measurement is by the highly specific fluorescence polarization or enzyme immunoassay techniques. The anti-arrhythmic quinidine metabolites are not measured by such specific assays and this may account for discrepancies occasionally observed between quinidine plasma concentration and antiarrhythmic effect. Quinidine elimination is grossly normal even in heart or renal failure, but the plasma half-life increases with age so that the dose should be reduced. Therapeutic blood levels are 2.3–5 μg/ml (= 3–5.5 μM/L) with specific assays and about 22 percent higher than with the earlier nonspecific assay.

Dose.   A test of 0.2 g of quinidine sulfate is traditionally given while the patient is monitored to check for drug idiosyncrasy including cardiovascular collapse, although such serious side-effects are seldom seen and the whole procedure is of unproven value. Then sustained oral therapy is started. One regimen is 0.2–0.3 g quinidine sulfate every 3–4 hours with a usual total dose of 1.2–1.6 g/day with a maximum of 2 g.[35] Doses over 1.6 g/day should be regulated by measurement of plasma levels and by repeated electrocardiograms (ECGs). Periodic blood counts are advisable during long-term therapy. Long-acting quinidine preparations (similar dose limits) are *quinidine gluconate* (multiples of 330 mg or 325 mg) and *quinidine polygalacturonate* (multiples of 275 mg as Cardioquin® 8–12–hourly).

The dose of these 3 preparations is the same, because quinidine sulfate has 83 percent (166 mg) of quinidine base; quinidine gluconate has 62 percent (200 mg) of quinidine base, and quinidine polygalacturonate has 80 percent (166 mg) of the base. Since bioavailability of quinidine gluconate is about 10 percent less than that of the sulfate, the systemic availability is nearly equivalent for the above doses of these 3 preparations.

Marked individual variations in half-life may require monitoring by plasma levels. When a long-acting preparation is started, a loading dose of quinidine sulfate 0.6–0.8 g, given 1 hour before the first long-acting dose, will produce an adequate blood level in 3 hours. *IV quinidine* is now rarely used because of hypotension (vasodilator effect) unless there are arrhythmias resistant to other drugs.

Side-effects.   Serious side-effects may develop soon after the first dose if there is idiosyncrasy or gradually from cumulative overdosage. They can therefore be lessened by adherence to the therapeutic blood level (see above section on pharmacokinetics and therapeutic levels).

Conduction delay and pro-arrhythmic effects are potentially serious. The major direct effect is depression of conduction with prolongation of QRS (consider dose reduction of quinidine if QRS duration widens by 50 percent or 25 percent in presence of intraventricular conduction defects, or if the total QRS duration exceeds 140 msec; these guidelines although reasonable are not well documented). The combination of depressed conduction and lengthened repolarization predisposes to heterogeneity in refractoriness, which heightens the risk of *torsades de pointes*,[14,48] the probable explanation of *quinidine syncope*. Quinidine is contraindicated when ventricular tachyarrhythmias are associated with QT-prolongation. **The risk of QT-prolongation may be lessened by selection of patients who have no initial hypokalemia and a QT-interval no longer than 400 msec;**[151a] in the absence of digitalis toxicity, the overall incidence of pro-arrhythmic effects with quinidine may only be as low as 2 percent.[120] Patients in the later series were treated only for premature ventricular complexes (PVCs); pro-arrhythmic events may be more common in the presence of more serious arrhythmias or heart disease. The QT-interval must be monitored throughout quinidine therapy; if it prolongs significantly, serum potassium, magnesium, and calcium must be checked and the dose of quinidine reduced. In patients with the *sick sinus syndrome*, a direct depressant effect of quinidine may be seen; in others nodal depression is overriden by the vagolytic effect.

Subjective side-effects were studied in a double-blind trial[25] when 139 patients took quinidine 300–400 mg every 6 hours. Most common were diarrhea (33 percent), nausea (18 percent), headache (13 percent), and dizziness (8 percent). Twenty-one patients dropped out because of these side-effects.

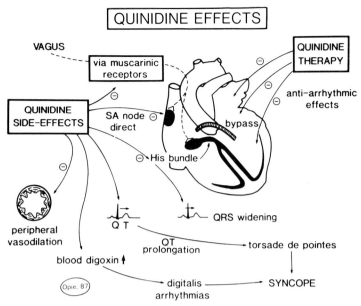

Fig. 4-2. Schematic proposal for therapeutic and side-effects of quinidine. See text for further details.

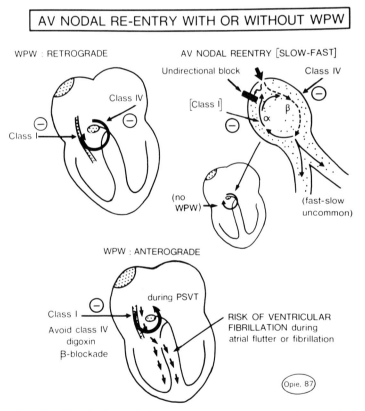

Fig 4-3. Site of effects of slow calcium channel blockers (verapamil and diltiazem) and of fast channel blockers in AV nodal re-entry tachycardia (panel A) or bypass re-entry (panel B). Slow channel blockers are used in most cases of paroxysmal supraventricular nodal tachycardia with or without overt bypass conduction, unless anterograde conduction down the bypass tract is expected (panel C). WPW = Wolff-Parkinson-White (Modified from Opie LH: The Heart. Physiology, Metabolism, Pharmacology and Therapy. London and Orlando, Florida, Grune & Stratton, 1984. With permission.)

Contraindications.   Prolonged QT-interval or QRS duration or clinical congestive heart failure (CHF) all require caution, with small initial doses and close monitoring. Other relative contraindications: sick sinus syndrome, bundle branch block, myasthenia gravis (see section on drug interactions below) and severe liver failure (altered pharmacokinetics).

Drug interactions.   Quinidine increases blood digoxin levels (decrease dose of digoxin, reassess blood levels). Quinidine may enhance the effects of other hypotensive agents, or agents inhibiting the sinus node (β-blockers and some calcium antagonists). The effect of coumarin anticoagulants may be enhanced by a hepatic interaction. Drugs such as phenytoin, phenobarbital, and rifampin (rifampicin), that induce hepatic enzymes, may markedly increase the hepatic metabolism of quinidine with decreased steady-state concentrations.[72,169] Conversely, cimetidine can decrease the metabolism of quinidine with opposite effects.[78] Interaction between the calcium channel blocking agents and quinidine have recently been observed. In one patient, coadministration of verapamil with quinidine appeared to cause an increase in quinidine plasma level accompanied by increased effect. This was attributed to a verapamil-induced decrease in quinidine clearance.[167a] Conversely, nifedipine has been reported to lower quinidine plasma concentration, particularly with poor left ventricular (LV) systolic function.[77a,84a,173a] This may be due to improved hemodynamics due to nifedipine resulting in enhanced quinidine disposition. Hypokalemia decreases quinidine efficacy and predisposes to QT-prolongation. Concomitant therapy with amiodarone or sotalol or other drugs prolonging the QT-interval requires great care.[22] Quinidine reduces the effects of procedures that enhance vagal activity such as carotid sinus massage by its vagolytic effect (this opposes some digitalis effects such as slowing of the heart). Quinidine also reduces the effects of anticholinesterases in myasthenia gravis (inhibition of muscarinic receptors) and enhances antibiotic-induced muscle weakness.

Treatment of toxicity.   Stop quinidine, reduce plasma potassium if elevated, and acidify urine to encourage excretion. Torsades de pointes or severely disorganised conduction may require temporary ventricular pacing and/or isoproterenol. Experimentally, glucagon benefits conduction block and bradycardia.

Quinidine—Summary

Quinidine, the prototype of Class IA antiarrhythmics, is the oldest antiarrhythmic agent. It is reasonably effective in suppressing ventricular premature systoles and recurrent ventricular tachycardia (VT). Quinidine has not been shown to reduce sudden death or to prolong survival. It is frequently used in attempted pharmacologic cardioversion of atrial flutter or fibrillation. About one-third of patients will suffer from gastrointestinal (GI) disturbances including nausea. Pro-arrhythmic effects (QRS and QT-prolongation) require monitoring of the ECG and elimination of hypokalemia, as well as great care when also using other drugs such as amiodarone that prolong the QT-interval. Numerous other drug interactions merit attention. Otherwise, long-term tolerance in those without early side-effects is excellent.

The salient features of quinidine and other antiarrhythmic agents are summarized in Tables 4-2 and 4-3.

Procainamide

Procainamide (Pronestyl®) is generally effective against a wide variety of supraventricular and ventricular arrhythmias, including VT. As in the case of quinidine, no effect on mortality or survival has been shown. Although usually given orally, IV procainamide is one of several agents that may be tried if lidocaine fails. The oral use is limited by a short half-life and the long-term danger of the lupus syndrome.

Electrophysiology.   Procainamide is a Class IA agent, like quinidine, but does not prolong the QT-interval to the same extent and also has less interaction with the muscarinic receptors.[117] Procainamide slows His-Purkinje conduction and prolongs atrial, His-Purkinje, ventricular and bypass tract effective refractory periods.

Pharmacokinetics. Oral procainamide has to be given frequently in high doses because of the rapid renal elimination (half-life, 3.5 hours with normal renal function). In the elderly with decreased renal function, the dose of procainamide should be reduced by about 50 percent.[150] In mild heart failure the dose should be reduced by a quarter. IV procainamide should not be given at a dose exceeding 24 mg/min (see side-effects). Plasma metabolism by acetylation yields the active N-acetyl procainamide (NAPA) with a half-life of 6–8 hours. *NAPA, the metabolite of procainamide, is also antiarrhythmic and increases disproportionately to procainamide blood levels in renal failure.* Electrophysiologically it differs from its parent in not altering depolarization and having a "pure" Class III activity. It has a longer half-life and lesser risk of lupus. In preliminary clinical testing, its antiarrhythmic potency has not been fully evaluated although relatively low in one study.[152]

Dose. An *oral* loading dose of procainamide 1 g is followed by up to 500 mg 3-hourly. A slow-release preparation of procainamide (Procan SR®) appears to allow 6-hourly dosing intervals. The *IV* dose is a 100 mg bolus over 2 minutes, then up to 20 mg/min to a maximum of 1 g in the first hour, then 2-6 mg/min. *Periodic procainamide*[49] is a new proposal to avoid the twin problems of short duration of action and immune-toxicity; high-dose oral procainamide (250 mg/kg, about 1750 mg) is given as a single dose after the onset of nonlife-threatening paroxysmal tachyarrhythmias to avoid recurrences.

Indications. In acute myocardial infarction (AMI), even when complicated by cardiac failure or low cardiac output,[58] procainamide can be given slowly intravenously and is much safer than IV quinidine. Continuous monitoring (blood pressure, ECG) is essential. Koch-Weser and associates[17] reported oral procainamide (oral loading dose 1 g) highly effective in prevention of ventricular arrhythmias early after infarction, but in the long-term, 500 mg every 6 hours was not effective.[18] Like other Class IA agents, procainamide is also effective against many supraventricular tachyarrhythmias, including those of the bypass tract.

If sustained VT remains inducible by electrophysiological testing after IV procainamide, it is unlikely that any other single conventional antiarrhythmic will result in noninducibility[146,182] although this correlation has not been observed by others.[163a]

Contraindications. Shock, severe heart failure, myasthenia gravis, heart block, and severe renal failure.

Side-effects. Hypotension is a common side-effect with IV administration (vasodilator effect) especially with doses exceeding 24 mg/min.[95] Heart block may develop or increase (Table 4-3). In atrial fibrillation or flutter the ventricular rate may increase as the atrial rate slows, so that concomitant digitalization is advisable. The vagolytic effect of procainamide is much weaker than that of quinidine.[117] Pro-arrhythmic effects (facilitation of electrophysiological induction of VT) may be dose-related.[182] During oral therapy,[18] 9 of 39 patients had early side-effects (rash, fever) and 14 of 16 had late side-effects (arthralgia, rash); fear of the lupus syndrome (likeliest in slow acetylators) limited therapy to 6 months at the most. Despite the efficacy of procainamide, the risk of lupus is about one-third of patients treated for over 6 months, and hence seriously limits the drug's long-term usage. It is possible that such patients in the future may be treated with NAPA (see pharmacokinetics) or the newer antiarrhythmic drugs. Agranulocytosis may be a late side-effect of procainamide, especially with the slow-release preparation.[76]

Drug interactions. Cimetidine inhibits the renal clearance of procainamide to prolong the elimination half-life so that the procainamide dose should be reduced.[68] Procainamide should normally not be combined with captopril (theoretical danger of enhanced immune effects).
Treatment of toxicity. As for quinidine.

Procainamide—Summary

Procainamide is effective against supraventricular and ventricular arrhythmias, although usually used for the latter. The short half-life and need for frequent dosing have limited its usefulness. New long-acting prepara-

TABLE 4-2   ANTIARRHYTHMIC DRUGS USED IN THERAPY OF VENTRICULAR ARRHYTHMIAS.

Agent	Dose	Pharmacokinetics	Comments, side-effects and precautions
Quinidine (Class IA)	Orally 1.2–1.6g/day in divided doses, 3–12-hourly depending on preparation. Not IV.	T½ 7–9 hr. Reduce dose in liver disease. Level 2.3–5μg/ml.	Many side-effects including torsades de pointes and hypotension. Vagolytic. Monitor QRS, QT, plasma K.
Procainamide (Class IA)	IV 100mg bolus over 2 min up to 20mg/min to 1g in first hr; then 2–6mg/min. Oral 1g, then up to 500mg 3-hourly.	T½ 3.5 hr. Level 4–10μg/mL. Toxic effects above 16μg/mL. (Reduce dose in renal or cardiac failure.)	Hypotension with IV dose. Limit oral use to 6 months (lupus). Note: N-acetylprocainamide (long half-life, less lupus).
Disopyramide (Class IA)	IV 0.5mg/kg over 5 min, repeat after 5 min (repeat twice more if needed), then 1mg/kg/hr from 0–3 hr and 0.4mg/kg/hr for 3–18 hr.	T½ 8 hr, prolonged in renal failure and after myocardial infarction. Level 3–6μg/mL; toxic > 7 μgmL.	Hypotension, QRS or QT prolongation, torsades, congestive heart failure. Prominent vagolytic and negative inotropic effects.
Lidocaine (Class IB)	IV 100–200mg; then 2–4mg/min for 24–30 hr.	Effect of single bolus lasts only few min, then T½ about 2 hr. Level 1.4–5.0μg/mL; toxic >9μg/mL.	Reduce dose by half if liver blood flow low (shock, β-blockade, cirrhosis, cimetidine, severe heart failure). High-dose CNS effects.
Tocainide (Class IB)	*IV 0.5–0.75mg/kg/min for 15 min. Oral loading 400–800mg, then 2–3× daily.	T½ 13.5 hr. Level 4–10μg/mL.	CNS, GI side-effects. Sometimes immune-based problems.
Mexiletine (Class IB)	*IV 100–250mg at 12.5mg/min, then 2.0mg/kg/hr for 3.5 hr, then 0.5mg/kg/hr. Oral 100–400mg 8-hourly, loading dose 400mg.	T½ 10–17 hr. Level 1–2μg/mL.	CNS, GI side-effects. Bradycardia, hypotension.

† Caution: For uses and doses approved in the USA, see text.

Drug (Class)	Dose	Pharmacokinetics	Side-effects
Phenytoin (Class IB)	IV 10–15mg/kg over 1 hr. Oral 1g; 500mg for 2 days; then 400–600mg daily.	T½ 24 hr. Level 10–18μg/mL. Hepatic or renal disease requires reduced doses.	Hypotension, vertigo, dysarthria, lethargy, gingivitis, macrocytic anemia, lupus, pulmonary infiltrates.
Flecainide (Class IC)	*IV 1–2mg/kg over 10 min, then 0.15–0.25mg/kg/hr. Oral 100–400mg 2× daily.	T½ 13–19 hr. Keep trough level below 0.2–1.0μg/mL.	QRS prolongation. Pro-arrhythmic. Depresses LV function. CNS side-effects.
Encainide (Class IC)	25–75 mg 3× daily	T½ 1–2 hr. No levels. Normal phenotype produces long-acting metabolites (3–12 hr).	QRS prolongation. CNS side-effects. Pro-arrhythmic.
Propafenone (Class IC)	*IV 2mg/kg then 2mg/min. *Oral 150–300mg 3× daily.	T½ variable 2–12 hr. Level 0.2–3.0μg/mL.	QRS prolongation. Modest negative inotropic effect. GI side-effects. Pro-arrhythmic.
β-Blockade (Class II)	Various schedules (Table 1-2).	Variable according to agent.	Myocardial depression, sinus bradycardia, AV block.
Amiodarone (Class III)	Oral loading dose 1200–1600mg daily; maintenance 200–400mg daily. *Occasional IV use (150–1000mg over 15–60 min).	T½ 25–110 days. Level 1.0–2.5μg/mL.	Complex side-effects including pulmonary fibrosis and QT-prolongation. S/E may be dose-related (keep dose low).
Bretylium tosylate (Class III)	IV 5–10mg/kg, repeat to max 30mg/kg, then IV 1–2mg/min or IM 5–10mg/kg 8-hourly at varying sites (local necrosis).	T½ 7–9 hr. Decrease dose in renal failure. Level 0.5–1.0μg/mL.	IV: hypotension. Initial sympathomimetic effects.

Compiled by LH Opie and modified from previous edition.

* Not in the USA

† Caution: For uses and doses approved in the USA; see text.

IV = intravenous; IM = intramuscular T½ = plasma half-life; level = therapeutic blood level.

TABLE 4-3

EFFECTS AND SIDE-EFFECTS OF ANTIARRHYTHMIC AGENTS AND OF DIGITALIS ON ELECTROPHYSIOLOGY AND HEMODYNAMICS

Agent	Sinus node	Sinus rate	Sick sinus syndrome	Atrial-His conduction	PR-interval (→ = prolong)	AV conduction block	His-Purkinje conduction	Accessory pathways in WPW	Effect on QRS (→ = widen)	Effect on QT (→ = lengthen)	Serious hemodynamic effects
Quinidine	→	↑	Avoid	0	0/→↑	0/	→	↓A/R	↑↑	↑↑	IV may cause
Procainamide	0	0/↑	0	0/↓	0/→↑	Probably avoid	→	↓A/R	↑ High dose	↑	IV may cause
Disopyramide	→	↑	Avoid	0	0/→↑	0	0/↓ can use in BBB	↓A/R	↑	↑↑	IV may cause
Lidocaine	0	0	0	0/↓	0	0	0	↓/0	0	0	Only with toxic doses
Phenytoin	0	0	Variable	↑/0	0	Use for digitalis toxicity	0	↓/0	0	↓	IV hypotension
Mexiletine	0	0	Avoid	↓/0	0	↓/0	↓/0	↓/0 ↑	0 ↑	0	Only with toxic doses
Tocainide	0	0	Probably avoid	↓/0	0	↓/0	↓/0	↓/0	0	0	Only with toxic doses

Flecainide	0	0	Probably avoid	↓↑	↑	Avoid	↓↑	↓A/R	↑↑	(Via QRS)	LV↓
Encainide	0	0	Probably avoid	↓↑	↑	Avoid	↓↑	↓A/R	↑↑	(Via QRS)	Only with toxic doses
β-Blockade	↓↑	↑	Avoid	→	↑	Avoid	0	↓/0	0	0	IV may cause
Amiodarone	→	→	Avoid	→	0/↑	Avoid	0/↓	↓A/R	0	↑↑	Slow IV safe vasodilator
Verapamil	↑	0/↓	Avoid	↓↑	↑	Avoid	0	↑A	0	0	IV if contraindicated
Digitalis	↓/0	↓/0	Care	→	(toxic)↑	Avoid	0	↑A	0	↓	No

See references 29 and 40 for further details.

WPW = Wolff-Parkinson-White syndrome; LV = left ventricle; R = retrograde; A = antegrade; BBB = bundle branch block; IV = intravenous; ↓depresses; ↑ = increases; ↑ = prolongs; ↓ = shortens.

tions are preferable. Nonetheless procainamide is not suited for long-term maintenance because of the risk of lupus erythematosus or other immune-related disorders. In contrast, other side-effects are less than with quinidine (GI, QRS or QT-prolongation, hypotension) and there is no interaction with digoxin.

Disopyramide

Disopyramide is a Class IA antiarrhythmic agent, electrophysiologically like quinidine, with a similar antiarrhythmic profile. Like quinidine, it may predispose to QT and QRS prolongation. The crucial differences lie in the side-effects: GI problems are fewer with disopyramide, but there is a much stronger anticholinergic effect because disopyramide is forty times more effective an inhibitor of the muscarinic receptors than is quinidine,[117] so that (1) **anticholinergic side-effects can become a major problem (urinary retention, worsening of glaucoma or myasthenia gravis, or constipation); and (2) there is a relative increase of sympathetic activity so that the direct depressant effects of disopyramide on nodal and conduction tissue may be masked.** Thus in the transplanted heart disopyramide prolongs QRS and His-ventricular interval (HV) conduction more than in the normally innervated heart.[51] A prominent and largely unexplained side-effect of disopyramide is the negative inotropic effect, so marked that disopyramide is now also used in the therapy of hypertrophic obstructive cardiomyopathy.[183]

Pharmacokinetics and therapeutic levels. The phosphate salt (Norpace®, Dirythmin®) and the free base (Rythmodan®) have similar bioavailability and pharmacokinetics. Most of the oral dose is bioavailable. About half is metabolized (not in the liver) by N-dealkylation and about half excreted unchanged in the urine. The usual half-life is about 8 hours. One metabolite is powerfully anticholinergic. Experimentally, anticholinergic and inotropic effects may be separated by the d and l-isomers.[140] Disopyramide reduces PVCs at a serum concentration of 3–8 μg/ml.[173] The higher the blood level, the lower the percentage bound to plasma proteins so that potential toxicity is enhanced.

Dose. The usual *oral dose* is 100–200 mg 6–hourly with an initial loading dose of 300 mg (omitted if CHF suspected). Several long-acting preparations, including Norpace CR®, Rythmodan Retard®, and Dirythmin SA® need only 12–hourly dosing. The dose should be reduced in severe renal failure and in the elderly (renal excretion of disopyramide) and in CHF (prolonged half-life). With the IV preparation (not in the USA) optimal blood levels can be rapidly achieved and maintained (Table 4-2).[99] In infants, the dose is about 10–30 mg/kg/day of disopyramide base; the dose decreases as the age increases towards adulthood.[170] To reduce anticholinergic side-effects, pyridostigmine may be used.[165]

Indications. Oral disopyramide is approved only for the treatment of *ventricular arrhythmias* in the USA. It prevents induction of VT/VF (ventricular fibrillation) in up to one-third of patients.[110] In paroxysmal VT and other ventricular arrhythmias, disopyramide may be effective when other Class IA agents such as quinidine or procainamide fail;[38] the logic for this observation is not clear, but may include minor electrophysiological differences[19] and a different side-effect profile so that relatively higher doses of disopyramide could be given to certain patients. Conversely, quinidine is sometimes effective when disopyramide fails.

In *supraventricular tachycardia*, oral or IV disopyramide may cause reversion to sinus rhythm,[57] especially if the arrhythmia is of recent onset. In the atrial arrhythmias of the WPW syndrome (Fig. 4-3), disopyramide acts by inhibition of both retrograde and antegrade conduction.[161] Disopyramide is about as effective as quinidine in reducing recurrent atrial fibrillation after direct current (DC) cardioversion.[11] Disopyramide is probably most effective in the prevention of recurrent atrial arrhythmias including fibrillation in patients without a history of CHF.

In *AMI*, IV disopyramide (not in the USA) is one of several agents used for lidocaine failures,[34] but the risk of myocardial depression with hypotension is much greater than with lidocaine. The role of oral disopyramide in the control of ventricular arrhythmias of late onset, or when lidocaine therapy is withdrawn, has not been critically evaluated.

In *hypertrophic cardiomyopathy*, disopyramide acts beneficially by its negative inotropic effect[183] and may be better than propranolol.[141]

Side-effects.   (1) Negative inotropic; (2) anticholinergic activity may be a serious side-effect especially in elderly men (prostatic obstruction) or in patients with threatened glaucoma or with myasthenia gravis or when constipation is a pre-existing problem (verapamil co-therapy); (3) QT-prolongation and torsades de pointes.[24] QRS-prolongation, prominent in the transplanted heart,[51] is normally obscured by the relative increase in sympathetic activity, as are negative effects on nodal and conduction tissue and the inotropic state; (4) occasional hypoglycemia[163] and cholestatic jaundice.

Contraindications.   Uncompensated CHF is an absolute contraindication, as are untreated urinary retention or glaucoma or hypotension. Relative contraindications are: (1) compensated CHF; (2) prostatism; (3) treated glaucoma or a family history of glaucoma; (4) severe constipation; and (5) sinus node dysfunction[20] and by analogy AV nodal block.[51,53] Bundle branch block is not normally a contraindication[4] except during β-blockade.

Precautions.   (1) ECG: QT-prolongation of greater than 25 percent of the corrected interval or significant widening (>25 percent) of the QRS, or the development of first degree heart block may all require discontinuation of disopyramide; the exact criteria are not known. Development of second or third degree AV block or uni-, bi- or trifascicular block requires discontinuation of the drug unless an artificial pacemaker is used. (2) Digitalization is indicated for borderline or suspected heart failure or for atrial flutter or fibrillation to avoid sudden acceleration of AV conduction. (3) Pregnancy—disopyramide may stimulate uterine contractions and is excreted in human milk.

> **Drug interactions.**   IV disopyramide can substantially *reduce cardiac output* in β-blocked patients, in those with chronic therapy by calcium antagonists and especially verapamil,[108] in patients with pre-existing myocardial depression and in patients with pre-existing therapy on other negatively inotropic drugs. Combinations with other *drugs likely to depress nodal tissue or conduction* such as quinidine, digoxin, β-blockade, and methyldopa are potentially dangerous. Disopyramide is ineffective in digitalis toxicity and should be avoided because of the possibility of added depressant effects on the AV and sinus nodes. There is no interaction between disopyramide and lidocaine. The concomitant use of *other type 1 antiarrhythmic agents and/or β-blockers* with disopyramide should be reserved for life-threatening arrhythmias, which are demonstrably unresponsive to single agent antiarrhythmic agents (risk of negative inotropic effects, prolonged conduction). Phenytoin or other inducers of hepatic enzymes may lower disopyramide plasma levels. Pyridostigmine bromide (Mestinon Timespan®, 90–180 mg 3× daily) *may reduce anticholinergic side-effects* of disopyramide by inhibition of cholinesterase activity.

Disopyramide—Summary

Disopyramide is a Class IA agent, in many ways electrophysiologically similar to quinidine and with a similar therapeutic efficacy. The choice between the two agents may be determined by the anticipated side-effects in a particular agent, with disopyramide particularly suited in patients with GI side-effects from quinidine or when nodal or conduction depression is anticipated; the vagolytic effect can usually overcome direct inhibition of nodal or conduction tissue. On the other hand, disopyramide is particularly unsuitable when there is myocardial depression or when cholinergic side-effects are likely to be troublesome.

CLASS IB: LIDOCAINE (LIGNOCAINE) AND SIMILAR COMPOUNDS

As a group, Class IB agents inhibit the fast sodium current (typical Class I effect) while shortening the action potential duration (Figs. 23–9, 23–11, see reference 134). The former has the more powerful effect while the latter might actually predispose to arrhythmias, but ensures that QT-prolongation does not occur. Class IB agents act selectively on diseased or ischemic tissue, where they are thought to promote conduction block, thereby interrupting re-entry circuits. They have a particular affinity for binding with inactivated sodium channels with rapid onset-offset kinetics.

Lidocaine (Lignocaine)

Lidocaine (Xylocaine®, Xylocard®) has become **the standard IV agent for suppression of arrhythmias associated with AMI and with cardiac surgery.** The drug does not have a major role in the control of chronic recurrent ventricular arrhythmias. The mode of action is complex and controversial but includes block of re-entry circuits in the ischemic myocardium. Lidocaine acts preferentially on the ischemic myocardium[9] and is more effective in the presence of a high external potassium; therefore hypokalemia must be corrected for maximum efficacy (also for other Class I agents).

Pharmacokinetics. The bulk of an IV dose of lidocaine is rapidly de-ethylated by liver microsomes. Hence two critical factors governing lidocaine efficacy are liver blood flow (decreased in old age and by heart failure, β-blockade, and cimetidine) and liver microsomal activity (enhanced by barbiturates and phenytoin). Since lidocaine is so rapidly distributed within minutes after an initial IV loading dose, there must be a subsequent infusion or repetitive doses to maintain therapeutic blood levels (1.4–5.0 μg/ml). Lidocaine metabolites circulate in high concentrations and may contribute to toxic and therapeutic actions. The effect of the mode of administration (IV versus intramuscular) on kinetics is shown in Figure 23–12 of reference 134.

Dose. A constant infusion would take 5–9 hours to achieve therapeutic levels (1.4–6.0 μg/ml) so standard therapy includes a loading dose of 100–200 mg intravenously[21,87] (see Table 4-2) or 400 mg intramuscularly.[104] Thereafter lidocaine is infused at 2–4 mg/min for 24–30 hours, aiming at 3 mg/min that prevents VF but may cause serious side-effects in about 15 percent of patients, in half of whom the lidocaine dose may have to be reduced.[21] Several other dosage schedules are designed to build up the blood level rapidly.[1] Poor liver blood flow (low cardiac output or β-blockade) or liver disease or cimetidine or halothane therapy calls for halved dosage. The dose should also be decreased for elderly patients in whom toxicity develops more frequently.

Side-effects. Lidocaine is generally free of hemodynamic depressive side-effects, even in patients with CHF, and it seldom impairs nodal function or conduction. The higher infusion rate of 3–4 mg/min may result in drowsiness, numbness, speech disturbances and dizziness, especially in patients over 60 years of age.[21] Minor adverse neural reactions can occur in about half the patients, even with 2–3 mg/min of lidocaine.[43] Although not usually used in patients with atrial arrhythmias, one patient with atrial flutter already receiving quinidine and digoxin developed 1:1 conduction with a high ventricular rate after 50 mg of IV lidocaine.[114]

Drug interactions. In patients receiving cimetidine,[7] propranolol,[132] or halothane,[54] the hepatic clearance of lidocaine is reduced and toxicity may occur more readily, so that the dose should be reduced. Sinoatrial arrest is predisposed to by co-administration of other agents potentially depressing nodal function.[97]

Lidocaine failure. If lidocaine apparently fails, is there hypokalemia? Are there technical errors? If none of these factors is present, a blood level is taken (if available) and the infusion rate can be increased cautiously until development of the central nervous system effects (confusion, slurred speech). Alternatively or thereafter, Class IA agents are tried (especially procainamide) before resorting to Class IC agents, β-blockers, or amiodarone.

Clinical use. Should lidocaine be administered routinely to all patients with AMI? The question has been asked for at least 8 years[87] and is still not fully resolved (see Fig. 4-4 for alternate schemes). In the pre-hospital phase, evidence for high-dose intramuscular lidocaine (400 mg) is good[104] but 250 pa-

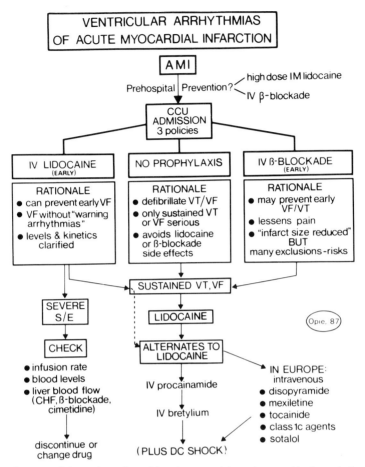

Fig. 4-4. Schematic and provisional approach to serious ventricular arrhythmias in patients with acute myocardial infarction. Compiled by DC Harrison, LH Opie, and T Mabin.

tients with suspected AMI had to be treated to save 1 from VF. In the Coronary Care Unit (CCU), data obtained by pooling of several studies, a marginally acceptable procedure, suggests that lidocaine should be used,[5] as does one well-conducted double-blind trial when patients seen within 6 hours of the onset of myocardial infarction were given a 100 mg bolus followed by an infusion of lidocaine 3 mg/min for 48 hours.[21] However, death in the untreated group did not occur and all patients could be resuscitated. Furthermore, since the incidence of primary VF is now so low (probably less than 5 percent), it is uncertain whether prophylactic lidocaine is cost-effective if given to all patients sustaining AMI. Many well-run CCUs in the USA and Europe have abandoned the routine use of lidocaine and consider prophylaxis only for selected patients.[2]

Lidocaine—Recommendations

Despite the controversy, it appears prudent to use lidocaine in patients admitted to CCUs within 6 hours of the onset of symptoms,[21] when the risk of VF is highest. An exception is when there is bradycardia or bradycardia plus ventricular tachyarrhythmias, when atropine (or pacing) is required. Now that early β-blockade is more common in patients with AMI, bradyarrhythmias may also become more common. β-Blockade reduces the liver blood flow to decrease the dose of lidocaine required. The aimed rate of infusion after the initial loading dose should be 3 mg/kg except in elderly patients, those with heart failure, or those receiving cimetidine or β-blockade, who all require reduced doses. The advantage of prophylactic lidocaine is that the prevention of VF even in a small number of patients facilitates management and makes for easier nursing, while the risk of serious side-effects is reasonably low. However, we recognize that it is perfectly legitimate not to give lidocaine or to opt instead for early IV β-blockade (see Fig. 4-4). Several of the authors of this chapter favor the use of prophylactic high-dose intramuscular lidocaine (400 mg) in the pre-hospital phase of myocardial infarction,[104] but the issue remains controversial.

Tocainide

Tocainide (Tonocard®) is an oral lidocaine analog, now available in the USA, with electrophysiologic properties similar to those of lidocaine[106] and a long plasma half-life.

Pharmacokinetics. The bioavailability of tocainide is virtually complete because of the absence of first-pass metabolism.[121] Peak plasma levels occur 2 hours after oral administration; optimal plasma levels appear to be 4–10 μg/ml.[121] Nearly half of an oral dose is recovered unchanged in the urine. There are no active metabolites. The plasma half-life is about 14 hours which is virtually unaltered in the presence of AMI,[84] but prolonged in severe renal disease.

Dose. The usual oral dose is 400–800 mg 3× daily; 2× daily administration may be effective. The dose should be decreased in renal failure (renal excretion) as well as in the elderly (low glomerular filtration rate [GFR]). The IV dose (not approved in the USA) is 250 mg over 2 minutes, 500 mg over 15 minutes and then 500 mg every 6 hours for 48 hours.[100a]

Indications. The approved indication in the USA is treatment of symptomatic ventricular arrhythmias. That includes those refractory to conventional antiarrhythmic agents such as quinidine, procainamide, and propranolol).[32,40,138] Its possible use in the WPW syndrome[179] needs further confirmation. When used as a first-line ventricular antiarrhythmic, it is much more likely to be effective than when used in patients with arrhythmias already resistant to more conventional drugs. In AMI, serious ventricular arrhythmias are reduced by combined IV and oral tocainide, but VF was not prevented.[63] There appears to be some relation between the response to IV lidocaine in patients with refractory arrhythmias and the subsequent response to oral tocainide.[92] Thus about two-thirds of those responding to lidocaine responded to oral tocainide, while few of those not responding to lidocaine did respond to oral tocainide.[40,138] IV tocainide is as good as IV lidocaine in AMI and may be followed by oral tocainide.[100a]

Contraindications. Hypersensitivity; second or third degree heart block in the absence of an artificial pacemaker. Like lidocaine, tocainide appears to have no significant direct negative inotropic effect, although occasional adverse reactions have been described in patients with complex cardiovascular disease. In the package insert, nondigitalized atrial flutter or fibrillation is mentioned as a relative contraindication because of the danger of ventricular acceleration, yet tocainide may mildly inhibit the AV node.[179]

Side-effects. Tocainide frequently causes dose-dependent nervous system (28 percent) and GI reactions (11 percent) including lightheadedness or dizziness, paresthesia or numbness in the extremities, tremor, and nausea, vomiting or diarrhea.[92] When tremor develops, that is a useful clinical indication that the maximum dose is being approached. According to the package insert, such side-effects cause discontinuation in about one-fifth of patients. Serious immune-based side-effects, such as pulmonary fibrosis, may occur. Polyarthritis and increased antinuclear factors are infrequent. Blood dyscrasias, such as leukopenia and thrombocytopenia, also occur and the relationship to tocainide is not clearly established. The incidence of pulmonary fibrosis and blood dyscrasias is not yet fully defined. As with other agents, a pro-arrhythmic effect may occur.

Precautions. Periodic blood counts are required. Patients should report bruising or bleeding or symptoms of infection (throat, chest).

Drug interactions and combinations. Tocainide may be used freely in digitalized patients with no change in digoxin levels. It has also been used in combination with β-blockers, other antiarrhythmic agents (without controlled studies), anticoagulants, and diuretics without evidence as yet of clinically significant interactions.[121]

Tocainide—Summary

Tocainide is an analog of lidocaine that can be given both orally and intravenously. Only the oral use is approved in the USA. Like lidocaine, it has little negative inotropic effect and is unlikely to aggravate CHF. Another advantage is shortening of the QT-interval (Class IB effect). Like mexiletine, the major side-effects are neurologic; GI side-effects are also frequent. Immune-based side-effects occur infrequently. For potentially lethal arrhythmias, the drug is about as effective as quinidine but has a different side-effect profile.[122]

Mexiletine

Mexiletine (Mexitil®) is an orally effective antiarrhythmic agent with Class IB activity, similar in structure to lidocaine, but not so rapidly metabolized by the liver. Like lidocaine, it has little or no negative inotropic effect in the therapeutic dose range.[154,162] It has recently been approved for use in the USA after wide use in Europe for many years.

Pharmacokinetics. Mexiletine is well absorbed with a high bioavailability and reaches peak plasma levels in 2–4 hours. The therapeutic blood level is 1–2 μg/ml. Ninety percent is metabolized in the liver to inactive metabolites and the rest excreted in the urine as unchanged mexiletine.[3] The half-life is 10–17 hours in normals. Higher than normal plasma levels are found in chronic liver disease but not in renal failure.[131] Mexiletine is lipophilic and enters the brain (central nervous side-effects).

Dose. The oral loading dose is 400 mg if high initial levels are required, followed by 300–1200 mg (given with food or antacid) in three divided daily doses, starting 2–6 hours after the loading dose. In the USA, the highest approved dose is 900 mg daily. The IV dose (not in the USA) is 100–250 mg (2.5 mg/kg) at 12.5 mg/min, then 2.0 mg/kg/hr for 3.5 hours, then 0.5 mg/kg/hr as long as needed. In Europe, sustained release capsules (Perlongets®) have a usual dose of 360 mg 2× daily. The dose of mexiletine should be reduced in severe liver disease and in CHF. In children, the dose should be titrated according to the blood level. In pregnant women, the drug seems safe although it crosses the placental barrier. In the elderly, the dose must be reduced because of possible central nervous system side-effects and because of lower hepatic blood flow.

Indications. In the USA, the major approved indication is treatment of symptomatic ventricular arrhythmias. In Europe, the major indications are the treatment and prevention of ventricular arrhythmias, and it is especially used in early myocardial infarction and postinfarction, as well as in digitalis-induced arrhythmias.

In the chronic oral prophylaxis of ventricular arrhythmias postinfarction, mexiletine 300 mg 8–hourly is as effective as procainamide.[62] A similar dose of mexiletine can be combined with quinidine (about 1 g daily) with a lower incidence of side-effects and better antiarrhythmic action than with higher doses of either agent alone.[6] In VT resistant to more conventional drugs, mexiletine alone gives only modest benefit.[154,181] Its use in WPW arrhythmias[167] needs confirmation.

In a major clinical trial on postinfarct patients, mexiletine reduced Holter-monitored arrhythmias in the first 6 months without improved mortality over 1 year; however, therapeutic blood levels (1–2 μg/ml) were not reached in the majority of patients[96] so that the trial was inconclusive.

Contraindications. Cardiogenic shock or second or third degree heart block without a pacemaker. Relative contraindications are: bradycardia, conduction defects in the presence of a pacemaker, hypotension, hepatic failure, and severe renal or myocardial failure. Caution in patients with liver damage or seizures.

Side-effects.   The major problem is a narrow therapeutic-toxic margin[135] so that in patients with ventricular arrhythmias resistant to conventional agents, an adequate antiarrhythmic effect was only obtained in 25 percent of patients without significant side-effects.[154]

Dizziness and mild disorientation may result from a single oral dose of 400 mg.[142] During chronic therapy, side-effects include indigestion in 40 percent, tremor or nystagmus (10 percent, higher in some series) and confusional states in less than 10 percent; severe side-effects occurred in about 35 percent of patients receiving 1 g or more per day.[59,60] In about 5 percent of patients bradycardia and hypotension may occur.[59,60] Prochloroperazine 12.5 mg IV can be given 5 minutes before the mexiletine injection to lessen dizziness and vomiting.[155] As with other antiarrhythmics, there may be a pro-arrhythmic effect. Liver damage occasionally occurs.

Drug interactions and combination therapy.   Narcotics delay the GI absorption of mexiletine. Rifampin (rifampicin) and phenytoin reduce plasma levels of mexiletine as a result of hepatic enzyme induction. Concurrent disopyramide predisposes to a negative inotropic effect.[55] The drug may be combined with quinidine,[6,85] β-adrenergic blockade[107] and amiodarone[180] provided contraindications are observed.

Mexiletine—Summary

Mexiletine, like lidocaine, is used chiefly against ventricular arrhythmias. Unlike lidocaine, it can be given orally. There are several arguments favoring it as one of several reasonable choices as a first-line antiarrhythmic in ventricular arrhythmias requiring therapy: (1) its comparable efficacy to quinidine; (2) little or no hemodynamic depression; (3) absence of QT-prolongation; and (4) absence of vagolytic effects. However, frequent GI and central nervous side-effects limit the dose and possible therapeutic benefit.

Phenytoin (Diphenylhydantoin)

Phenytoin (Dilantin®, Epanutin®) has three specific uses. First, in digitalis-toxic arrhythmias, it maintains conduction or even enhances it especially in the presence of hypokalemia; it also inhibits delayed afterdepolarizations.[41] Second, phenytoin is effective against the ventricular arrhythmias occurring after congenital heart surgery.[39] Third, phenytoin is used in the congenital prolonged QT-syndrome when β-blockade alone has failed; here, reliable comparable studies have not been done. Why phenytoin is so effective in the ventricular arrhythmias of young children is not known.

The IV dose is 10–15 mg/kg over 1 hour followed by oral maintenance of 400–600 mg/day (2–4 mg/kg/day in children). The long half-life allows once daily dosage with, however, the risk of serious side-effects including dysarthria, pulmonary infiltrates, lupus, gingivitis, and macrocytic anemia.

Phenytoin is an inducer of hepatic enzymes and therefore alters the dose requirements of many other drugs used in cardiology, including quinidine, lidocaine and mexiletine.

Ethmozine

Ethmozine (Moricizine®) is a phenothiazine derivative, originally from the USSR, and currently under investigation in the USA.[118,136] Electrophysiologically, it has both lidocaine-like Class IB properties and also prolongs the PR and QRS times while leaving the QT-interval unchanged. Therefore ethmozine may represent a "mixed" Class IB/IC agent. Clinically, it is effective for the treatment of both ventricular and supraventricular arrhythmias, acting in the former by slowing conduction in the fast limb of the AV nodal re-entrant tachycardia or decreasing conduction along the bypass tract.[65,66,143] The phenothiazine-like structure (which could perhaps predispose to QT-prolongation) also suggests a third antiarrhythmic mechanism through a central nervous system effect. Ethmozine is rapidly and extensively metabolized in the liver with a half-life of approximately 2–5 hours that is prolonged in renal insufficiency. The average dose is 200 mg 3× daily. Neurologic side-effects, most evident during IV infusion, include nervousness, dizziness, and vertigo. Generally, during oral therapy, side-effects are slight. A pro-arrhythmic effect has been found.[95] Ethmozine has only mildly depressant effects on LV function, yet further studies on side-effects are required to see whether the drug really is "extraordinarily well tolerated with only minor side-effects."[143] Whether ethmozine is as powerfully antiarrhythmic as its properties theoretically suggest, also remains to be evaluated.

CLASS IC AGENTS

Such agents, recently subcategorized by Harrison,[88] have three major electrophysiological effects. First, they are powerful inhibitors of the fast sodium channel causing a marked depression of the upstroke of the cardiac action potential. Second, they have a marked inhibitory effect on His-Purkinje tissue with QRS widening. Third, they have relatively little effect on the action potential duration except in Purkinje fibers where there is marked shortening. From the kinetic point of view, Class IC drugs are slower than Class IA or Class IB.[61] Class IC agents are all potent antiarrhythmics used largely in the control of resistant ventricular tachyarrhythmias, although their effect on induced VT may be modest. Their markedly depressant effect on conduction may explain their significant pro-arrhythmic action. However, they do not directly prolong the QT-interval (indirect prolongation caused by QRS widening).

Flecainide

Flecainide acetate (Tambocor®) is effective for a broad spectrum of arrhythmias and has recently been approved for use in the USA.

Pharmacology. As a Class I agent, flecainide inhibits the fast sodium current. Powerful inhibition of His-Purkinje conduction and prolongation of the QRS interval (Class IC effect) explains QT-prolongation.[77] Flecainide also inhibits the sinus node in the presence of the sick sinus syndrome[176] and inhibits the fast AV nodal pathway in some AV nodal re-entrant arrhythmias[90] as well as the bypass tract.[130]

Pharmacokinetics. Flecainide is well absorbed with a bioavailability as high as 95 percent, and peak plasma levels at 2–4 hours. When feasible, plasma levels should be monitored and kept below 0.2–1.0 μg/ml (trough levels) to avoid myocardial depression.[149] The plasma half-life is 13–19 hours. Flecainide is two-thirds metabolized by the liver to inactive metabolites while about one-third is excreted unchanged by the kidneys and a small amount (5 percent) in the feces.

Dose. The oral dose of flecainide is 100–400 mg 2× daily; the IV dose (not approved in the USA) is 1–2 mg/kg over 10 minutes followed by an infusion of 0.15–0.25 mg/kg/hr. Lower doses are required for patients with poor LV function or severe renal failure; an initial dose of 100 mg 2× daily is increased at about 4–day intervals to 200 mg 2× daily (flecainide plasma levels should be checked if required, particularly in the presence of CHF).

Indications. Symptomatic VT.[42] It is also effective in WPW arrhythmias[130] and in AV nodal re-entrant arrhythmias.[90]

Contraindications. Significant conduction delay, sick sinus syndrome[77] and myocardial depression. A relative contraindication is renal disease.

Side-effects. Cardiac side-effects include aggravation of ventricular arrhythmias in 5–12 percent,[28,79,119,149] or possibly even more in the presence of pre-existing LV failure. The pro-arrhythmic effect may be related to nonuniform slowing of conduction rather than to QRS-prolongation.[28] Monitoring the QRS-interval is logical[102] but "safe limits" are not established. In patients with pre-existing sinus node or AV conduction problems, there may be worsening. IV flecainide (2 mg/kg over 30 minutes; not in the USA) has a negative inotropic effect even in postinfarct patients without heart failure[109] with a fall in ejection fraction and a rise in pulmonary capillary wedge pressure, sometimes to very high levels, so that clinical heart failure may be precipitated.[98]

Extracardiac side-effects are common,[25] especially those related to the central nervous system (blurred vision, dizziness, headache, nausea, paresthesias, fatigue, tremor, and nervousness). Yet in one trial over a mean of 100 days, only 2 of 36 patients receiving flecainide at a mean daily dose of 300 mg had the drug discontinued.[149] Rash, abdominal pain, diarrhea, and impotence may be nonspecific.

Drug interactions and combinations. Additive inhibitory effects require great care when flecainide is combined with other agents inhibiting sinus or AV nodal function (β-blockers, verapamil, diltiazem, digitalis), when there are additive negative inotropic effects (β-blockers, verapamil, disopyramide) or when there may be combined effects on His-Purkinje conduction (quinidine, procainamide, and to a lesser extent disopyramide). Amiodarone increases flecainide plasma levels (decrease flecainide dose by one-third).[158a]

Flecainide—Summary

Flecainide is a powerful new drug, effective for the treatment of both supraventricular and ventricular arrhythmias. However it prolongs the PR and QRS times. The negative inotropic effect limits its use in ischemic heart disease or dilated cardiomyopathy. In patients with life-threatening arrhythmias, the potentially serious pro-arrhythmic effect requires that this drug should only be started under careful observation preferably in the hospital, using a gradually increasing low oral dose with checks of serum levels. In an emergency IV flecainide (not in the USA) can be very effective for supraventricular or ventricular tachycardias. Thus, with care, flecainide will be very effective in some selected patients with severe ventricular arrhythmias but without LV failure.[95]

Encainide

Encainide (Enkaid®), under consideration for use in the USA, has a spectrum of action and electrophysiologic effects similar to flecainide. However, encainide has little negative inotropic effect[168] so that it may be given to patients with poor LV function.[158] There are two phenotypes for metabolism, normal metabolizers (over 90 percent) produce two active metabolites with a much longer half-life than the parent compound (Table 4-2) whereas in nonmetabolizers the half-life of encainide itself is prolonged. The dose of encainide in both phenotypes is, however, 25–75 mg 3× daily (4× daily doses sometimes given). Such doses do not depress LV function.[75,168] Slowly accumulating metabolites may be important in the antiarrhythmic activity of encainide so that the oral route is more effective than the IV. Cimetidine increases plasma concentrations of encainide. Routine measurements of plasma levels are not available.

Side-effects include vertigo, visual disturbances, and headache as well as lengthening of the PR and QRS intervals.[75] "Minor" side-effects may limit the use of encainide before a therapeutic effect is reached.[50]

Encainide may have pro-arrhythmic effects[184] especially in patients with potentially lethal or lethal arrhythmias and cardiomyopathy (17 percent pro-arrhythmic events according to package insert). Initial low doses, increasing upwards only every 4 days to a limit of 200 mg daily, and careful monitoring are required in such patients. With more benign arrhythmias, encainide can be started as out-patient therapy.[123] The full spectrum of drug interactions of encainide is not yet known, but may come to resemble those of flecainide.

Propafenone

Propafenone (Rytmonorm®, not in the USA) has complex additional properties besides Class IC actions, such as mild nonspecific β-blockade, perhaps one-fortieth that of propranolol at peak concentrations of propafenone.[160] Widely used in Europe and investigational in the USA, propafenone is regarded as relatively safe in suppressing ventricular and supraventricular arrhythmias including those of the WPW syndrome. Propafenone seems to have a low pro-arrhythmic potential (unlike flecainide and encainide), although strict comparisons are lacking.

Electrophysiology. In keeping with its Class IC effects, propafenone blocks the fast inward sodium channel, has a potent membrane stabilizing activity and increases PR and QRS times without effect on the QT-interval.[145]
Pharmacokinetics. Oral propafenone is rapidly absorbed with a bioavailability of about 50 percent, reaching peak blood levels within 2 hours.[95] Therapeutic plasma concentrations (highly variable) are 0.2–3.0 μg/ml.[71] There is variable and sometimes almost complete liver metabolism to 5–hydroxypropafenone, also antiarrhythmic. The poor correlation between plasma levels and therapeutic response and the variable plasma half-life (2–12 hours) may be explained by genetic variations in the propafenone metabolism.[160]

Dose.   Oral: 150–300 mg 3× daily. IV: 2 mg/kg followed by an infusion of 2 mg/min.

Indications.   Ventricular and supraventricular arrhythmias including those of the WPW syndrome. In this way, propafenone resembles amiodarone.[67] In ventricular arrhythmias, propafenone inhibits PVCs, couplets, VT, and induced VT.[71,91,103,139,145,160] Failure to prevent induced VT does not preclude long-term benefit. In supraventricular tachycardias with AV nodal or bypass re-entry, propafenone is fully effective in about 40 percent of patients.[56]

Contraindications.   Pre-existing sinus, AV or bundle branch abnormalities, or depressed LV function are relative contraindications.
Side-effects.   Cardiac side-effects include PR and QRS-prolongation and conduction block.[91] Occasionally CHF is precipitated[139] by a modest negative inotropic effect.[47,139] A pro-arrhythmic effect has been reported,[129] but may not be frequent.
  Extracardiac side-effects are relatively uncommon and are chiefly GI, including abdominal discomfort and alteration in taste or smell.[139] Hepatitis is rare.[56,71]

Drug interactions and combinations.   Like other Class IC agents, propafenone is likely to interact adversely with drugs depressing nodal function or intraventricular conduction, or the inotropic state. Propafenone has been combined with quinidine or procainamide at reduced doses of both drugs in the treatment of PVCs.[103] Propafenone substantially increases serum digoxin levels.[91]

Propafenone—Summary

Propafenone is a new antiarrhythmic drug, widely used in Europe, of predominant Class IC properties. Usually well tolerated, the spectrum of activity and some of the side-effects resemble those of Class IC agents, including a pro-arrhythmic effect. Marked interindividual variations in its metabolism mean that dose must be individualized and that plasma levels may not be a good guide to the expected therapeutic benefit.

Other Class IC Agents

Lorcainide, not yet approved for use in the USA, has been widely used in Europe. Like flecainide, it has the advantages of both IV and oral administration. A recent American trial showed that IV lorcainide (loading dose 2 mg/kg at 2 mg/min followed by 8 mg/hr) compared well with a standard lidocaine infusion.[43]

Indecainide likewise is investigational.

CLASS II AGENTS: β-ADRENERGIC ANTAGONISTS

β-Blockade is used especially for inappropriate or unwanted sinus tachycardia, for paroxysmal atrial tachycardia provoked by emotion or exercise, for exercise-induced ventricular arrhythmias, in the arrhythmias of pheochromocytoma (combined with α-blockade to avoid hypertensive crises), in the hereditary prolonged QT-syndrome, and possibly in the arrhythmias of mitral valve prolapse. In AMI, the cardiodepressant effects argue against the use of β-blockers as antiarrhythmic agents of choice, but in appropriate dosage and in patients without manifest heart failure β-blockade may be used to prevent and control supraventricular and ventricular arrhythmias. A common denominator to most of these indications is increased sympathetic β-adrenergic activity. β-Blockers suppress chronic ventricular ectopic beats in about 50 percent of patients, but are seldom used unless there is an added indication such as angina or hypertension. The mechanism of benefit of β-blockade in postinfarct patients is uncertain, possibly but not certainly being antiarrhythmic.[82,133]

The antiarrhythmic activity of the various β-blockers is reasonably uniform, the critical property being of β-adrenergic blockade, with any associated properties such as membrane depression (local anesthetic action), cardioselectivity, and intrinsic sympathomimetic activity (ISA) having no major influence on the antiarrhythmic potency. There is one exception: the additional Class III effect of sotalol (next section).

CLASS III AGENTS: AMIODARONE, BRETYLIUM AND SOTALOL

Class III compounds basically act by prolonging the action potential duration and must inevitably prolong the QT-interval to be effective.[166] In the presence of added hypokalemia or other specific factors, QT-prolongation may predispose to torsades de pointes. By acting only on the repolarization phase of the action potential, they leave conduction unchanged, a critical difference from Class IC agents that are also potent antiarrhythmics. Here, however, it should be noted that amiodarone, bretylium, and sotalol all have additional antiarrhythmic properties that might modify the effect on conduction— amiodarone is also a significant sodium channel inhibitor, sotalol is a β-blocker, and bretylium initially releases catecholamines besides blocking adrenergic neurones.

> Other important electrophysiological properties of Class III agents include the capacity to make more uniform the action potential pattern throughout the myocardium, thereby opposing electrophysiological heterogeneity that underlies some serious ventricular arrhythmias. Furthermore, as a group these compounds have little or no negative inotropic effect (sotalol, a β-blocker, is by definition negatively inotropic). The efficacy of amiodarone is generally thought to exceed that of other antiarrhythmic compounds although strict comparisons between amiodarone and Class IC agents such as flecainide are lacking.
>
> Despite these common electrophysiological features, Class III agents are structurally, pharmacokinetically, and electrophysiologically dissimilar so that neither the antiarrhythmic effects nor the clinical indications are interchangeable. In the USA, IV bretylium has long been available and oral amiodarone has recently been approved for use for refractory ventricular arrhythmias. Investigational studies with sotalol are under way. In Europe, amiodarone is the drug of choice for severe refractory arrhythmias, with sotalol increasingly being seen as a safe albeit probably less powerful agent.

Amiodarone

Amiodarone (Cordarone®), initially used in Europe as a coronary vasodilator and antianginal agent, is a unique antiarrhythmic compound[30,36] with four remarkable properties—a wide spectrum of antiarrhythmic effect against both supraventricular and ventricular tachyarrhythmias (including VF), little or no negative inotropism, an exceedingly long elimination half-life and a complex interrelation with thyroid metabolism. To offset its positive qualities, is a high incidence of serious side-effects that restrict the use of amiodarone especially in the USA (see package insert); in the UK, amiodarone is much more widely used.

Pharmacology.   Amiodarone lengthens the effective refractory period by prolonging the action potential duration in all cardiac tissues including the bypass tract. It also has a powerful Class I antiarrhythmic effect inhibiting inactivated sodium channels at high stimulation frequencies.[115,185] Amiodarone also noncompetitively blocks β-adrenergic receptors.[111] A calcium antagonist effect might explain coronary and peripheral vasodilator actions, as well as bradycardia and AV nodal inhibition.[10] Amiodarone is therefore a complex antiarrhythmic agent that shares at least some of the properties of each of the four electrophysiologic classes of antiarrhythmics.[185]

> *Pharmacokinetics.*   After variable (30–50 percent) and slow GI absorption, amiodarone is very slowly eliminated with a half-life of about 25–110 days.[13,15] The onset of action after oral administration is delayed and a steady-state drug effect ("amiodaronization") may not be established for several months unless large loading doses are used.[15] Even when given intravenously, its full electrophysiologic effect is delayed. Amiodarone is lipid-soluble and extensively distributed in the body and highly concentrated in many tissues especially in the liver and lungs. A correlation between the clinical effects and serum concentrations of the drug or its metabolite desethylamiodarone (pharmacologically active[185]) has not been clearly

shown,[13] although there is a direct relation between the oral dose and the plasma concentration.[159] The therapeutic level, not well defined, may be between 1.0 and 2.5 μg/ml, almost all of which (95 percent) is protein bound. Amiodarone is not excreted by the kidneys but rather by the lacrimal glands, skin, and biliary tract.

Dose.   When reasonably rapid control of an arrhythmia is needed, the initial loading regime is 1200–1600 mg in two divided doses usually given for 7–14 days that is then reduced to 600–800 mg/day for a further 1–3 weeks, and thereafter to a maintenance dose that rarely needs to exceed 200–400 mg/day, given as a single dose. The loading dose is essential because of the slow onset of full action with a delay of about 10 days.[159] Downward dose adjustment may be required during prolonged therapy to avoid development of side-effects while maintaining optimal antiarrhythmic effect. However, at a fixed dose, the overall success rate may fall off between 12–24 months of therapy.[80] The maintenance doses for supraventricular arrhythmias are generally lower than those needed for serious ventricular arrhythmias. IV administration (not in the USA) may be used for intractable arrhythmias (150 mg given slowly over 5 minutes, then 600 mg over 24 hours for 3–4 days, then 600 mg orally daily); when thus given, the β-blocking properties could be of importance[111] and there is still a latent period to the onset of full action.

Indications.   In the prophylactic control of life-threatening ventricular tachyarrhythmias and in recurrent cardiac arrest,[12,125] amiodarone is one of the most effective agents available. Amiodarone is highly effective in preventing recurrences of paroxysmal atrial fibrillation or flutter and of paroxysmal supraventricular tachycardias (PSVTs),[23,94,137] and in WPW arrhythmias.[30] For such supraventricular arrhythmias (use not approved in the USA), a very low dose (<200 mg/day after loading) may be strikingly effective with few side-effects. Amiodarone may be tried for variant angina[31] complicated by severe ventricular arrhythmias. For atrial fibrillation in AMI, slow IV amiodarone seems better than digoxin.[71a]

Serious side-effects.   The recent use of amiodarone in higher doses has revealed an unusual spectrum of toxicity, the most serious being pneumonitis[153] potentially leading to pulmonary fibrosis and occurring in up to 10 percent of some series, although only 1–5 percent in others. If recognized early (check diffusion capacity[175]) and if amiodarone is discontinued and steroids given, pulmonary complications usually regress. Pulmonary toxicity may be dose-related.[70,156] A pro-arrhythmic effect may result from QT-prolongation plus hypokalemia (see drug interactions).

Proximal muscle weakness, peripheral neuropathy, and neural symptoms (tremors, impaired memory, insomnia) rarely occur, although regarded as common (20 percent) in one series.[80] Increased liver function enzymes may occur in 10–20 percent of patients.[156] Amiodarone also has a complex effect on the metabolism of thyroid hormones (it contains iodine and shares a structural similarity to thyroxine), the main action being to inhibit the peripheral conversion of T_4 to T_3 with a rise in the serum level of T_4 and a small fall in the level of T_3; serum reverse T_3 is increased as a function of the dose and duration of amiodarone therapy.[27] In most patients thyroid function is not altered by amiodarone; in about 3–5 percent hypothyroidism or hyperthyroidism may develop. At a low dose of amiodarone (200–400 mg daily), there may be biochemically documented but clinically silent alterations in thyroid function in 10 percent of patients.[70]

Less serious side-effects.   Corneal microdeposits develop in nearly all adult patients given prolonged amiodarone. They are rarely associated with symptoms or impairment of visual acuity. Halovision, when encountered, responds to reduced dosage. Photosensitivity of exposed areas is frequently seen and in over 10 percent of patients a slate-grey or bluish skin discoloration develops after prolonged therapy, usually exceeding 18 months. The pigmentation regresses slowly on drug withdrawal.

Drug interactions.   (1) The most serious interaction[22] is an additive pro-arrhythmic effect with other drugs prolonging the QT-interval such as Class IA antiarrhythmic agents, phenothiazines, tricyclic antidepressants, thiazide diuretics, and sotalol (Fig. 4-5). (2) Amiodarone prolongs the prothrombin time

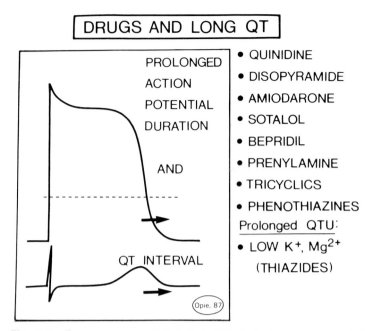

Fig. 4-5. Therapeutic agents including antiarrhythmics may cause QT-prolongation. Hypokalemia causes QTU not QT-prolongation. Some agents act at least in part chiefly by prolonging the action potential duration, such as amiodarone and d-sotalol. QT-prolongation is therefore an integral part of their therapeutic benefit. On the other hand, QT-prolongation, especially in the presence of hypokalemia and other electrolyte disturbances or when there is co-therapy with one of the other agents prolonging the QT-interval, may precipitate torsades de pointes.

and may cause bleeding in patients on warfarin, perhaps by a hepatic interaction.[86] (3) Amiodarone increases the plasma digoxin concentration[126] predisposing to digitalis toxic effects (not arrhythmias because amiodarone protects); this interaction may explain nonspecific neural side-effects of amiodarone. (4) Amiodarone, by virtue of its weak β-blocking and calcium antagonist effect, tends to inhibit nodal activity and may therefore interact adversely with β-blocking agents and calcium antagonists.[22] When amiodarone is added, the dose of digoxin should be decreased by about half, that of warfarin and flecainide by about one-third, and Class IA antiarrhythmics (quinidine, disopyramide, procainamide) should be avoided. Careful electrocardiographic monitoring should obviate adverse interactions with β-blockers or calcium antagonists.

Precautions.   To initiate therapy, the patient may require hospitalization and possible pro-arrhythmic effects monitored (most common in first 7 days). Plasma electrolytes should be normal and drug interactions considered. During chronic therapy the ECG and Holter recordings are monitored and periodic lung functions, chest x-rays, and thyroid tests are required.

Amiodarone—Summary

Amiodarone is a "wide spectrum" antiarrhythmic agent acting through multiple mechanisms. Its benefits need to be balanced against, first, the slow onset of action of oral therapy that may in turn require large oral loading doses. Even IV use (not in the USA) in truly urgent life-threatening arrhythmias may not give a full effect rapidly. Second, the serious side-effects, especially pulmonary infiltrates, mean that there must be a fine balance between the maximum antiarrhythmic effect of the drug and the potential for the side-effects caused by high doses and prolonged therapy. Third, there are a large number of potentially serious drug interactions some of which predispose to torsades de pointes. In recurrent supraventricular arrhythmias, low-dose amiodarone may be strikingly effective with little risk of side-effects. Otherwise, the use of amiodarone in as low a dose as possible should be restricted to patients with refractory ventricular arrhythmias failing to respond to other less toxic agents and after careful evaluation and with an adequate knowledge of its side-effect profile.

Sotalol

Although still not available in the USA, sotalol (Sotacor®) is now widely used in Europe and in American investigational centers for control of ventricular arrhythmias resistant to other measures. Sotalol has combined Class II and III activities; only the latter is found with the d-isomer.[100,112] Sotalol seems much safer than amiodarone, but may not be as effective. The chief hazard is a prolonged QT-interval and torsades de pointes, so that it is important that sotalol should not be given with thiazide diuretics[116] or with any other agent prolonging the QT-interval (see p 81). The major indication for sotalol is its antiarrhythmic capacity rather than its β-blocking antihypertensive effect (it is the only β-blocker with risk of torsades). On the other hand, it is the only antiarrhythmic with simple pharmacokinetics, being totally lipid-insoluble (Fig. 1-7). Sotalol should be especially effective when a combined β-blocking and antiarrhythmic potency is required as in some postinfarct patients, hypertrophic cardiomyopathy, and hypertension with symptomatic arrhythmias; all these possibilities require testing. A limited number of studies have shown the superiority of sotalol to other β-blockers in inducible-VT,[151] and its efficacy in patients with recurrent VT/VF.[128] The oral antiarrhythmic dose is 160–480 mg $2\times$ daily, i.e. higher than the β-blocking doses; the usual contraindications to β-blockade (Table 1-1) apply, but are joined by hypokalemia and co-therapy with other agents likely to produce QT-prolongation.

Bretylium tosylate

Bretylium tosylate (Bretylol®) differs from all other antiarrhythmics in being concentrated in the terminal sympathetic neurons, where it accumulates initially to release stored norepinephrine (NE) and then to inhibit further release of NE with a "chemical" sympathectomy.[33] The latter effect also results in hypotension. Bretylium is an agent used acutely and intravenously for serious VT and VF in patients not responding to other IV agents such as lidocaine and procainamide.

Pharmacology. The antiarrhythmic effect may be due only in part to the chemical sympathectomy because bretylium has Class III activity in Purkinje fibers but less in ventricular muscle and none in atrial tissue. Experimentally, bretylium is better than lidocaine in lessening the current required to defibrillate anesthetized dogs.[46,164] There is little inhibitory effect on nodal or conduction tissue.[73]

Pharmacokinetics. After IV administration, bretylium is widely distributed to various tissues and then excreted almost entirely by the kidneys by active tubular secretion. There is no liver metabolism and the elimination half-life is 7–9 hours (much prolonged in renal failure).

Dose. The initial dose of 5 mg/kg can be increased to 10 mg/kg in the absence of hypotension (which is the major problem with its use). In emergencies, the drug is given undiluted by rapid IV injection, although it is preferable to dilute bretylium 1:4 to a minimum of 50 ml with 5 percent dextrose or sodium chloride and to infuse it over 10–30 minutes to minimize nausea and vomiting.[95] A further dose may be repeated at 1–2-hour intervals if required. Following the loading dose, a constant infusion of 1–2 mg/min may be given.

Indications. Bretylium may have a special use in patients subject to defibrillation and external cardiac massage. In 7 patients with VF after AMI,[33] bretylium 5–10 mg/kg was given intravenously as soon as fibrillation was detected, the patient's arm was raised above the heart, and resuscitation was continued as needed. In 5 patients, defibrillation ensued without DC shock. In a series of 27 patients treated by a hospital cardiac arrest team, VF was resistant to 30 minutes of conventional electric and pharmacologic procedures (lidocaine plus one or more of the following: procainamide, propranolol, and phenytoin),[93] yet after a single IV bolus of bretylium tosylate (5 mg/kg), 20 patients were successfully defibrillated by DC shock. In another series,[44] bretylium 300–400 mg was given intravenously over 10–20 minutes to 17 patients in VF while external cardiac massage and ventilation were continued. Drug defibrillation was achieved in 10 patients. A recent randomized clinical trial of 147 patients compared bretylium and lidocaine in the management of VF occurring outside the hospital, and showed that the two drugs were equally effective.[89]

Side-effects.   The major side-effect is drug-induced hypotension. Severe hypotension can be treated by vasopressor catecholamines or by protriptyline (5 mg every 6 hours) that pharmacologically antagonizes the hypotensive effect.[148] With bretylium, initial sympathomimetic effects (transient hypertension and increased arrhythmias) probably result from transient discharge of NE from the terminal neurons. Nausea and vomiting are common after rapid IV bolus injection.

Drug interactions.   Experimentally, bretylium may worsen digitalis-induced VT.[83] Nonetheless the drug may be life-saving in patients with digitalis-induced recurrent VF.[177]

Bretylium—Summary

Bretylium is generally limited to recurrent VF or VT after lidocaine and DC cardioversion have failed.

CLASS IV AGENTS: VERAPAMIL AND DILTIAZEM

Verapamil is a major advance in the acute therapy of supraventricular arrhythmias (see Chapter 3). Nifedipine is devoid of this effect. Diltiazem is of similar value to verapamil, but neither available in the IV form nor licensed for an antiarrhythmic effect in the USA.

PHYSIOLOGIC ANTIARRHYTHMICS

Hypokalemia predisposes to ventricular arrhythmias especially in the context of AMI and during the use of agents prolonging the action potential duration when torsades becomes a risk. In such situations, *potassium* infusions may be required. It is prudent always to check plasma potassium during antiarrhythmic therapy or during digoxin therapy.

Magnesium salts are reported of benefit in the therapy of torsades[171] and also in the arrhythmias of early AMI.[147]

Adenosine and ATP, given intravenously, are increasingly used to inhibit the AV node in re-entrant tachycardias. They are physiologic "calcium antagonists".

COMPARATIVE STUDIES

Although comparative studies are fraught with hazards (see reference 186), such trials are now becoming increasingly sophisticated with careful definition of patient population, the exact end-points and with increasing use of double-blind techniques.[122,127] All such comparisons, although to be taken with reserve, nevertheless give an indication of the probable efficacy of a drug in a given dose in relation to its possible side-effects.

Quinidine is approximately equally as effective as propafenone against PVCs[74] and likewise about as effective as mexiletine against PVCs and VT, although with different side-effects (for quinidine: diarrhea 11/17; for mexiletine: nausea 7/17 and tremor or nervousness 7/17).[6] Quinidine seems to be much less effective than flecainide in suppressing complex ventricular arrhythmias,[25] while flecainide caused many more ECG changes.

Procainamide was less effective than mexiletine in PVC suppression in a double-blind comparison[127] without any real difference in the side-effect profile.

Disopyramide appeared to be about equipotent with quinidine in the therapy of ventricular and supraventricular arrhythmias, with however a different side-effect profile.[45] Compared with other Class I agents such as flecainide[102] and encainide[64] as well as ethmozine,[144] disopyramide seems less effective with in each case a different pattern of side-effects for the two drugs. When compared with IV lidocaine, IV disopyramide (not available in the USA) seems about equally effective.[34]

Mexiletine—the major comparative trials are (1) in the chronic oral prophylaxis of ventricular arrhythmias after myocardial infarction, mexiletine 300 mg 8-hourly is about as effective as procainamide;[62] (2) in comparison with quinidine a mean mexiletine dose of 950 mg daily is about as effective as quinidine at a mean dose of 1042 mg daily although with a different side-effect profile.[6] The combination of the two agents with a mean mexiletine dose of 800 mg daily and a mean quinidine dose of 820 mg daily produced a better antiarrhythmic response; (3) in a prolonged study with repetitive trials on 114 patients, mexiletine had to be discontinued for side-effects less frequently than quinidine and arrhythmia aggravation occurred more frequently in quinidine-treated than in mexiletine-treated patients, according to a preliminary communication.[81] During a 14 month follow-up period, mexiletine was as effective as quinidine in arrhythmia control. Amiodarone worked in all cases in which mexiletine failed.

Tocainide—oral tocainide and quinidine were compared in a large multicenter double-blind study. They were about equally effective in potentially lethal ventricular arrhythmias.[122] Between one-third to one-half of patients responded to either drug, and about one-quarter required discontinuation because of side-effects. Dizziness was more common during tocainide and diarrhea during quinidine. The QT-interval was prolonged by quinidine and slightly shortened by tocainide. Logically, tocainide (Class IB) and quinidine (Class IA) should be suitable for combination therapy,[88] although untested.

Flecainide was better than disopyramide in suppressing PVCs and complex ventricular arrhythmias,[102] while causing more QT-prolongation as a result of QRS widening. In comparison with quinidine, flecainide was much more effective against complex ventricular arrhythmias, while simultaneously causing much more prolongation of the PR and QRS-intervals.[25]

Encainide was better tolerated and superior to quinidine or disopyramide with PVCs as end-point.[64,157] In potentially lethal ventricular arrhythmias, encainide (100–200 mg daily) was equipotent with quinidine (800–1600 mg daily) with fewer side-effects (less diarrhea and fever) although with more QRS widening.[123]

Propafenone was similar to quinidine in a low dose (propafenone 300 mg 12–hourly, quinidine 200 mg 6–hourly) and in higher doses (propafenone 300 mg 8–hourly, quinidine 400 mg 6–hourly) with no difference in side-effects in suppressing PVCs.[74] There are no data on complex ventricular arrhythmias.

Ethmozine reduced PVCs more than disopyramide without QT-prolongation or other side-effects of disopyramide.[144]

Amiodarone is generally regarded as a powerful antiarrhythmic, possibly the most potent, yet few comparative studies are available. Generally amiodarone has been used after other agents have failed. One careful study[127] took 21 patients failing to respond to mexiletine after dose ranging and in 15 there was a good response to amiodarone (usually 200–400 mg daily). In an actuarial comparison in a similar group of patients (no strict comparisons), amiodarone was more successful than encainide, but the benefit of both drugs rapidly decreased with time.[80] In patients with paroxysmal atrial fibrillation resistant to quinidine, amiodarone helps in over half.[94]

COMBINATION THERAPY

A combination of antiarrhythmic agents is increasingly used on the supposition that added antiarrhythmic potency may be achieved while side-effects are minimized. Some such combinations are: quinidine and procainamide,[101] mexiletine plus quinidine or procainide,[85] quinidine plus verapamil (with the risk of added hypotension[113]), verapamil and disopyramide (in experimental animals[108]), and propafenone with quinidine or procainamide.[103] Drug interactions merit careful attention (Table 4-4). At present, a useful guide is not to combine agents of the same class or subclasses, nor to combine agents with potentially additive side-effects such as the added risk of QT-prolongation with Class IA and Class III agents, or the added risk of arrhythmias with Class IA and Class IC agents.[88] Such "rules," although helpful, do not always apply because of the complex mode of action of many antiarrhythmic agents.[186]

INTERMITTENT THERAPY

Some patients with recurrent tachyarrhythmias that are not potentially lethal can be treated by drugs given "on demand" after the onset of arrhythmias. For supraventricular arrhythmias, a single dose of propranolol-diltiazem may be effective and "periodic procainamide" is likewise worth trying for

TABLE 4-4

INTERACTION OF ANTIARRHYTHMIC DRUGS

Drug	Interaction with	Result
Quinidine	digoxin other Type 1 antiarrhythmics β-blockers, verapamil amiodarone, sotalol diuretics verapamil nifedipine warfarin other interactions	Increased digoxin level Added negative inotropic effect and/or depressed conduction Enhanced hypotension, nega- tive inotropic effect Increased risk of torsades If hypokalemia, risk of torsades Increased quinidine level Decreased quinidine level Enhanced anticoagulation See text
Procainamide	few interactions captopril	See text ? avoid (possible immune effects)
Disopyramide	Other Type 1 antiarrhythmics β-blockers, verapamil anticholineragics pyridostigmine	Enhanced negative inotropic effect and/or depressed con- duction Enhanced hypotension, nega- tive inotropic effect Exaggerated anticholinergic effect Decreased anticholinergic effect
Lidocaine	β-blockers cimetidine halothane	Reduced hepatic clearance of lidocaine; toxicity
Tocainide	few interactions	See text
Mexiletine	few interactions disopyramide	See text Negative inotropic potential
Flecainide	agents inhibiting SA or AV nodes (β-blockers, verapamil, dil- tiazem, digoxin) agents with negative inotropic effects (β-blockers, quinidine, disopyr- amide) agents with depressed HV con- duction (quinidine, procainamide) amiodarone	SA and AV nodal depression Depressed myocardium Conduction delay Increased flecainide levels
Propafenone	as for flecainide but amiodarone interaction not reported digoxin	Enhanced SA, AV and myocar- dial depression Digoxin level increased
Sotalol	diuretics, Class 1A agents, amiodarone, tricyclics, phenothiazines	Risk of torsades
Amiodarone	as for sotalol digoxin flecainide	Risk of torsades Digoxin level increased Flecainide level increased
Verapamil	β-blockers, excess digoxin, myocardial depressants, quinidine	See Table 3-3

ventricular arrhythmias. Clearly, intermittent therapy can only be considered for selected arrhythmias.

PRO-ARRHYTHMIC EFFECTS OF ANTIARRHYTHMIC COMPOUNDS

Unfortunately all agents with an antiarrhythmic effect also have pro-arrhythmic potential, varying between 5–15 percent.[174] The precise mechanisms, not fully established, may include: (1) either inhomogeneities in conduction between the normal and abnormal myocardium or (2) prolongation of the action potential duration with early afterdepolarization, thereby predisposing to torsades de pointes. It is often difficult to distinguish between the pro-arrhythmic effects and lack of efficacy of an agent acting on a background of recurrent variable arrhythmias. A pro-arrhythmic effect may be suspected by: (1) a marked prolongation of the QRS time (100 percent or greater, but see reference 120) or by prolongation of the QT-interval (see next section); (2) the appearance of ventricular pauses and postpause T-wave changes; and (3) the appearance of a new arrhythmia not previously detected on Holter monitoring. Patients with more severe heart disease such as cardiomyopathy may develop more pro-arrhythmic effects. Pro-arrhythmic effects must be suspected when therapy seems to fail.

QT-PROLONGATION AND TORSADES DE POINTES

Delayed repolarization is a mechanism for controlling arrhythmias (Class III and IA agents) that at the same time predisposes to potentially life-threatening arrhythmias. It is clinically recognized by a prolonged QT (500–600 msec[16,120]) or QTU interval (QTc, corrected for heart rate exceeding 440 msec).[26] The prolonged QT-syndrome may either be acquired or be a congenital abnormality (Romano-Ward and related conditions). The recent realization that quinidine, disopyramide and related Class IA agents, Class III agents and others (Fig. 4-5) can all prolong the QT-interval, has led to a reassessment of the mode of use of such agents in antiarrhythmic therapy. Prolongation of the QT-interval may be an essential part of the antiarrhythmic effect of amiodarone.[166] Serious problems may arise when QT-prolongation is combined with bradycardia, hypokalemia, hypomagnesemia, hypocalcemia, intense or prolonged diuretic therapy, or combined Class IA and Class III therapy. Sotalol, with added diuretic therapy especially when accompanied by hypokalemia, may prolong the QT-interval in hypertensives (blood pressure not stated) and result in torsades de pointes.[116] When sotalol is given to patients not receiving diuretics or other drugs, nor hypokalemic and without pre-existing QT-prolongation, torsades is very rare and one case occurring in a patient with a borderline pretreatment QT-prolongation has been reported.[105]

Prevention. **Probably the most effective way to avoid the drug-induced QT-syndrome is by regular monitoring of the ECG for the appearance of ventricular pauses, postpause T-wave changes and late cycle PVCs,[52] as well as QT-prolongation, while checking blood potassium, magnesium and calcium, and using a potassium-sparing diuretic whenever possible. All these precautions are essential when using type IA or type III antiarrhythmics.**

Treatment. Torsades de pointes is best treated by agents that shorten the QT-interval such as isoproterenol or temporary cardiac pacing. Isoproterenol is contraindicated in ischemic heart disease and the congenital prolonged QT-syndrome. A recent report stresses the value of IV magnesium sulphate.[171] If the QT-interval is not markedly prolonged, torsades de pointes is excluded and therapy with conventional ventricular antiarrhythmic agents is acceptable.[8] When the QT-interval is congenitally prolonged, the underlying cause may be an imbalance of the sympathetic drive coming from the left and right sympathetic chains. The therapy now becomes full dose β-blockade, with added phenytoin if needed.[26]

SOME PRINCIPLES OF THERAPY

Paroxysmal Supraventricular Tachycardia

The management of PSVT of the re-entrant type is reasonably well established and falls into two categories: (1) conversion of the acute tachyarrhythmia and (2) prevention of recurrences. For acute conversion, IV verapamil (or diltiazem) is the drug of choice when vagal maneuvers fail. Such conversion occurs by block of anterograde AV nodal conduction. IV digoxin, β-blockers or edrophonium may be used but their effects are less consistent. In the future, IV adenosine may be an agent of choice. Fast-channel blockers (IV procainamide, disopyramide, and others) may also be effective by producing block of the retrograde limb of the tachycardia circuit, but they are seldom used in clinical practice.

In the prophylaxis of PSVT, therapy is aimed either at inhibition of the trigger mechanism (PVCs or premature atrial complexes), or at prolonging the refractory period of the tachycardia circuit in either the anterograde (verapamil, diltiazem, β-blockers, digoxin alone or in combination) or the retrograde direction (fast-channel blockers). In refractory cases, complex agents such as amiodarone may be used in low doses before contemplating ablative therapy.

Wolff-Parkinson-White Syndrome

In this syndrome (Fig. 4-3), the most important point to stress is that digoxin may sometimes dangerously accelerate anterograde conduction and is best avoided in all patients with overt forms of the WPW syndrome (delta wave, short PR-interval on the ECG) unless electrophysiological studies have shown that digoxin is safe in a particular patient. IV verapamil and diltiazem are safe unless atrial fibrillation and flutter are suspected and the QRS complexes during the tachycardia are wide. In such instances with anterograde conduction down the bypass tract, inhibition of the AV node by these agents or β-blockade may predispose to anterograde conduction. During an attack of atrial fibrillation or flutter, the delta waves may not be obvious and it is the very rapid ventricular response that should alert the clinician to the possibility of an underlying WPW. Immediate therapy of choice is electrical conversion. In contrast, verapamil is routinely used for terminating orthodromic PSVT with or without manifest features of the WPW syndrome.

Ventricular Tachycardia

This complex area cannot be simplified (see pp 199–200). First optimal cardiac and electrolyte status are required. There is no unanimity of cardiological opinion on the principles and indication for antiarrhythmic therapy.[178] Nonetheless, some guidelines are useful and are given in Fig. 4-6. Logically, only one compound of one category should be tried, i.e. quinidine, disopyramide, or procainamide. In reality, side-effects may limit the effective dose with one drug (e.g. GI effects of quinidine) to allow another drug of the same class to be effective unless also limited by side-effects (e.g. disopyramide and vagolytic side-effects). Furthermore, many antiarrhythmic mechanisms are complex and not simply explained by effects on the action potential.[186] Also, the experience of any given physician is likely to be limited to a small number of drugs. Hence the "progression" in Fig. 4-6 is only hypothetical. For each category of agent, the profile of electrophysiologic and hemodynamic side-effects shown in Table 4-3 needs to be matched against the clinical situation in the individual patient. In Europe, the trend is away from quinidine towards initial use of Class IB and IC agents. The potential for pro-arrhythmic events and the lack of firm evidence for prevention of sudden death by antiarrhythmics needs stressing. Exceptions to these statements appear to be (1) prehospital lidocaine or very early IV propranolol that reduces VF in AMI; (2) postinfarct β-blockade that prolongs life and reduces sudden death; and (3) therapy of truly life-threatening, serious symptomatic ventricular arrhythmias.

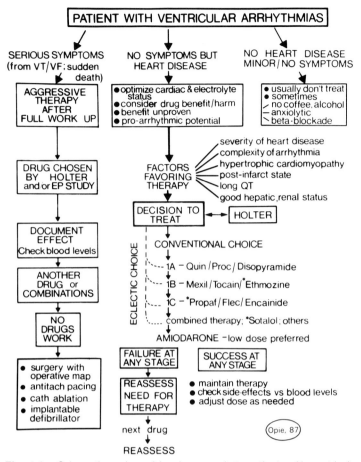

Fig. 4-6. Schematic and provisional approach to patients with ventricular arrhythmias. Note that considerable controversy exists and there is no unanimity of cardiological opinion. Specific individual consideration is required for each patient, because in each the exact nature of the ventricular arrhythmia and its significance may be different. Compiled by LH Opie, DC Harrison and T Mabin.
* = not in the USA.

Ventricular Arrhythmias of AMI

Here too, there is no widely accepted general policy. Again, some guidelines are given in Fig. 4-4. By far the most important drug is lidocaine, with procainamide and the new Class IC agents increasingly used. Bretylium is the standard agent when all else fails.

SUMMARY

The complexity of the numerous agents available and the ever-increasing problems with side-effects underline the requirement for careful cardiological evaluation and monitoring in patients receiving such drugs. In terms of drug effects, the therapy of supraventricular arrhythmias is assuming an increasingly rational basis with a prominent role for verapamil in supraventricular tachycardia with AV nodal re-entry. Sodium blockers can inhibit the bypass tract or retrograde fast AV nodal fibers. The therapy of ventricular arrhythmias remains a controversial and constantly evolving area of development and antiarrhythmic drug therapy may be only one avenue of overall management. In AMI, IV lidocaine remains the agent of choice and prophylaxis of VF by prehospital intramuscular lidocaine or by very early β-blockade are new approaches not yet fully established as routine procedures. In other patients, whether or not ventricular arrhythmias should be treated largely depends on the nature and severity of the underlying heart disease and the nature of the arrhythmia. All symptomatic arrhythmias need therapy; whether asymptomatic arrhythmias should be treated is a moot point, even if they look "premalignant" and "life-threatening." As yet, there has been no definite proof that treatment of asymptomatic arrhythmias improves mortality. Patients with recurrent symptomatic VT or aborted sudden death should ideally be referred for electrophysiologic evaluation and therapy. Potential pro-arrhythmic effects and drug interactions add to the problems of therapy. Patients with the WPW syndrome or those with refractory supraventricular arrhythmias may also need full electrophysiologic work-up. To summarize: only in cases of supraventricular tachycardia or atrial fibrillation is therapy usually relatively simple.

REFERENCES

References from Previous Edition

For details see previous edition of Opie et al, Drugs for the Heart, American Edition. Orlando, FL, Grune & Stratton, 1984, pp 65–98.

1. Campbell NPS, Kelly JG, Adgey AJ, et al: Br Heart J 40:1371–1375, 1978
2. Carruth JE, Silverman ME: Am Heart J 104:545–550, 1982
3. Chew CYC, Collett J, Singh BN: Drugs 17:161–181, 1979
4. Desai JM, Scheiman M, Roberts RW, et al: Circulation 59:215–225, 1979
5. De Silva RA, Hennekens CH, Lown B, et al: Lancet ii:855–858, 1981
6. Duff HJ, Roben D, Primm RK, et al: Circulation 67:1124–1128, 1983
7. Feely J, Wilkinson GR, McAllister CB, et al: Ann Intern Med 96:592–594, 1982
8. Fontaine G, Frank R, Grosgogeat Y: Mod Concepts Cardiovasc Dis 51:103–108, 1982
9. Gerstenblith G, Scherlag BJ, Hope RR, et al: Am J Cardiol 42:587–591, 1978
10. Gloor HO, Urthaler F, James TN: J Clin Invest 71:1457–1466, 1983
11. Hartel G, Louhija A, Konttinen A: Clin Pharmacol Ther 15:551–555, 1974
12. Heger J, Prystowsky EN, Jackman WM, et al: New Engl J Med 305:539–546, 1981
13. Holt DW, Tucker GT, Jackson PR, et al: Am Heart J 106:840–847, 1983
14. Jenzer HR, Hagemaijer F: Eur J Cardiol 4:447–451, 1976
15. Kannan R, Nademanee K, Hendrickson JA, et al: Clin Pharmacol 31:438–451, 1982
16. Keren A, Tzivoni D, Gavish D, et al: Circulation 64:1167–1174, 1981
17. Koch-Weser J, Klein SW, Foo-Canto LL, et al: New Engl J Med 281:1253–1260, 1969
18. Kosowsky BD, Taylor J, Lown B, et al: Circulation 47:1204–1210, 1973
19. Kus T, Sasyniuk BI: Can J Physiol Pharmacol 56:326–331, 1978
20. LaBarre A, Strauss HC, Scheinman MM, et al: Circulation 59:226–235, 1979
21. Lie KI, Wellens HJ, Van Capelle FJ, et al: New Engl J Med 291:1324–1326, 1974
22. Marcus FI: Am Heart J 106:924–930, 1983
23. Marcus FI, Fontaine GH, Frank R, et al: Am Heart J 101:480–493, 1981
24. Meltzer RS, Robert EW, McMorrow M, et al: Am J Cardiol 42:1049–1056, 1978
25. Morganroth J, Panadis I, Lee G, et al: Circulation 67:1117–1123, 1983
26. Moss AJ, Schwartz PJ: Mod Concepts Cardiovasc Dis 51:85–90, 1982
27. Nademanee K, Singh BN, Hendrickson JA, et al: Ann Intern Med 98:577–587, 1983
28. Nathan AW, Hellestrand KJ, Bexton RS, et al: Am Heart J 107:222–228, 1984
29. Roos JC, Paalman ACA, Dunning AJ: Br Heart J 38:1262–1271, 1976
30. Rosenbaum MB, Chiale PA, Halpern MS, et al: Am J Cardiol 38:934–944, 1976
31. Rutitzky B, Girotti AL, Rosenbaum MB: Am Heart J 103:38–43, 1982
32. Ryan W, Engler R, Lewinter M, et al: Am J Cardiol 43:285–291, 1979
33. Sanna G, Arcidiancono R: Am J Cardiol 32:982–987, 1973
34. Sbarbaro JA, Rawling DA, Fozzard HA: Am J Cardiol 44:513–520, 1979
35. Selzer A, Wray HW: Circulation 30:17–26, 1964
36. Singh BN, Vaughan Williams EM: Br J Pharmacol 39:675–687, 1970
37. Singh BN, Vaughan Williams M: Cardiovasc Res 6:109–119, 1972
38. Vismara LA, Vera Z, Miller RR, et al: Am J Cardiol 39:1027–1034, 1977
39. Webb Kavey RE, Blackman MS, Sondheimer HM: Am Heart J 104:794–798, 1982
40. Winkle RA, Mason JW, Harrison DC: Am Heart J 180:1031–1036, 1980
41. Wit AL, Rosen MR, Hoffman BF: Am Heart J 90:397–404, 1975

New References

42. Anderson JL, Lutz JL, Allison SB: Electrophysiologic and antiarrhythmic effects of oral flecainide in patients with inducible ventricular tachycardia. J Am Coll Cardiol 2:105–114, 1983

43. Anderson JL, Anastasiou-Nana M, Lutz JR, et al: Comparison of intravenous lorcainide with lidocaine for acute therapy of complex ventricular arrhythmias. J Am Cardiol 5:333–341, 1985

44. Arcidiancono R: Use of bretylium tosylate in ventricular fibrillation. Clin Ther 84:253–266, 1978

45. Arif M, Laidlaw JC, Oshrain C, et al: A randomized, double-blind, parallel group comparison of disopyramide phosphate and quinidine in patients with cardiac arrhythmias. Angiology 34:393–400, 1983

46. Babbs CF, Yim GKW, Whistler SJ, et al: Elevation of ventricular defibrillation threshold in dogs by antiarrhythmic drugs. Am Heart J 98:345–350, 1979

47. Baker BJ, Dinh H, Kroskey D, et al: Effect of propafenone on left ventricular ejection fraction. Am J Cardiol 54:20D-22D, 1984

48. Bauman JL, Bauerfeind RA, Hoff JV, et al: Torsade de pointes due to quinidine: observations in 31 patients. Am Heart J 107:425–430, 1984

49. Benson DW, Dunnigan A, Green TP, et al: Periodic procainamide for paroxysmal tachycardia. Circulation 72:147–152, 1985

50. Berchtold-Kanz E, Schwarz G, Hust M, et al: Increased incidence of side effects after encainide: a newly developed antiarrhythmic drug. Clin Cardiol 7:493–497, 1984

51. Bexton RS, Hellestrand KG, Cory-Pearce R, et al: The direct electrophysiologic effects of disopyramide phosphate in the transplanted human heart. Circulation 67:38–44, 1983

52. Bhandari AK, Scheinman M: The long QT syndrome. Mod Concepts Cardiovasc Dis 54:45–49, 1985

53. Birkhead S, Vaughan Williams EM: Dual effect of disopyramide on atrial and atrioventricular conduction and refractory periods. Br Heart J 39:657–660, 1977

54. Boyce JR, Cervenko FW, Wright FJ: Effects of halothane on the pharmacokinetics of lidocaine in digitalis-toxic dogs. Canad Anaes Soc J 25:323–328, 1978

55. Breithardt G, Selpel L, Abendroth RR: Comparative cross-over study of the effects of disopyramide and mexiletine on stimulus-induced ventricular tachycardia. Circulation 62 (suppl III):III-153, 1980

56. Breithardt G, Borggrefe M, Wiebringhaus E, et al: Effect of propafenone in the Wolff-Parkinson-White syndrome: Electrophysiologic findings and long-term follow-up. Am J Cardiol 54:29D-39D, 1984

57. Brugada P, Wellens HJJ: Effects of intravenous and oral disopyramide on paroxysmal atrioventricular nodal tachycardia. Am J Cardiol 53:88–92, 1984

58. Burton JR, Mathew MT, Armstrong PW: Comparative effects of lidocaine and procainamide on acutely impaired hemodynamics. Am J Med 61:215–219, 1976

59. Campbell NPS, Pantridge JF, Adgey AAJ: Mexiletine in the management of ventricular arrhythmias. Eur J Cardiol 6:245–258, 1978

60. Campbell NPS, Pantridge JF, Adgey AAJ: Long-term oral antiarrhythmic therapy with mexiletine. Br Heart J 40:796–801, 1978

61. Campbell TJ: Kinetics of onset of rate-dependent effects of Class I antiarrhythmic drugs are important in determining their effects on refractoriness in guinea-pig ventricles, and provide a basis for their subclassification. Cardiovasc Res 17:344–352, 1983

62. Campbell RWF, Dolder MA, Prescott LF, et al: Comparison of procainamide and mexiletine in prevention of ventricular arrhythmias after acute myocardial infarction. Lancet i:1257–1260, 1975

63. Campbell RWF, Hutton I, Elton RA, et al: Prophylaxis of primary ventricular fibrillation with tocainide in acute myocardial infarction. Br Heart J 49:557–563, 1983

64. Caron JF, Libersa CC, Kher AR, et al: Comparative study of encainide and disopyramide in chronic ventricular arrhythmias: A double-blind placebo-controlled crossover study. J Am Coll Cardiol 5:1457–1463, 1985

65. Chazov EI, Shugushev KK, Rosenshtraukh LV: Ethmozine. I. Effects of intravenous drug administration on paroxysmal supraventricular tachycardia in the ventricular pre-excitation syndrome. Am Heart J 108:475–482, 1984

66. Chazov EI, Rosenshtraukh LV, Shugushev KK: Ethmozine. II. Effects of intravenous drug administration on atrioventricular nodal reentrant tachycardia. Am Heart J 108:483–489, 1984

67. Chilson DA, Heger JJ, Zipes DP, et al: Electrophysiologic effects and clinical efficacy of oral propafenone therapy in patients with ventricular tachycardia. J Am Coll Cardiol 5:1407–1413, 1985

68. Christian CO Jr, Meredith CG, Speeg KV Jr: Cimetidine inhibits procainamide clearance. Clin Pharmacol Ther 36:221–227, 1984

69. Colatsky TJ: Mechanisms of action of lidocaine and quinidine on action potential duration in rabbit cardiac Purkinje fibers. An effect on steady state sodium currents Circ Res 50:17–22, 1982

70. Collaborative Group for Amiodarone Evaluation: Multicenter controlled observation of a low-dose regimen of amiodarone for treatment of severe ventricular arrhythmias. Am J Cardiol 53:1564–1569, 1984

71. Connolly SJ, Kates RE, Lebsack CS, et al: Clinical pharmacology of propafenone. Circulation 68:589–596, 1983

71a. Cowan JC, Gardiner P, Reid DS, et al: A comparison of amiodarone and digoxin in the treatment of atrial fibrillation complicating acute myocardial infarction. J Cardiovasc Pharmacol 8:252–256, 1986

72. Dada JL, Wilkinson GR, Nies AJ: Interaction of quinidine with anticonvulsant drugs. New Engl J Med 294:699–702, 1976

73. Dhurandhar RW, Bakersmith D: Bretylium tosylate, in Gould LA (ed): Drug Treatment of Cardiac Arrhythmias. Mount Kisco, New York, Futura Publishing Company, 1983, pp 299–324

74. Dinh HA, Murphy ML, Baker BJ, et al: Efficacy of propafenone compared with quinidine in chronic ventricular arrhythmias. Am J Cardiol 55:1520–1524, 1985

75. Dumoulin P, Jaillon P, Kher A, et al: Long-term efficacy and safety of oral encainide in the treatment of chronic ventricular ectopic activity: Relationship to plasma concentrations—a French multicenter trial. Am Heart J 110:575–581, 1985

76. Ellrodt AG, Murata GH, Riedinger MS, et al: Severe neutropenia associated with sustained-release procainamide. Ann Intern Med 100:197–201, 1984

77. Estes NAM, Garan H, Ruskin JN: Electrophysiologic properties of flecainide acetate. Am J Cardiol 53:26B-29B, 1984

77a. Farringer JA, Green JA, O'Rourke RA, et al: Nifedipine-induced alterations in serum quinidine concentrations. Am Heart J 108:1570–1572, 1984

78. Farringer JA, McWay-Hess K, Clementi WA: Cimetidine-quinidine interaction. Clin Pharmacol 3:81–83, 1984

79. Flecainide Ventricular Tachycardia Study Group: Treatment of resistant ventricular tachycardia with flecainide acetate. Am J Cardiol 57:1299–1304, 1986

80. Fogoros RN, Anderson KP, Winkle RA, et al: Amiodarone—clinical efficacy and toxicity in 96 patients with recurrent drug-refractory arrhythmias. Circulation 68:88–94, 1983

81. Frank MJ, Russell SL, Watkins LO, et al: Relative efficacy of mexiletine and quinidine in consecutive trials. Circulation 72 (suppl III):III-164, 1985

82. Friedman LM, Byington RP, Capone RJ, et al: Effect of propranolol in patients with myocardial infarction and ventricular arrhythmia. J Am Coll Cardiol 7:1–8, 1986

83. Gillis RA, Clancy MM, Anderson RJ: Deleterious effects of bretylium in cats with digitalis-induced ventricular tachycardia. Circulation 47:974–983, 1973

84. Graffner C, Conradson T-B, Hofvendahl S, et al: Tocainide kinetics after intravenous and oral administration in healthy subjects and in patients with acute myocardial infarction. Clin Pharmacol Ther 27:64–71, 1980

84a. Green JA, Clementi WA, Porter C, et al: Nifedipine-quinidine interaction. Clin Pharm 2:461–465, 1983

85. Greenspan AM, Spielman SR, Webb CR, et al: Efficacy of combination therapy with mexiletine and a Type 1A agent for inducible ventricular tachyarrhythmias secondary to coronary artery disease. Am J Cardiol 56:277–284, 1985

86. Hamer A, Peter T, Mandel WJ, et al: The potentiation of warfarin anticoagulation by amiodarone. Circulation 65:1025–1029, 1982

87. Harrison DC: Should lidocaine be administered routinely to all patients after acute myocardial infarction. Circulation 58:581–583, 1978

88. Harrison DC: Antiarrhythmic drug classification: New science and practical applications. Am J Cardiol 56:185–187, 1985

89. Haynes RE, Chinn TL, Copass MK, et al: Comparison of bretylium tosylate and lidocaine in management of out of hospital ventricular fibrillation: A randomized clinical trial. Am J Cardiol 48:353–360, 1981

90. Hellestrand KJ, Nathan AW, Bexton RS, et al: Cardiac electrophysiologic effects of flecainide acetate for paroxysmal reentrant junctional tachycardias. Am J Cardiol 51:770–776, 1983

91. Hodges M, Salerno D, Granrud G: Double-blind placebo-controlled evaluation of propafenone in suppressing ventricular ectopic activity. Am J Cardiol 54:45D-50D, 1984

92. Hohnloser SH, Lange HW, Raeder EA, et al: Short- and long-term therapy with tocainide for malignant ventricular tachyarrhythmias. Circulation 73:143–149, 1986

93. Holder DA, Smiderman AD, Fraser G, et al: Experience with bretylium tosylate by a hospital cardiac arrest team. Circulation 55:541–544, 1977

94. Horowitz LN, Spielman SR, Greenspan AM, et al: Use of amiodarone in the treatment of persistent and paroxysmal atrial fibrillation resistant to quinidine therapy. J Am Coll Cardiol 6:1402–1407, 1985

95. Huang SK, Marcus FI: Antiarrhythmic drug therapy of ventricular arrhythmias. Current Problems in Cardiology 11:179–240, 1986

96. IMPACT Research Group: International mexiletine and placebo antiarrhythmic coronary trial: I. Report on arrhythmia and other findings. J Am Coll Cardiol 4:1148–1163, 1984

97. Jeresaty RM, Kahn AH, Landry AB Jr: Sinoatrial arrest due to lidocaine in a patient receiving quinidine. Chest 61:683–685, 1972

98. Josephson MA, Kaul S, Hopkins J, et al: Hemodynamic effects of intravenous flecainide relative to the level of ventricular function in patients with coronary artery disease. Am Heart J 109:41–45, 1985

99. Karim A, Nissen C, Azarnoff DL: Clinical pharmacokinetics of disopyramide. J Pharmacokinet Biopharm 10:465–494, 1982

100. Kato R, Ikeda N, Yabek SM, et al: Electrophysiologic effects of the levo- and dextrorotatory isomers of sotalol in isolated cardiac muscle and their in vivo pharmacokinetics. J Am Coll Cardiol 7:116–125, 1986

101. Kim SG, Seiden SW, Matos JA, et al: Combination of procainamide and quinidine for better tolerance and additive effects for ventricular arrhythmias. Am J Cardiol 56:84–88, 1985

102. Kjekshus J, Bathen J, Orning OM, et al: A double-blind, crossover comparison of flecainide acetate and disopyramide phosphate in the treatment of ventricular premature complexes. Am J Cardiol 53:72B-78B, 1984

103. Klein R, Huang SK, and the Southwest Cardiology Research Group: Combination therapy of propafenone with quinidine or procainamide: enhanced efficacy and reduced side-effects. J Am Coll Cardiol 5 (abs):423, 1985

104. Koster RW, Dunning AJ: Intramuscular lidocaine for prevention of lethal arrhythmias in the prehospitalization phase of acute myocardial infarction. New Engl J Med 313:1105–1110, 1985

105. Kuck KH, Kunze KP, Roewer N, et al: Sotalol-induced torsade de pointes. Am Heart J 107:170–180, 1984

106. Kutalek SP, Morganroth J, Horowitz LN: Tocainide: a new oral antiarrhythmic agent. Ann Intern Med 103:381–391, 1985

107. Leahey EB, Heissenbuttel RH, Giardina EGV, et al: Combined mexiletine and propranolol treatment of refractory ventricular tachycardia. Br Med J 2:357–358, 1980

107a. Leak D: Intravenous amiodarone in the treatment of refractory life-threatening cardiac arrhythmias in the critically ill patient. Am Heart J 111:456–462, 1982

108. Lee JT, Davy J-M, Kates RE: Evaluation of combined administration of verapamil and disopyramide in dogs. J Cardiovasc Pharmacol 7:501–507, 1985

109. Legrand V, Vandormael M, Collignon P, et al: Hemodynamic effects of a new antiarrhythmic agent, flecainide (R-818), in coronary heart disease. Am J Cardiol 51:422–426, 1983

110. Lerman BB, Waxman HL, Buxton AE, et al: Disopyramide: evaluation of electrophysiologic effects and clinical efficacy in patients with sustained ventricular tachycardia or ventricular fibrillation. Am J Cardiol 51:759–764, 1983

111. Lubbe WF, McFadyen ML, Muller CA, et al: Protective action of amiodarone against ventricular fibrillation in the isolated perfused rat heart. Am J Cardiol 43:533–540, 1979

112. Lynch JJ, Coskey LA, Montgomery DG, et al: Prevention of ventricular fibrillation by dextrorotatory sotalol in a conscious canine model of sudden coronary death. Am Heart J 109:949–958, 1985

113. Maisel AS, Motulsky HJ, Insel PA: Hypotension after quinidine plus verapamil. New Engl J Med 312:167–171, 1985

114. Marriott HJL, Bieza CF: Alarming ventricular acceleration after lidocaine administration. Chest 61:682–683, 1972

115. Mason JW, Hondeghem LM, Katzung BG: Block of inactivated sodium channels and of depolarization-induced automaticity in guinea pig papillary muscle by amiodarone. Circ Res 55:277–285, 1984

116. McKibbin JK, Pocock WA, Barlow JB, et al: Sotalol, hypokalemia, syncope and torsade de pointes. Br Heart J 51:157–162, 1984

117. Mirro MJ, Manalan AS, Bailey JC: Anticholinergic effects of disopyramide and quinidine on guinea pig myocardium. Circ Res 47:855–865, 1980

118. Morganroth J, Pearlman AS, Dunkman WB, et al: Ethmozine: A new antiarrhythmic agent developed in the USSR. Efficacy and tolerance. Am Heart J 98:621–628, 1979

119. Morganroth J, Horowitz LN: Flecainide: Its proarrhythmic effect and expected changes on the surface electrocardiogram. Am J Cardiol 53:89B-94B, 1984

120. Morganroth J, Horowitz LN: Incidence of proarrhythmic effects from quinidine in the outpatient treatment of benign or potentially lethal ventricular arrhythmias. Am J Cardiol 56:585–587, 1985

121. Morganroth J, Nestico PF, Horowitz LN: A review of the uses and limitations of tocainide—a class IB antiarrhythmic agent. Am Heart J 110:856–863, 1985

122. Morganroth J, Oshrain C, Steele PP: Comparative efficacy and safety of oral to-cainide and quinidine for benign and potentially lethal ventricular arrhythmias. Am J Cardiol 56:581–585, 1985

123. Morganroth J, Somberg JC, Pool PE, et al: Comparative study of encainide and quinidine in the treatment of ventricular arrhythmias. J Am Coll Cardiol 7:9–16, 1986

124. Motulsky HJ, Maisel AS, Snavely MD, et al: Quinidine is a competitive antagonist at α_1- and α_2-adrenergic receptors. Circ Res 55:376–381, 1984

125. Nademanee K, Hendrickson JA, Cannom DS, et al: Control of refractory life-threatening ventricular tachyarrhythmias by amiodarone. Am Heart J 101:759–768, 1981

126. Nademanee K, Kannan R, Hendrickson J, et al: Amiodarone-digoxin interaction: clinical significance, time course of development, potential pharmacokinetic mechanisms and therapeutic implications. J Am Coll Cardiol 4:111–116, 1984

127. Nademanee K, Feld G, Hendrickson J, et al: Mexiletine: double-blind comparison with procainamide in PVC suppression and open-label sequential comparison with amiodarone in life-threatening ventricular arrhythmias. Am Heart J 110:923–931, 1985

128. Nademanee K, Feld G, Hendrickson J, et al: Electrophysiologic and antiarrhythmic effects of sotalol in patients with life-threatening ventricular tachyarrhythmias. Circulation 72:555–564, 1985

129. Nathan AW, Bexton RS, Hellestrand KJ, et al: Fatal ventricular tachycardia in association with propafenone, a new Class IC antiarrhythmic agent. Postgrad Med J 60:155–156, 1984

130. Neuss H, Buss J, Schlepper M, et al: Effects of flecainide on electrophysiological properties of accessory pathways in the Wolff-Parkinson-White syndrome. Eur Heart J 4:347–353, 1983

131. Nitsch J, Steinbeck G, Luderitz B: Increase of mexiletine plasma levels due to delayed hepatic metabolism in patients with chronic liver disease. Eur Heart J 4:810–814, 1983

132. Ochs HR, Carstens G, Greenblatt DJ: Reduction in lidocaine clearance during continuous infusion and by coadministration of propranolol. New Engl J Med 303:373–377, 1980

133. Olsson G, Rehnqvist N: Ventricular arrhythmias during the first year after acute myocardial infarction: Influence of long-term treatment with metoprolol. Circulation 69:1129–1134, 1984

134. Opie LH: The Heart. Physiology, metabolism, pharmacology and therapy. London and Orlando, Grune & Stratton, 1984

135. Palileo EV, Welch W, Hoff J, et al: Lack of effectiveness of oral mexiletine in patients with drug-refractory paroxysmal sustained ventricular tachycardia. Am J Cardiol 50:1075–1081, 1982

136. Podrid PJ, Lyakishev A, Lown B, et al: Ethmozine, a new antiarrhythmic drug for suppressing ventricular premature complexes. Circulation 61:450–457, 1980

137. Podrid PJ, Lown B: Amiodarone therapy in symptomatic, sustained refractory atrial and ventricular tachyarrhythmias. Am Heart J 101:374–379, 1981

138. Podrid PJ, Lown B: Tocainide for refractory symptomatic arrhythmias. Am J Cardiol 49:1279–1286, 1982

139. Podrid PJ, Cytryn R, Lown B: Propafenone: Noninvasive evaluation of efficacy. Am J Cardiol 54:53D-59D, 1984

140. Pollick C, Giacomini KM, Blaschke TF, et al: The cardiac effects of d- and l-disopyramide in normal subjects: A noninvasive study. Circulation 66:447–453, 1982

141. Pollick C, Detsky A, Ogilvie RI, et al: Disopyramide and propranolol in hypertrophic cardiomyopathy: double-blind randomised trial. Circulation 72 (suppl III):III-155, 1985

142. Pottage A: Oral dosage schedules for mexiletine. Postgrad Med J 53 (suppl 1):155–157, 1977

143. Pratt CM, Yepsen SC, Taylor AA, et al: Ethmozine suppression of single and repetitive ventricular premature depolarizations during therapy: Documentation of efficacy and long-term safety. Am Heart J 106:85–91, 1983

144. Pratt CM, Young JB, Francis MJ, et al: Comparative effect of disopyramide and ethmozine in suppressing complex ventricular arrhythmias by use of a double-blind, placebo-controlled, longitudinal crossover design. Circulation 69:288–297, 1984

145. Prystowsky EN, Heger JJ, Chilson DA, et al: Antiarrhythmic and electrophysiologic effects of oral propafenone. Am J Cardiol 54:26D-28D, 1984

146. Rae AP, Sokoloff NM, Webb CR, et al: Limitations of failure of procainamide during electrophysiological testing to predict response to other medical therapy. J Am Coll Cardiol 6:410–416, 1985

147. Rasmussen HS, McNair P, Norregard P, et al: Intravenous magnesium in acute myocardial infarction. Lancet i:234–236, 1986

148. Reele S, Woosley RL, Oates JA: Pharmacologic reversal of the hypotensive effect that complicates therapy with bretylium. Circulation 58 (suppl II):II-962, 1978

149. Reid PR, Griffith LSC, Platia EV, et al: Evaluation of flecainide acetate in the management of patients at high risk of sudden cardiac death. Am J Cardiol 53:108B-111B, 1984

150. Reidenberg MM, Campcho M, Kluger J, et al: Aging and renal clearance of procainamide and N-acetyl procainamide. Clin Pharmacol Ther 28:732-735, 1980

151. Rizos I, Senges J, Jauernig R, et al: Differential effects of sotalol and metoprolol on induction of paroxysmal supraventricular tachycardia. Am J Cardiol 53:1022-1027, 1984

151a. Roden DM, Woosley RL, Primm RK: Incidence and clinical features of quinidine-associated long QT syndrome. Am Heart J 111:1088-1093, 1986

152. Rodman JH, Hurst A, Gaarder T, et al: N-acetylprocainamide kinetics and clinical response during repeated dosing. Clin Pharmacol Ther 32:378-386, 1982

153. Rotmensch HH, Liron M, Tupilski M, et al: Possible association of pneumonitis with amiodarone therapy. Am Heart J 100:412-413, 1980

154. Rutledge JC, Harris F, Amsterdam EA: Clinical evaluation of oral mexiletine therapy in the treatment of ventricular arrhythmias. J Am Coll Cardiol 6:780-784, 1985

155. Salem HH: Persistent supraventricular tachycardia treated with mexiletine. Lancet ii:94, 1977

156. Salerno JA, Bressan MA, Vigano M, et al: Medical and surgical treatment of sustained and recurrent post-infarction ventricular tachycardia. Eur Heart J 6:1054-1062, 1985

157. Sami M, Harrison DC, Kraemer H, et al: Antiarrhythmic efficacy of encainide and quinidine: Validation of a model for drug assessment. Am J Cardiol 48:147-156, 1981

158. Sami MH, Derbekyan VA, Lisbona R: Hemodynamic effects of encainide patients with ventricular arrhythmia and poor ventricular function. Am J Cardiol 52:507-512, 1983

158a. Shea P, Lal R, Kim SS, et al: Flecainide and amiodarone interaction. J Am Coll Cardiol 7:1127-1130, 1986

159. Siddoway LA, McAllister CB, Wilkinson GR, et al: Amiodarone dosing: A proposal based upon its pharmacokinetics. Am Heart J 106:951-956, 1983

160. Siddoway LA, Roden DM, Woosley RL: Clinical pharmacology of propafenone: Pharmacokinetics, metabolism and concentration- response relations. Am J Cardiol 54:9D-12D, 1984

161. Spurrell RAJ, Thorburn CW, Camm J, et al: Effects of disopyramide on electrophysiological properties of specialized conduction system in man and on accessory atrioventricular pathway in Wolff-Parkinson-White syndrome. Br Heart J 37:861-867, 1975

162. Stein J, Podrid P, Lown B: Effects of oral mexiletine on left and right ventricular function. Am J Cardiol 54:575-578, 1984

163. Strathman I, Schubert EN, Cohen A, et al: Hypoglycemia in patients receiving disopyramide phosphate. Drug Intell Clin Pharm 17:635-638, 1983

163a. Swiryn S, Palileo E, Rosen KM: Prediction of response to Class I antiarrhythmic drugs during electrophysiologic study of ventricular tachycardia. Am Heart J 104:43-50, 1982.

164. Tacker WA, Niebauer MJ, Babbs CF, et al: The effect of new antiarrhythmic drugs on defibrillation threshold. Crit Care Med 8:177-180, 1980

165. Teichman SL, Fisher JD, Matos JA, et al: Disopyramide- pyridostigmine: Report of a beneficial drug interaction. J Cardiovasc Pharmacol 7:108-113, 1985

166. Torres V, Tepper D, Flowers D, et al: QT prolongation and the antiarrhythmic efficacy of amiodarone. J Am Coll Cardiol 7:142-147, 1986

167. Touboul P, Gressard A, Kirrorian G, et al: Effects of mexiletine in Wolff-Parkinson-White syndrome. Arch Mal Coeur 74:1315-1323, 1981

167a. Trohman RG, Estes DM, Castellanos A, et al: Increased quinidine plasma concentrations during administration of verapamil: A new quinidine-verapamil interaction. Am J Cardiol 57:706-707, 1986.

168. Tucker CR, Winkle RA, Peters FA, et al: Acute hemodynamic effects of intravenous encainide in patients with heart disease. Am Heart J 104:209-215, 1982

169. Twum-Barima Y, Carruthers SG: Quinidine-rifampcin. New Engl J Med 304:1466-1469, 1981

170. Tynan M, Keaton BR, Hayler AM, et al: The dosage of disopyramide in infants and children. Br J Clin Pract (Symp Suppl 11):40-42, 1981

171. Tzivoni D, Keren A, Cohen AM, et al: Magnesium therapy for torsades de pointes. Am J Cardiol 53:528-530, 1984

172. Ueda CT, Hirschfield DS, Scheinman MN, et al: Disposition kinetics of quinidine. Clin Pharmacol Ther 19:30-36, 1976

173. Ueda CT, Dzindzio BS, Vosik WM: Serum disopyramide concentrations and suppression of ventricular premature contractions. Clin Pharmacol Ther 36:326-336, 1984

173a. Van Lith RM, Appleby DH: Quinidine-nifedipine interaction. Drug Intell Clin Pharm 19:829–830, 1985.
174. Velebit V, Podrid P, Lown B, et al: Aggravation and provocation of ventricular arrhythmias by antiarrhythmic drugs. Circulation 65:886–894, 1982
175. Veltri EP, Reid PR, Platia EV, et al: Amiodarone in the treatment of life-threatening ventricular tachycardia: Role of Holter monitoring in predicting long-term clinical efficacy. J Am Coll Cardiol 6:806–813, 1985
176. Vik-Mo H, Ohm O-J, Lund-Johansen P: Electrophysiologic effects of flecainide acetate in patients with sinus nodal dysfunction. Am J Cardiol 50:1090–1094, 1982
177. Vincent JL, Dufaye P, Berre J, et al: Bretylium in severe ventricular arrhythmias associated with digitalis intoxication. Am J Emerg Med 2:504–506, 1984
178. Vlay SC: How the university cardiologist treats ventricular premature beats: A nationwide survey of 65 University Medical Centers. Am Heart J 110:904–912, 1985
179. Waleffe A, Bruninx P, Mary-Rabine L, et al: Effects of tocainide studied with programmed electrical stimulation of the heart in patients with reentrant tachyarrhythmias. Am J Cardiol 43:292–299, 1979
180. Waleffe A, Mary-Rabine L, Legrand V, et al: Combined mexiletine and amiodarone treatment of refractory recurrent ventricular tachycardia. Am Heart J 100:788–793, 1980
181. Waspe L, Waxman HL, Buxton AE, et al: Mexiletine for control of drug-resistant ventricular tachycardia: Clinical and electrophysiologic results in 44 patients. Am J Cardiol 51:1175–1181, 1983
182. Waxman HL, Buxton AE, Sadowski LM, et al: The response to procainamide during electrophysiological study of sustained ventricular tachyarrhythmias predicts the response to other medications. Circulation 67:30–37, 1983
183. Wigle ED, Sasson Z, Henderson MA, et al: Hypertrophic cardiomyopathy. The importance of the site and the extent of hypertrophy. A review. Prog Cardiovasc Dis 28:1–83, 1985
184. Winkle RA, Mason JW, Griffin JC, et al: Malignant ventricular tachyarrhythmias associated with the use of encainide, clinical investigations. Am Heart J 102:857–864, 1981
185. Yabek SM, Kato R, Singh BN: Effects of amiodarone and its metabolite, desethylamiodarone, on the electrophysiologic properties of isolated cardiac muscle. J Cardiovasc Pharmacol 8:197–207, 1986
186. Zipes DP: A consideration of antiarrhythmic therapy. Circulation 72:949–956, 1985

Reviews

Huang SK, Marcus RI: Antiarrhythmic drug therapy of ventricular arrhythmias. Curr Probl Cardiol 11:179–240, 1986
Keefe DL, Miura D, Somberg JS: Supraventricular tachycardias. Their evaluation and therapy. Am Heart J 111:1150–1161, 1986
McGovern B, Schoenfeld MH, Ruskin JN, et al: Ventricular tachycardia. Historical perspective. PACE 9:449–462, 1986

F. I. Marcus
L. H. Opie
E. H. Sonnenblick

5

Digitalis, Sympathomimetics, and Inotropic-Dilators

DIGITALIS

The crucial question with digitalis (as with any other drug) is whether the proposed benefits outweigh the possible harmful effects. This question is particularly pertinent because of the narrow therapeutic-toxic ratio of digitalis. Thus, does the patient really need digitalis? What are the indications and contraindications? If digitalis is needed, what dose? If the patient is already on digitalis, is that the correct dose (any sign of toxicity?) and is the treatment effective? Also, the physician needs to consider which other drugs the patient is receiving and their possible interaction with digitalis.

Digoxin is now the most widely used agent because its shorter half-life allows easier treatment of toxicity, and because plasma digoxin assays are so widely available. Digitoxin, the alternative agent, is considered separately.

Role of Digitalis in Congestive Heart Failure (CHF)

Digitalis compounds, together with diuretics, remain the basis of the therapy of CHF. Digitalis has two main effects: (1) the heart rate is slowed especially when there is atrial fibrillation so that ventricular filling is improved; and (2) there is a positive inotropic effect. The bradycardiac effect is universally regarded as beneficial unless there is digitalis toxicity; the inotropic effect has potential for both harm (increasing the work of the heart and the oxygen demand in the face of myocardial disease) and benefit (decreasing the heart size decreases the myocardial oxygen demand). Nonetheless **the combined inotropic-bradycardiac action of digitalis is unique when compared to the many sympathomimetic inotropes that all tend to cause tachycardia.** Furthermore, no sympathomimetics are currently approved for oral use in the USA. Therefore digitalis, whatever its defects, remains the basic inotrope despite the narrow therapeutic-toxic margin and the "intensifying myriad of interactions."[74]

Pharmacologic Properties

Structure. All cardiac glycosides share an aglycone ring wherein the pharmacologic activity resides, combined with one to four molecules of sugar that modify the pharmacokinetic properties. Digoxin is a polar compound with an OH group binding to the steroid nucleus, whereas digitoxin is nonpolar with lesser central nervous penetration.

Mechanism of action. The *cellular effect* of digitalis occurs when it binds to the cardiac receptor, which is the sodium pump (Na/K-ATPase) where digitalis inhibits the pump.[1] The result is an enhanced transient increase in intracellular sodium close to the sarcolemma, which in turn enhances calcium influx by the sodium–

Drugs for the Heart, Second Expanded Edition
Copyright © 1987 by Grune & Stratton, Inc.

ISBN 0-8089-1840-0

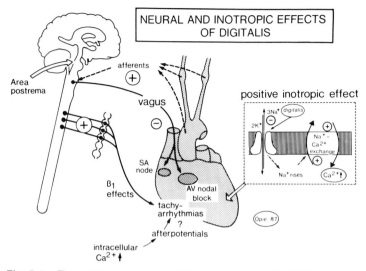

Fig. 5-1. The inotropic effect of digitalis is best explained by inhibition of the sodium pump. Slowing of the heart rate and inhibition of the atrioventricular node is explained by vagal stimulation (a direct effect on nodal tissue may also play a role). Toxic arrhythmias are less well understood, but may be caused by a combination of sympathomimetic stimulation (β_1 = beta$_1$ adrenoceptor stimulation) and the development of calcium-dependent afterpotentials.

calcium exchange mechanism, so that an increased cytosolic calcium ion concentration results.[68] The result is enhanced myocardial contractility.

The *autonomic nervous system* is involved in both the therapeutic and toxic effects of digitalis. Parasympathetic activation results in two therapeutic effects—sinus slowing and atrioventricular (AV) nodal inhibition; thus the inhibitory effect on the AV node depends partly on the degree of vagal tone, which varies from person to person;[24] an ill-understood direct depression of nodal tissue may account for those effects of digitalis still found after vagal blockade.[64]

High serum digoxin levels may have sympathomimetic effects, which probably facilitate the development of toxic arrhythmias. The site of this effect is near the floor of the fourth ventricle.[80]

The *hemodynamic effects* of IV digoxin were first described in a classic paper by McMichael and Sharpey-Schafer,[35] who showed that acute digitalization improved cardiac output and heart failure. The fall in the venous pressure they found is probably best explained by a decreased sympathetic drive as heart failure improves; the direct effect of digitalis on peripheral veins and arteries is mild vasoconstriction (increase of intracellular calcium). The action of digitalis on AV conduction which it slows, and on the AV refractory period which it prolongs, is primarily dependent on vagal tone and only to a minor extent on the direct inhibitory effect of digitalis.[43] Thus the inhibitory effect on the AV node and on the inotropic state occur by different mechanisms (Fig. 5-1) and at different doses, the inotropic effect usually being observed first.[24]

Pharmacokinetics of digoxin (Table 5-1). The serum half-life is 1.5 days. The major portion is ultimately excreted by the kidneys unchanged. About 18–28 percent is excreted by nonrenal routes (stools, hepatic metabolism) in patients with normal renal function.[77] Multiple pharmacokinetic factors influence the blood level obtained with a given dose of digoxin (Tables 5-2, 5-3). If renal function is subnormal, excretion is impaired and the maintenance dose is lower. The body weight governs the loading dose because a low skeletal mass means less binding to skeletal muscle receptors so that the blood level for any given loading dose is higher as, for example, in a thin old man.

Dose of digoxin. Various nomograms have been designed for calculation of the dose, taking into account lean body mass and renal function,[19,51] but none appears to be more effective than the experienced physician's intuitive estimation of the correct digoxin dosage.[21]

A *loading dose* may be required for urgent indications because a certain amount of digoxin is required to saturate the skeletal muscle receptors throughout the body and for tissue penetration until equilibrium is reached.

TABLE 5-1

DIGOXIN PHARMACOKINETICS

1. 75 percent of oral dose rapidly absorbed; rest inactivated in lower gut to digoxin reduction products by bacteria.

2. Circulates in blood, unbound to plasma proteins; "therapeutic level" 1–2 ng/mL; blood half-life about 36 hr.

3. Binds to tissue receptors in heart and skeletal muscle.

4. Lipid-soluble; brain penetration.

5. Most of absorbed digoxin excreted unchanged in urine (tubular excretion and glomerular filtration).

6. In chronic renal failure, reduced volume of distribution.

7. In small lean body mass, reduced total binding to skeletal muscle.

TABLE 5-2

CAUSES OF LOW SERUM DIGOXIN LEVEL

Dose too low or not taken.

Poor absorption
  Hyperthyroidism (real mechanism unknown)
  Malabsorption, high bran diet
  Unknown causes
  Drug interference: cholestyramine, sulfasalazine, neomycin, PAS, kaolin-pectin, rifampin (= rifampicin)

Enhanced renal secretion
  Improved GFR* as vasodilator therapy enhances renal blood flow

*GFR = glomerular filtration rate

Thus the loading dose is governed by the lean body weight (reduced in old age and severe renal insufficiency). The usual IV loading dose of digoxin is 0.75–1 mg that gives peak plasma digoxin levels as high as 95 ng/ml without toxic effects, which usually only arise when steady-state levels exceed 2 ng/ml. An oral loading dose of 1 mg produces peak blood levels of over 1 ng/ml in about 1–5 hours and a maximum inotropic effect at 4–6 hours.

Digitalization is now commonly started with multiple doses over a longer period (0.5 mg 2× daily for 2 days or 0.5 mg 3× daily for 1 day followed by 0.25 mg daily) to allow for variable gastrointestinal (GI) absorption, variable cardiac responses, and possible drug interactions. When no loading dose is given, steady-state plasma and tissue concentrations are achieved in 5–7

TABLE 5-3

CAUSES OF HIGH SERUM DIGOXIN LEVELS

Excess initial dose for body mass (small lean body mass)

Decreased renal excretion
  Depressed GFR (elderly patients, renal disease)
  Severe hypokalemia (<3 mEq/L)
  Concurrent cardiac drugs (quinidine, verapamil, amiodarone)
  K-retaining diuretics (spironolactone)
  Depressed renal blood flow (congestive heart failure, β-blockers)

Decreased nonrenal clearance
  Cardiac drugs (quinidine, verapamil, amiodarone)
  K-retaining diuretics (spironolactone, triamterene, amiloride)

Decreased conversion in gut to digoxin reduction products
  Antibiotics destroying bacteria converting digoxin to inactive reduction products (erythromycin, tetracycline)

Mechanism unknown
  Propafenone (degree of interaction not clear)

days. *Rapid digitalization* can be achieved with a combination of IV digoxin (0.5 mg IV, followed by oral digoxin 0.25 mg, one or two doses) to a total of 0.75–1.0 mg.

The usual *maintenance dose* remains 0.25 mg daily, even with a wide range of renal and hepatic function.[8] The optimal dose required varies from 0.1–0.75 mg daily[18] and renal function is the most important determinant.[8] We advise a *single evening dose* to allow a steady-state situation for blood digoxin assays in the morning; timing in relation to meals is not important.

Each patient's dose must be individually adjusted. In *atrial fibrillation*, the aim is for a resting apical rate less than 90 beats/min and a mild postexercise rise. (Added verapamil or diltiazem may be needed, see p 198).

Digitalis Indications and Contraindications

Indications.   The indications for digitalis are shrinking, particularly for the treatment of acute heart failure. The introduction of dopamine, dobutamine, and vasodilators has lessened the need for digitalis in acute heart failure with sinus rhythm,[34] while for acute management of supraventricular tachycardias, calcium-blocking agents such as verapamil (or diltiazem when available in IV form) are usually preferred when there is no myocardial failure.

Atrial fibrillation—the most solid indication for digitalis is still the combination of chronic CHF with atrial fibrillation. It is also used for atrial fibrillation from other causes and sometimes for the treatment of acute supraventricular tachycardias. In such arrhythmias, it may be used alone or in combination with verapamil, diltiazem or β-blocking drugs (it is preferred to these other drugs if there is heart failure).

In *mitral stenosis with sinus rhythm*, "prophylactic" digitalis is sometimes used to avoid the harmful effects of sudden atrial fibrillation and to slow the sinus rate to improve ventricular filling. However, (1) the acute onset of atrial fibrillation is usually accompanied by a rapid ventricular response despite prophylactic digitalis; and (2) the inhibitory effect on the sinus node is not very powerful and not as effective as β-blockade.

In *low-output heart failure* with sinus rhythm, the beneficial effects of chronic digitalis therapy is being disputed and the old dictum "once on digitalis, always on digitalis" can no longer be upheld.[11] It is now acceptable to start treatment of chronic CHF with a diuretic[34] adding digitalis when needed. Yet at least some of the inotropic effect of digitalis is maintained chronically. If digitalis is discontinued in patients with symptomatic heart failure, an exacerbation of CHF may follow,[3,25] unless the patients are optimally managed by diuretics and/or vasodilators. Since *some but not all patients with chronic CHF benefit from long-term digitalis therapy*, the challenge for future investigators is to identify the patients who will benefit from long-term digitalization. **Long-term digitalis is still frequently given without good reason,** as shown by a recent survey in Boston.[56]

Acute left ventricular (LV) failure is generally treated by more potent inotropic drugs such as dopamine, dobutamine, amrinone, or diuretics before digitalis is considered. In valvular heart disease with failure, digitalization is conventionally the first line of treatment, but patients with regurgitation may do better with vasodilators.

In *children*, digitalis is preferred to diuretics as first-line treatment of heart failure even in high-output states with left or right shunts.[4] Nevertheless, its efficacy is not without dispute.[53]

Contraindications.   (1) *Hypertrophic obstructive cardiomyopathy* (hypertrophic subaortic stenosis, asymmetrical septal hypertrophy) is a contraindication (unless there is atrial fibrillation and severe myocardial failure), because the inotropic effect can worsen outflow obstruction. (2) The possibility of *digitalis toxicity* is a frequent contraindication, pending a full history of digitalis dosage, renal function tests and measurement of serum digoxin. (3) In some cases of *Wolff-Parkinson-White* (WPW) syndrome (Fig. 4-3, p 82), digitalization may accelerate antegrade conduction over the bypass tract to precipitate ventricular tachycardia (VT) or ventricular fibrillation (VF);[44] expert evaluation is needed before digitalis is considered in these patients. (4) Significant *AV nodal heart block*. Intermittent complete heart block or second degree AV block may be worsened by digitalis, especially if there is a history of Stokes-Adams attacks or when conduction is likely to be unstable as in acute myocardial infarction (AMI) or acute myocarditis. (5) Hypertensive cardiomegaly but without impairment of systolic function (normal or high ejection fraction).

> *Relative contraindications.*   (1) If a poor response can be expected as when low-output states are caused by valvular stenosis, in chronic pericarditis, in chronic cor pulmonale, or high-output states[33] or when atrial fibrillation is caused by thyrotoxicosis; (2) all conditions increasing digitalis sensitivity to apparently therapeutic levels such as hypokalemia, chronic pulmonary disease, myxedema, acute hypoxemia; (3) AMI (see p 6); (4) renal failure—a lower dose, monitoring of plasma potassium, and a watch for digitalis toxicity are needed; (5) sinus bradycardia or sick sinus syndrome—occasional patients will show a marked fall in sinus rate or sinus pauses.[41] A prolonged PR-interval is usually not a contraindication;[5] (6) combination with other drugs causing sinus bradycardia such as β-blockade, diltiazem, amiodarone, reserpine, methyldopa, and clonidine; (7) other drugs inhibiting AV conduction (verapamil, diltiazem, β-blockers, amiodarone); here IV digoxin may be hazardous; (8) heart failure accompanying acute glomerulonephritis because renal excretion of digoxin is impaired; (9) severe myocarditis may predispose to digitalis-induced arrhythmias and decreased digitalis effect; (10) cardioversion—ideally the digoxin dose should be reduced to avoid post-conversion ventricular arrhythmias, but there is risk of an undue increase in the ventricular response. If digitalis toxicity is suspected, elective cardioversion should be delayed. If cardioversion is required, the energy level should be minimal at first and only carefully increased.

Clinical States Altering Digitalis Activity

Digitalis in the Elderly

Dall[7] suggested that three-quarters of elderly British patients receiving digoxin did not need it; often the dose was too high, more often it was too low and compliance was poor. There is much to be said for withdrawing digitalis in the elderly unless it is obviously needed (as in atrial fibrillation with LV failure) while the patient is carefully observed for any clinical deterioration.

> The pharmacokinetics of digitalis in the elderly have been well studied.[2] Digoxin absorption is delayed but not decreased. A decreased skeletal muscle and lean body mass causes increased digoxin levels (Table 5-4). The latter are also promoted by a decreasing glomerular filtration rate (GFR), especially after the fifth and sixth decades. Creatinine clearance may be substantially reduced before a rise in serum creatinine alerts the clinician. Digoxin half-life is prolonged to a mean of 73 hours in the elderly. There is no solid evidence of any alteration in myocardial sensitivity or response to cardiac glycosides in older individuals.

Digoxin and Renal Function

The most important determinant of the daily digoxin dosage in all age groups is renal function (creatinine clearance or radionuclide methods). The clinician usually relies upon measurement of the blood urea nitrogen or serum creatinine. These parameters are influenced by factors other than glomerular filtration. For example, serum creatinine may be normal in an elderly patient with a GFR that is half normal if there is a marked decrease in muscle mass, because the amount of creatinine released daily is diminished. Even the GFR provides only a rough estimate of the renal excretion of digoxin, since it is also excreted by tubular secretion. In severe renal insufficiency, there is a decrease in the volume of distribution of digoxin,[14,22] so that it is not exact to use a nomogram to estimate the maintenance dose based on creatinine clearance.[23] One practical policy is to start with a maintenance dose of 0.125 mg/day in patients with severe renal insufficiency and rely on serum digoxin levels for dose adjustment.

> In less severe renal insufficiency, a "guestimate" of the digoxin dose can be made as follows: the creatinine clearance can be estimated from age, sex, body weight and serum creatinine if direct measurement is impractical. In elderly patients with renal impairment, the following approximations hold:[38]

Creatinine clearance	Approximate digoxin dose
10–25 mL/min	0.125 mg/day
26–49 mL/min	0.1875 mg/day
50–79 mL/min	0.25 mg/day

As an example, for a 70 kg male aged 70, the "guestimated" digoxin dose is 0.25 mg for serum creatinine up to about 1.5 mg/dL (140 μmole/L) and 0.125 mg when the creatinine exceeds about 3.0 mg/dL (275 μmole/L). These values are rough approximations, stressing the important role of renal function in determining digoxin dosage. In this situation, nothing can improve on regular monitoring of blood digoxin levels. Digitoxin, without renal elimination, is an alternative, given in maintenance doses of 0.1 mg 5 days a week.

Digitalis and Pulmonary Heart Disease

Not only is digitalis not beneficial in patients with right heart failure due to cor pulmonale, but it may be especially hazardous since such patients may exhibit a sensitivity to digitalis intoxication even in the absence of hypokalemia because of hypoxia, electrolyte disturbances, and sympathetic discharge.[37] When right ventricular failure is accompanied by LV failure and diuretics alone do not succeed, digitalis is again indicated.[11]

Digitalis and Myocardial Infarction

When *atrial fibrillation or flutter* develops with a rapid ventricular response, digitalis is the drug of choice because these arrhythmias frequently either accompany or precipitate CHF. Verapamil more quickly reduces the ventricular rate and may be used while awaiting the effect of digitalis.

When mild to moderate *CHF* that persists for several days complicates AMI, digitalis exerts a modest but detectable inotropic effect. This benefit may be achieved without decreasing myocardial perfusion or an apparent increase in infarct size.[37]

Combination therapy may, however, be used since (1) the inotropic effects of digoxin 0.5 mg IV can be magnified by vasodilator therapy with nitroprusside;[40] (2) added β-receptor stimulation may achieve more marked hemodynamic effects.[55]

Contraindications to digoxin in AMI are (1) the absence of clinical cardiac failure, because peripheral vasoconstriction caused by digoxin may depress LV function;[6] and (2) severe LV failure with acute pulmonary edema or shock, because the inotropic effect is only mild and other drugs such as dopamine or dobutamine are more effective.[32]

TABLE 5-4
FACTORS ALTERING DIGITALIS SENSITIVITY TO APPARENTLY THERAPEUTIC LEVELS

Systemic factors or disorders
  Renal failure (reduced volume of distribution and excretion)
  Low lean body mass (reduced binding to skeletal muscle)
  Chronic pulmonary disease (hypoxia, acid–base changes)
  Myxedema (prolonged half-life)
  Acute hypoxemia (sensitizes to digitalis arrhythmias)

Electrolyte disorders
  Hypokalemia (sensitizes to toxic effects)
  Hyperkalemia (protects from digitalis arrhythmias)
  Hypomagnesemia (sensitizes to toxic effects)
  Hypercalcemia (increases sensitivity to digitalis)
  Hypocalcemia (decreases sensitivity)

Cardiac disorders
  Acute myocardial infarction (may cause increased sensitivity)
  Acute rheumatic or viral carditis (danger of conduction block)
  Thyrotoxic heart disease (decreased sensitivity)

Concomitant drug therapy
  Diuretics with K⁺ loss (increased sensitivity)
  Drugs with added effects on SA or AV nodes (verapamil, diltiazem, β-blockers, clonidine, methyldopa, or amiodarone)

Postinfarct Digoxin

Several studies have suggested that postinfarct digoxin may increase mortality, presumably acting by induction of arrhythmias or by increasing the myocardial oxygen demand. In the absence of a randomized controlled trial, finality cannot be reached. It is prudent to use digoxin in postinfarct patients only when strictly required and with frequent checks of serum digoxin levels and K[+].

Chronic Ischemic Heart Disease and β-Blockade

In anginal patients with cardiomegaly, acute digitalization may avert the precipitation of cardiac failure by β-blockade,[46] but chronic digitalization might be less effective. In the large dilated hearts of chronic ischemic cardiomyopathy, the response of digitalis is variable.

Inhibition of Premature Ventricular Complexes (PVCs)

Protection by digitalis against PVCs is variable[31] and cannot be predicted by the ejection fraction.[17,78]

Ideal Serum Digoxin Levels

Can serum digoxin levels help assessment of the therapeutic effect? The usual therapeutic level ranges between 1 and 2 ng/mL ($=1.3$–2.6 nmole/L).[19,47,51] Although values above that range may indicate digitalis toxicity and values below may indicate underdigitalization, there are numerous problems in relating digoxin levels to digoxin therapy (Table 5-4). For example, digitalis-induced arrhythmias can arise in the presence of hypokalemia even when serum levels are well within the therapeutic range, whereas with a normal potassium, serum digoxin levels of 2.0 ng/mL or more are usually required (Fig. 5-2).[45,47] In supraventricular arrhythmias being treated with digoxin, a serum level of 2–4 ng/mL (achieved by a higher dose) may be needed

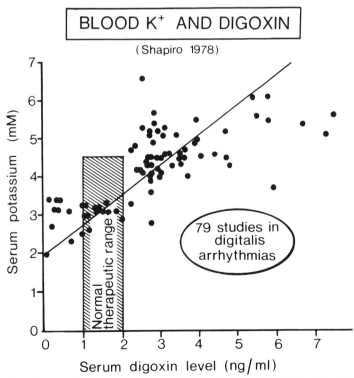

Fig. 5-2. As the serum potassium falls the heart is sensitized to the arrhythmias of digitalis toxicity. Conversely, as the serum potassium rises a higher serum digoxin level is tolerated. (Modified from Shapiro W: Correlative studies of serum digitalis levels and the arrhythmias of digitalis intoxication. Am J Cardiol 41: 852–859, 1978. With permission.)

to stimulate the vagus enough to control the ventricular rate; addition of oral verapamil or diltiazem or β-adrenergic blocking drugs seems preferable to pushing digoxin so high. Conversely, patients with acute hypoxia as in cor pulmonale may get digitalis arrhythmias at lower serum levels.

The pharmacokinetics of digoxin also influence interpretation of serum levels. The blood should not be taken less than 4 hours after an IV dose or 6–8 hours after an oral dose, or 10–12 hours after an intramuscular dose. Because of the multiplicity of factors altering the effects of any given digoxin level (Table 5-4), it is best to decide whether the level is inappropriately high or low for the particular patient. Absolute levels are not correlated tightly with effects.

Drug Interactions with Digoxin

The *quinidine-digoxin* interaction is best known. The concomitant adminis-tration of quinidine causes the blood digoxin level approximately to double, probably by reducing both renal and extrarenal clearance; such patients should be given about half the previous dose of digoxin, and the clinical course and plasma digoxin should be monitored. *Quinine*, an agent some-times used in the therapy of muscle cramps, acts likewise. The *verapamil-digoxin* interaction is equally important; similar rules apply. However, verapamil does not alter the volume of distribution of digoxin so that the loading dose of digoxin is unaltered.[76] Other calcium antagonists (exception: tiapamil, a vera-pamil congener) have less or no effect so that adjustment of the digoxin dose with diltiazem or nifedipine is seldom necessary. *Amiodarone* and propafenone (Chapter 4) also elevate serum digoxin levels. With quinidine, verapamil, amiodarone, and possibly propafenone (Chapter 4), digitalis toxicity is more likely to be precipitated. In the case of quinidine, tachyarrhythmias become more likely; in the case of amiodarone and verapamil, the ventricular arrhyth-mias of digitalis toxicity seem to be suppressed, so that bradycardia and AV block become more likely.[74] Other antiarrhythmics, including procainamide, have no interaction with digoxin (Table 5-5).

Diuretics may induce hypokalemia which (1) sensitizes to digitalis toxicity and (2) nearly shuts off the tubular secretion of digoxin when the plasma K falls to below 2–3 mEq/L. *Potassium-depleting corticosteroids* may act likewise. *Potassium-sparing diuretics*, such as amiloride, triamterene, and spironolac-tone, may all through diverse mechanisms decrease digoxin clearance by about 20–30 percent; hence the blood digoxin level needs to be rechecked.[74]

Drugs altering GI absorption of digoxin include the following. First, *cholestyramine* decreases digoxin levels, probably by binding of digoxin to the resin with impaired uptake from the GI tract; this interaction can be minimized by giving the digoxin several hours before the resin or by prescribing digoxin solution in a gelatin capsule (Lanoxicaps®; 0.2 mg = 0.25 mg of digoxin; same precautions as di-goxin). The latter preparation likewise reduces the risk of (1) kaolin-pectate-induced reduction of GI uptake of digoxin; and (2) *antibiotic-induced increase* in digoxin level (mechanism: erythromycin and tetracycline inhibit the GI flora that convert digoxin to inactive digoxin reduction products). *Cancer chemotherapeutic agents* also depress the GI uptake of digoxin, probably by damaging the intestinal mucosa. *Antacid gels* and a *high bran* diet may also impair the GI uptake of digoxin; here the remedy is to give the digoxin at a different time. Agents altering the *motility of the gut* such as propantheline (Pro-Banthine®) do not alter digoxin

TABLE 5-5

ANTIARRHYTHMIC DRUGS THAT HAVE NO PHARMACOKINETIC INTERACTION   WITH DIGOXIN

Class I agents:	procainamide, disopyramide
Class IB agents:	lidocaine, phenytoin, tocainide, mexiletine, ethmozine
Class IC agents:	flecainide, encainide
Class II agents:	β-blockade, unless renal blood flow critical
Class III agents:	sotalol (not amiodarone)
Class IV agent:	diltiazem (modest elevation may occur)

uptake,[74] contrary to the package insert. The *antimicrobial* agents, neomycin, sulfasalazine, and paraaminosalicylic acid (PAS) all delay digoxin uptake by the gut; this effect cannot be avoided by giving digoxin at a different time.

Rifampin (rifampicin) accelerates the metabolism of many drugs, including digoxin; this may cause a marked reduction in digoxin levels in patients with renal failure where nonrenal clearance becomes important. *Cimetidine* may decrease digoxin levels (controversial). *Vasodilators* (hydralazine, nitroprusside) by enhancing renal blood flow may increase renal excretion of digoxin.

Digitalis Toxicity

The typical patient with digitalis toxicity (Table 5-6) is usually elderly with advanced heart disease and atrial fibrillation, often associated with pulmonary disease and abnormal renal function. Digitalis toxicity should, however, be considered in any patient receiving digitalis who presents with a new GI, ocular, or central nervous system complaint, or in whom a new arrhythmia or AV conduction disturbance develops. Symptoms do not necessarily precede serious cardiac arrhythmias. The cellular mechanism of digitalis toxicity resides in part in (1) intracellular calcium overload that predisposes to calcium-dependent delayed afterdepolarizations which in turn may develop into ventricular automaticity; (2) excessive vagal stimulation, predisposing to AV block; (3) an added "direct" depressive effect of digitalis on nodal tissue, and (4) sympathetic stimulation.

Typical Digitalis Arrhythmias

A slow pulse, although a traditional indicator of digitalis toxicity, is only a useful alerting signal.[52] Digitalis toxicity may result in second or third degree AV block and increases the automaticity of junctional and His-Purkinje tissue. **Thus accelerated junctional or ventricular arrhythmias may result and when combined with AV nodal block are highly suggestive of digitalis toxicity.** The most common cardiac arrhythmias[9] are PVCs including bigeminy (total, 45 percent), AV junctional escape beats or tachycardia (40 percent), second or third degree heart block (25 percent), atrial tachycardia with block (15 percent), VT (10 percent), and SA node or sinus arrest (5 percent; all figures rounded off).

The *diagnosis* of digitalis toxicity is confirmed if the arrhythmias resolve when the drug is discontinued; and/or if the digoxin blood level is inappropriately high for the patient in the presence of suspicious clinical features. Provided that hypokalemia is excluded (Fig. 5-2), an inappropriately low plasma digoxin level strongly suggests that an arrhythmia or conduction disturbance is not due to digitalis toxicity.

Treatment of Digitalis Toxicity

Much depends on the clinical severity. With only suggestive symptoms, withdrawal of digoxin is sufficient while awaiting confirmation by elevated plasma levels. With dangerous arrhythmias and a low plasma potassium, potassium chloride may be infused intravenously as 30–40 mEq in 20–50 ml of saline at 0.5–1 mEq/min into a large vein through a plastic catheter (infiltration of potassium solution can cause tissue necrosis and infusion into small veins causes local irritation and pain). *Oral potassium* (4–6 g of potassium chloride, 50–80 mEq) may be given orally in divided doses when arrhythmias are not urgent (e.g. PVCs). Potassium is contraindicated if AV conduction block or hyperkalemia are present, because potassium further increases AV block.[10]

TABLE 5-6

FEATURES OF DIGITALIS TOXICITY

System	Symptoms and Signs
Gastrointestinal	Anorexia, nausea, vomiting, diarrhea
Neurologic	Malaise, fatigue, confusion, facial pain, insomnia, depression, vertigo, colored vision (green or yellow halos around lights)
Cardiologic	Palpitations, arrhythmias, syncope
Blood	High digoxin level especially with low potassium; check magnesium, urea, creatinine

Lidocaine is usually chosen for ventricular ectopy since it does not impair the AV conduction frequently present. Phenytoin, in addition, reverses the high degree AV block, possibly acting by a central mechanism.[13] Class IA agents, such as quinidine, disopyramide, and procainamide, all depress automaticity and may enhance AV block. Quinidine is seldom given intravenously and disopyramide can have a marked negative inotropic effect.

If the patient is already receiving any drugs elevating the blood digoxin, these should be stopped (verapamil, quinidine) as also should β-blockade. On the other hand, because of the long half-life, there is little point in stopping amiodarone.

Temporary transvenous ventricular pacing may be required for marked sinus bradycardia or advanced heart block not responsive to atropine.

Digoxin-specific antibodies are effective therapy for life-threatening digitalis intoxication; the reversal of toxicity is rapid and not accompanied by adverse effects except that anaphylactic shock is theoretically possible. This therapy is usually reserved for the management of toxicity unresponsive to conventional measures, but specialized centers are using it more and more.[83]

Digitoxin

The pharmacokinetics include virtually complete absorption, so that the oral and IV digitalizing doses are the same. Because it is chiefly metabolized or excreted in the gut, **blood levels are not much altered by poor renal function.** However, hypokalemia predisposes to toxicity as for digoxin. The great disadvantage is the long half-life (6–7 days compared with 36 hours for digoxin) that complicates the treatment of toxicity.

Digitalization is usually started with a loading dose since otherwise it would take over a month to achieve a steady-state plasma level or serum level. The loading dose ranges from 0.8–1.2 mg in 24 hours given in four divided doses 6 hours apart. The maintenance dose is usually 0.1–0.15 mg of digitoxin daily. As with digoxin, the dose may need individual adjustment (usual range 0.05–0.20 mg, the smaller dose is preferred in the elderly). Therapeutic levels are 15–25 ng/mL and toxic levels over 35 ng/mL.

The management of digitalis toxicity changes in patients given digitoxin because of (1) the much longer half-life than that of digoxin, (2) the enterohepatic circulation with 25 percent recycled so that activated charcoal can be given to promote excretion of digitoxin by the gut.[39]

Digitalis—Summary

These compounds, by their unique combination of a positive inotropic effect and bradycardia with inhibition of AV nodal conduction, remain the oral inotropic agents of choice. A thorough understanding of their pharmacokinetics, numerous interactions with other drugs, and correct use in various clinical situations is mandatory. Chronic digitalis therapy should only be undertaken for clearly defined indications, in the absence of which the benefit will be limited yet with the risk of digitalis toxicity.

SYMPATHOMIMETIC INOTROPES AND VASODILATORS

Adrenergic Receptors and Inotropic Effects

Norepinephrine (NE) is the endogenous catecholamine that is synthesized and stored in granules in adrenergic nerve endings in the myocardium. When sympathetic nerves to the heart are activated, NE is released from its stores and stimulates specific sites on the myocardial cell surface, termed β_1-*adrenergic receptors* (Fig. 1-1). Stimulation of these β_1-receptors increases the rate of discharge of the sinoatrial node, thereby augmenting heart rate, enhances AV conduction, and increases the force and speed of contraction of atrial and ventricular myocardium. Most of the released NE is subsequently taken up by the same adrenergic nerve endings and stored for renewed release. Smaller amounts are metabolized. NE also has effects that are exerted largely on the peripheral arterioles, termed α-receptors, and these cause vasoconstriction, raise the blood pressure and cause reflex bradycardia.

Another type of β-sympathomimetic effect, termed β_2, causes dilation of the smooth muscles of the bronchi, blood vessels, and uterus. A subpopulation of β_2-*receptors* is also found in the heart with effects similar to those of the β_1-receptors; in severe CHF β_2-receptors dominate.[55a] Sympathomimetic agents could thus benefit the failing heart: β_1-stimulation by an inotropic effect, β_2-stimulation by afterload reduction (peripheral arterial vasodilation), and α-stimulation by restoring pressure in hypotensive states. Experimental work unfortunately shows that catecholamine stimulation as exemplified by NE infusion should be used with caution in the low output state of AMI, because β_1-effects may precipitate arrhythmias and tachycardia, which can potentially increase ischemia, while excessive α-effects increase the afterload as the blood pressure rises beyond what is required for adequate perfusion. While β_2-stimulation achieves beneficial vasodilation and also mediates some inotropic effect, β-stimulation also causes hypokalemia with enhanced risk of arrhythmias. A new problem is that prolonged or vigorous β-stimulation leads to receptor downgrading with a diminished inotropic response. Consequently, there is an ongoing search for catecholamine-like agents, including phosphodiesterase inhibitors, that lack the undesirable effects.

α-Adrenergic stimulation may also induce a limited calcium-mediated inotropic effect, to contribute to the total effect of adrenergic stimulation.

Inotropic Effect versus Vasodilation

An intracellular elevation of cyclic AMP, the second messenger of β-adrenergic stimulation, causes the inotropic effect, the chronotropic effect, and peripheral vasodilation. The therapeutic effects that are generally needed are the inotropic and vasodilatory effects. Specific β_1-stimulation will not have a pure inotropic effect without direct vasodilation. β_2-Stimulators and phosphodiesterase inhibitors will generally increase cyclic AMP in the heart and in peripheral vessels to cause both vasodilation and a positive inotropic effect. Dopamine, by releasing NE, has mixed β-receptor stimulatory effects and in addition causes specific vasodilation by enhancing the activity of dopaminergic receptors. **Compounds such as dopamine and the phosphodiesterase inhibitors are mixed inotropic-vasodilators ("inodilators").** The properties of some of these agents are highlighted in Tables 5-7 and 5-8.

β_1-SELECTIVE STIMULATION

Dobutamine

Dobutamine (Dobutrex®), a synthetic analog of dopamine, is a β-adrenergic stimulating agent. It acts directly on β_1-adrenergic receptors so as to cause a stronger inotropic than chronotropic effect.[20,48] Dobutamine does not directly release NE as does dopamine, nor does it affect the dopamine receptors. Effects on β_2-receptors are less than those of isoproterenol and effects on α-receptors are less than those of NE. **Dobutamine can be used cautiously as an inotropic agent in heart failure to increase cardiac output while reducing ventricular filling pressures.** It may also be used in selected cases of evolving myocardial infarction with heart failure and low output, without great risk of increasing infarct size or inducing arrhythmias.[15] Dobutamine directly stimulates the β_1-receptor and does not require the presence of NE stores that may be depleted in chronic heart failure. Dobutamine also causes modest peripheral vasodilation. The mechanism is unlikely to be via direct stimulation of the vascular β-receptors (β_2) but rather by relief of sympathetic discharge following improvement in heart failure.

Pharmacokinetics. An infusion is rapidly cleared (half-life 2.4 minutes).
Dose. The standard IV dose is 2.5–10 μg/kg/min, occasionally up to 40 μg/kg/min.[16] The drug can be infused for up to 72 hours with monitoring. There is no oral preparation.
Indications. Refractory heart failure; severe acute forward failure (AMI, after cardiac surgery); cardiogenic shock; excess β-blockade.
Side-effects. In severe CHF, dobutamine causes tachycardia,[16] but there is a dose-related increase in cardiac output.[20] Although there may be less tachycardia

TABLE 5-7

PROPOSED CLASSIFICATION OF INODILATORS

Agent	Receptor stimulation involved in inodilation	Mechanism
Possible receptors involved	DA_1, DA_2, β_1, β_2	DA_1 = vasodilatory DA_2 = inhibition of presynaptic NE release β_1 = inotropic β_2 = vasodilator
β-agonists isoprenaline (isoproterenol)	$\beta_1 + \beta_2$	Increase of myocardial and vascular cyclic AMP (disadvantage: tachycardias and arrhythmias; receptor downgrading).
epinephrine	$\beta_1 > \beta_2$	Myocardial > vascular cyclic AMP. May show disadvantages of isoproterenol.
pirbuterol	$\beta_2 > \beta_1$	Vascular > myocardial cyclic AMP.
albuterol (salbutamol)	$\beta_2 > \beta_1$	Vascular > myocardial cyclic AMP.
PDE inhibitors amrinone milrinone enoximone	No receptors involved	Inhibition of PDE leads to accumulation of cyclic AMP in myocardium and vasculature.
Dopaminergic agents levodopa	$DA_1 + DA_2 + \beta_1$	Vascular cyclic AMP increased, decreased neuronal release of norepinephrine, myocardial cyclic AMP increase.
ibopamine	$DA_1 + DA_2 + \beta_1$	Vascular cyclic AMP increased, decreased neuronal release of norepinephrine, myocardial cyclic AMP increase.
propyldopamine	$DA_1 + DA_2 + \beta_1$	Vascular cyclic AMP increased, decreased neuronal release of norepinephrine, myocardial cyclic AMP increase.
bromocriptine	$DA_1 + DA_2$	Vasodilator without direct inotropic effect.

Adapted from Opie LH: Inodilators. Lancet i:1336, 1986. With permission.
PDE = phosphodiesterase
DA_1 = dopaminergic postsynaptic vasodilatory
DA_2 = dopaminergic presynaptic, inhibition of NE release
β_1 = β-adrenergic type 1 receptors
β_2 = β-adrenergic type 2 receptors

and arrhythmias than with dopamine or isoproterenol, all inotropic agents have risk of enhanced arrhythmias.

Precautions.   Dilute in sterile water or dextrose or saline, not in alkaline solutions. Use within 24 hours. Hemodynamic monitoring of patient required. Check blood potassium.

Clinical use.   The ideal candidate for dobutamine therapy is the patient who has severely depressed LV function with a low cardiac index and elevated LV filling pressure, but in whom extreme hypotension is not present (mean arterial BP not < 70 mmHg).[12,26,30,50] The potential disadvantages of dobutamine are (1) that in severe CHF the β-receptors may be downgraded so that dobutamine may not be as effective as anticipated, (2) prolonged therapy with dobutamine itself could cause receptor downgrading, and (3) dobutamine is not specifically vasodilatory, although relief of CHF may improve peripheral blood flow and enhance renal function indirectly.

An interesting concept for chronic CHF is that infusion of dobutamine for only 4 hr/week may produce a "conditioning effect" with enhanced exercise tolerance and increased functional classification.[27] Possibly intermittent inotropic therapy may improve β-receptor activity as CHF improves, while at the same time avoiding drug-induced receptor downgrading. Another new strategy is a 3–day infusion of dobutamine.[81]

TABLE 5-8

OVERALL PROPERTIES OF β-STIMULANTS AND INOTROPIC VASODILATORS ("INODILATORS")

	β_1-Stimulation	Mixed β_1-β_2 effects	Mixed β_1-agonist-antagonists	PDE Inhibitors	Dopaminergic
Drug examples	Dobutamine (also some β_2)	Epinephrine	Xamoterol [†]	Amrinone Milrinone	Dopamine
Inotropic effect	++	++	Variable, 0/++	+	++
Arteriolar vasodilation	+	+	0	++	++
Chronotropic effect	0/+	++	0/+	++	0/+
Direct diuretic effect	0	0	0	0	++
Arrhythmia risk	+/++	+++	0	+/++	0; + (high dose)
Use in CHF	++	0	+	++	++

† Not in the USA

CHF = congestive heart failure; PDE = phosphodiesterase

103

MIXED β_1-β_2-RECEPTOR STIMULATION

Epinephrine

Epinephrine (Adrenaline®) gives mixed β-stimulation with some added α-mediated effects. It is used chiefly when combined inotropic/chronotropic stimulation is urgently desired as in cardiac arrest when the added α-stimulatory effect helps to maintain the blood pressure despite the peripheral vasodilation achieved by β_2-receptor stimulation.

MIXED AGONIST–ANTAGONIST EFFECT (β-Blockers with High ISA)

β-Blockers that also have a high degree of β-receptor stimulation (high intrinsic sympathomimetic activity [ISA], Fig. 1-6) have significant β-mediated inotropic effect. Oral prenalterol has now been withdrawn because of carcinogenicity in animals. *Xamoterol* (Corwin, in Europe) is as good as dobutamine in LV failure of acute myocardial experimental ischemia[82] and under trial in idiopathic cardiomyopathy. These agents have complex and sometimes unpredictable effects dependent on the level of sympathetic tone in CHF. They are orally active and do not increase the heart rate (β-blocking effect). Possible receptor downgrading during prolonged use requires caution.[58]

MIXED INOTROPIC-VASODILATOR AGENTS ("INODILATORS")

Dopamine

Dopamine (Intropin®) is a catecholamine-like agent used for therapy of severe heart failure and cardiogenic shock. Physiologically it is both the precursor of NE and releases NE from the stores in the nerve-endings in the heart (Fig. 5-3). However, in the periphery this effect is overridden by the activity of the **prejunctional dopaminergic DA$_2$-receptors, inhibiting NE release and thereby helping to vasodilate.**[63] Theoretically, dopamine has the valuable

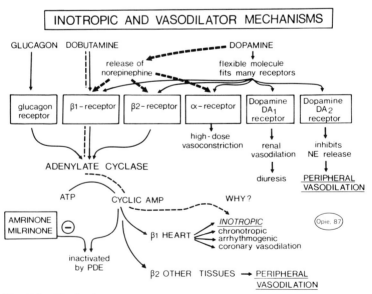

Fig. 5-3. The basic mechanisms for an inotropic or vasodilator effect are (1) stimulation of adenylate cyclase to elevate cyclic AMP that has a positive inotropic and vasodilatory effect; (2) modulation of release of norepinephrine (NE = noradrenaline) by dopamine receptor stimulation; and (3) inhibition of phosphodiesterase (PDE) that increases myocardial and vascular cyclic AMP.

property in severe CHF or shock of specifically increasing blood flow to the renal,[75] mesenteric, coronary, and cerebral beds by activating the specific postjunctional dopamine DA_1-receptors. However, at high doses dopamine causes α-receptor stimulation with peripheral vasoconstriction; the peripheral resistance increases and renal blood flow falls.[16] The dose should therefore be kept as low as possible to achieve the desired ends; a combination of dopamine and vasodilator therapy or dopamine and dobutamine would be better than increasing the dose of dopamine.[36]

Pharmacology.   The prejunctional DA_2-receptors inhibit NE release and thereby cause vasodilation. The prejunctional DA_1-receptors cause direct vasodilation in renal, mesenteric, coronary, and cerebral vascular beds.[63] Dopamine, a "flexible molecule," also fits into many receptors to cause direct β_1 and β_2-receptor stimulation as well as α-stimulation.

Pharmacokinetics.   Dopamine is inactive orally. IV dopamine is metabolized within minutes by dopamine β-hydroxylase and monoamine oxidase.

Dose and indications.   In *refractory cardiac failure*, dopamine can only be given intravenously, which restricts its use to short-term treatment.[16] The dose starts at 0.5–1 μg/kg/min and is raised until an acceptable urinary flow, blood pressure or heart rate is achieved; vasoconstriction begins at about 10 μg/kg/min and calls for an α-blocking agent or sodium nitroprusside. In a few patients vasoconstriction can begin at doses as low as 5 μg/kg/min. In *cardiogenic shock* or *AMI*, 5 μg/kg/min of dopamine is enough to give a maximum increase in stroke volume, while renal flow reaches a peak at 7.5 μg/kg/min, and arrhythmias may appear at 10 μg/kg/min.[28] In *septic shock*, dopamine has an inotropic effect and increases urine volume.[29] Dopamine is widely used for *myocardial failure* after cardiac surgery.[16] It is sometimes given in *acute renal failure* for diuresis.

Precautions.   Dopamine must not be diluted in alkaline solutions. Blood pressure, electrocardiogram, and urine flow must be monitored constantly with intermittent measurements of cardiac output and pulmonary wedge pressure if possible. For oliguria, first correct hypovolemia; add furosemide.

Side-effects and interactions.   Dopamine is contraindicated in ventricular arrhythmias, in pheochromocytoma, and during the use of cyclopropane or halogenated hydrocarbon anesthetics. Extravasation can cause sloughing, prevented by infusing the drug into a large vein through a plastic catheter, and treated by local infiltration with phentolamine. If the patient has recently taken a monoamine-oxidase inhibitor, the rate of dopamine metabolism by the tissue will fall and the dose should be cut to one-tenth of the usual.

Clinical use.   Comparison of dopamine and dobutamine after cardiac surgery suggests that dobutamine may be best for the patient with depressed cardiac output with only mild to moderate hypotension, particularly when the patient has sinus tachycardia or ventricular arrhythmias. Dopamine, on the other hand, is preferred in the patient who requires both a pressor effect and increase in cardiac output, and who does not have marked tachycardia or ventricular irritability.[49,65] **Dopamine is especially beneficial when renal blood flow is impaired in severe CHF.**[75] Infusion of equal concentrations of dopamine and dobutamine may afford more advantages than either drug singly in cardiogenic shock.[42] Dopamine can further increase the cardiac output in patients treated by nitroprusside.[36]

Levodopa

An oral dopamine-like agent would be useful and levodopa has been tried after IV dopamine therapy.[16] It can be increased slowly from 250 mg–2000 mg 4× daily over 7 days with 50 mg pyridoxine (required to decarboxylate levodopa). However, the ideal oral dopamine-like agent would not cross the blood-brain barrier, thereby avoiding the centrally induced nausea and vomiting that may occur with levodopa.

New Dopaminergic Agents

Bromocriptine, fenoldopam, and *dopexamine* are vasodilators without direct inotropic effect. Agents such as ibopamine stimulate both types of dopamine receptors and are "inodilators" (Table 5-7). *Ibopamine*[60] is orally active, already available in Europe (Inopamil®, Scandine®), and under investigation elsewhere. Chemically, it is a butyric acid ester of methyldopamine (the latter is also called epinine). Once absorbed, the ester is hydrolyzed by nonspecific esterases in the bloodstream to release epinine, which has effects very similar to those of IV dopamine. There is a desirable hemodynamic profile with a fall in the peripheral vascular resistance, a modest direct inotropic effect, and almost no increase in the heart rate. The added diuretic effect is also a potential benefit. The dose is 50–100 mg orally 2–3× daily.

Long-term studies of these new dopaminergic agents are required to show (1) a sustained benefit; (2) the absence of drug tolerance; and (3) the absence of serious side-effects such as arrhythmias. Some early evidence, suggests (1) a possible antiarrhythmic effect by reduced release of NE, and (2) attenuation of the hemodynamic benefit during chronic therapy.[78a]

PHOSPHODIESTERASE INHIBITORS

These agents, epitomized by amrinone and milrinone, were initially regarded as pure inotropes. Now their "inodilator" properties are increasingly recognized. The added dilator component may explain relative conservation of the myocardial oxygen consumption.[65a]

Amrinone

Amrinone (Inocor Lactate®) is a phosphodiesterase inhibitor with both inotropic and vasodilating properties. The IV preparation has recently been approved by the Food and Drug Administration (FDA) for patients with severe CHF, not adequately responsive to digitalis, diuretics and/or vasodilators. Although orally active, a recent multicenter investigation[61] showed no improvement in cardiac function beyond that provided by standard treatment (see acute versus chronic effects of sympathomimetics and vasodilators).

Pharmacology and pharmacokinetics.   By inhibition of phosphodiesterase III, a combined inotropic and vasodilator effect can be obtained. In patients with severe CHF, the vasodilator effect dominates with a variable direct positive inotropic contribution.[62,66,67a,84] IV amrinone is rapidly distributed in the circulation with a half-life of 5 minutes and elimination half-life of 4 hours (prolonged in CHF). About 20–40 percent is plasma bound and the therapeutic plasma level about 3 μg/mL. Most is excreted unchanged in the urine, some is metabolized and some excreted in the feces.

Dose.   Intravenously, therapy is initiated with 0.75 mg/kg bolus over 2–3 minutes followed by an infusion of 5–10 μg/kg/min. An added bolus dose may be given 30 minutes later. Higher infusion doses have also been used (10–20 μg/kg/min).[66] Orally (not approved in the USA) amrinone may be given as 100 mg 8–hourly.

Precautions.   Amrinone ampoules should be protected from the light and amrinone should not be mixed with glucose (dextrose) for infusion. Predrug and frequently repeated platelet counts are required (decrease drug or discontinue if platelets fall below 150,000/mm³). Monitor fluid balance and blood potassium (risk of added hypokalemia). Monitor liver and renal function.

Indications.   Severe CHF resistant to conventional therapy; acute LV failure; AMI with cardiogenic shock when dopamine or dobutamine are ineffective (but see contraindications).

Contraindications.   AMI (risk of arrhythmias); aortic or pulmonic stenosis (as for all vasodilators); hypertrophic cardiomyopathy (may aggravate obstruction).

Serious side-effects.   Serious side-effects include: thrombocytopenia, ventricular arrhythmias, hepatotoxicity (rare with IV use), hypotension, and possibly hypersensitivity reactions. Other side-effects include nausea and vomiting that may sometimes be severe. However, during acute use adverse effects may be slight.[72]

Drug interactions.   Vasodilation may exaggerate negative inotropic effects of other drugs such as disopyramide.

Combination therapy.   Amrinone has been combined with digitalis (check blood levels for arrhythmias), diuretics (monitor blood K⁺) and vasodilators such as captopril, hydralazine, and nitrates (watch for additive hypotension). The combined inotropic-vasodilator effects of amrinone are additive with the effects of dobutamine (different mechanisms of stimulating formation of cyclic AMP), dopamine (different mechanisms of vasodilation), and hydralazine.[72]

Amrinone—Summary

Although amrinone in the oral form is no longer used, the IV preparation with its major "inodilator" and vasodilator effects should be especially useful in patients with β-receptor downgrading, such as those in severe CHF or prior prolonged therapy with dobutamine or other β_1-stimulants. Although in practice, amrinone is usually confined to acutely ill patients requiring IV therapy, not responding to more conventional inotropes such as dobutamine and dopamine, the full potential of this drug as a "first-line" inodilator requires elucidation especially in strict comparison with other inotropes and inodilators. Despite the significant reservations expressed,[58] amrinone is likely to find a place in the management of the short-term therapy of heart failure.

Milrinone

Milrinone is $20\times$ more potent than amrinone with a similar mechanism of action, also with a prominent vasodilatory component[57,71] and seemingly better tolerated. When given acutely, its inotropic and vasodilatory effect is combined with an increase in heart rate.[54] Milrinone gives added benefit to patients already receiving captopril.[70] When given chronically, only some patients benefit[79] and there is risk of arrhythmias.[67] A major limitation in the assessment of the possible effects of chronic milrinone is the downhill course of heart failure that limits survival despite hemodynamic benefits. This problem explains why chronic oral milrinone therapy (25–30 mg daily initial dose) given over 2½ years improved symptoms in about half without altering the high baseline mortality of 63 percent after about 1 year.[53a] Yet only 11 percent of patients had drug-related side-effects.

ACUTE VERSUS CHRONIC EFFECTS OF SYMPATHOMIMETICS AND VASODILATORS

In *acute LV failure*, these agents may achieve dramatic short-term benefits to remedy the added deterioration that usually accompanies and promotes the condition. Together with loop diuretics and nitrates, the positive inotropes or inodilators frequently save the patient from "drowning in his own secretions." In contrast, in *chronic severe heart failure*, the major limitation is the underlying state of the myocardium, which is usually damaged beyond repair so that all therapy has inherent limitations.[69] Therapy is now aimed at improving the peripheral circulation[73] so that it is vasodilating rather than inotropic properties that become more important. In a third and intermediate situation, *chronic mild to moderate CHF*, the myocardium is still theoretically capable of at least some response to inotropic stimulation, and may also be better able to withstand possible side-effects of inotropic agents such as arrhythmias and aggravation of ischemia. It is in this category that there is most potential for new oral inotropic agents.

SUMMARY

In acute and chronic heart failure, the aims of therapy differ. In acute heart failure, reduction of pulmonary capillary pressure and right atrial filling pressure is sought along with an elevation of cardiac output if the latter is also reduced. These aims can be achieved by a variety of inotropes including dopamine, dobutamine, amrinone, and their newer derivatives. Some of these, such as dopamine and amrinone, have a prominent vasodilator component to their action ("inodilators"). Such inotropic-dilator therapy should be combined with diuretics and sometimes with digitalis.

In chronic heart failure, the aim of therapy is to translate the hemodynamic benefits of inotropic-vasodilator therapy into improved functional capacity, without shortening the duration of life or impairing its quality. Digoxin, a weak inotropic drug, only partially fulfils these criteria. Digoxin does, however, slow the heart rate and decreases the size of the failing heart, thus lessening myocardial oxygen demands. Clearly, the use of digoxin requires thorough knowledge of the multiple factors governing its efficacy and toxicity including numerous drug interactions. Today, digoxin is no longer the first line of therapy for acute severe heart failure, but still usually prescribed for chronic LV failure especially after full therapy by diuretics.

In mild to moderate heart failure, the search for an orally active and effective agent with prolonged inotropic and vasodilatory properties is still under way; two promising developments are the new dopamine-like agents and milrinone. The role of the new the positively inotropic "mixed" β-blocker-stimulators is under investigation. In severe heart failure, the peripheral component progressively dominates, so that vasodilator therapy becomes more logical, especially because the primary myocardial process limits any response to inotropic therapy.

REFERENCES

References from Previous Editions

For details see previous edition of Opie et al: Drugs for the Heart, American Edition. Orlando, FL, Grune & Stratton, 1984, pp 99–128.

1. Akera T, Brody TM: Pharmacol Rev 29:187–218, 1978
2. Algeo S, Fenster PE, Marcus FI: Geriatrics 38:93–101, 1983
3. Arnold SB, Byrd RC, Meister W, et al: New Engl J Med 303:1443–1448, 1980
4. Berman WR Jr, Yebak SM, Dillon T, et al: New Engl J Med 308:363–366, 1983
5. Blumgart HL, Altschule MD: Am J Med Sci 198:455–463, 1939
6. Creager MA, Halperin JL, Klein MD, et al: Clin Pharmacol Ther 32:736–743, 1982
7. Dall JLC: Br Med J 2:705–706, 1970
8. Dobbs SM, Mawer GE, Rodgers EM, et al: Br J Clin Pharmacol 3:231–237, 1976
9. Ewy GA, Marcus FI, Fillmore SJ, et al: In Melmon KL (ed): Cardiovascular Drug Therapy. Philadelphia, Davis Co, 1974, pp 153–174
10. Fisch C, Martz BL, Priebe FH: J Clin Invest 39:1885–1893, 1960
11. Fleg JL, Gottlieb SH, Lakatta EG: Am J Med 73:244–250, 1982
12. Francis GS, Sharma B, Hodges M: Am Heart J 103:995–1000, 1982
13. Garan H, Ruskin JN, Powell WJ Jr: Am J Physiol 241:H67–H72, 1981
14. Gault MH, Churchill DN, Kalras J: Br J Clin Pharmacol 9:593–597, 1980
15. Gillespie TA, Ambos HT, Sobel BE, et al: Am J Cardiol 39:588–594, 1977
16. Goldberg LI, Hsieh Y-Y, Resnekov L: Prog Cardiovasc Dis 19:327–340, 1977
17. Gradman AH, Cunningham M, Harbison M, et al: Am J Cardiol 51:765–769, 1983
18. Hoechsen RJ, Cuddy TE: Am J Cardiol 35:469–472, 1975
19. Jelliffe RW, Brooker G: Am J Med 57:63–68, 1974
20. Jewitt DE, Birkhead J, Mitchell A, et al: Lancet ii:363–367, 1974
21. Johnston GD: Drugs 20:494–499, 1980
22. Jusko WG, Weintraub M: Clin Pharmacol Ther 18:449–454, 1974
23. Keller F, Molzahn M, Ingerowski R: Eur J Clin Pharmacol 18:433–441, 1980
24. Kim YI, Noble RJ, Zipes DP: Am J Cardiol 36:459–467, 1975
25. Lee DC, Johnson RA, Bingham JB, et al: New Engl J Med 306:699–705, 1982
26. Leier CV, Heban PT, Huss P, et al: Circulation 58:466–475, 1978
27. Leier CV, Huss P, Lewis RP, et al: Circulation 65:1382–1387, 1982
28. Levine PA, McGillavray M, Klein MD: Circulation 51/52 (abs):208, 1975
29. Loeb HS, Winslow EBJ, Rahimtoola SH, et al: Circulation 44:163–173, 1971
30. Loeb HS, Bredakis J, Gunnar RM: Circulation 55:375–381, 1977
31. Lown B, Grayboys TB, Podrid PJ, et al: New Engl J Med 296:301–306, 1977
32. Marcus FI: Circulation 62 (editorial):17–19, 1980
33. Mathur PM, Powles P, Pugsley SO, et al: Ann Intern Med 95:283–288, 1981
34. McHaffie D, Purcell H, Mitchell-Heggs P, et al: Q J Med 47:401–419, 1978
35. McMichael J, Sharpey-Schafer EP: Q J Med 53:123–135, 1944
36. Miller RR, Awan NA, Joye JA, et al: Circulation 55:881–884, 1977
37. Morrison J, Caromilas J, Robins M, et al: Circulation 62:8–16, 1980
38. Opie LH: Lancet i:912–918, 1980
39. Pond S, Jacobs M, Marks J, et al: Lancet ii:1177–1178, 1981
40. Raabe DS Jr: Am J Cardiol 43:990–994, 1979
41. Reiffel JH, Bigger JT Jr, Cramer M: Am J Cardiol 43:983–994, 1979
42. Richard C, Ricome JL, Rimailho A, et al: Circulation 67:620–626, 1983
43. Schaal SF, Sugimoto T, Wallace AG, et al: Cardiovasc Res 2:356–359, 1968

44.   Sellers TD Jr, Bayshore TM, Gallagher JJ: Circulation 56:260–267, 1977
45.   Shapiro W: Am J Cardiol 41:852–859, 1978
46.   Sharma B, Majid PA, Meeran MK, et al: Br Heart J 34:631–637, 1972
47.   Smith TW, Haber E: New Engl J Med 289:945–952, 1010–1015, 1063–1072, 1125–1129, 1973
48.   Sonnenblick EH, Frishman WH, LeJemtel TH: New Engl J Med 300:17–22, 1979
49.   Steen PA, Tinker JH, Pluth JR, et al: Circulation 57:378–384, 1978
50.   Stoner JD, Bolen JL, Harrison DC: Br Heart J 39:536–539, 1977
51.   Sumner DJ, Russell AJ, Whiting B: Br J Clin Pharmacol 3:221–229, 1976
52.   Williams P, Aronson J, Sleight P: Lancet ii:1340–1342, 1978

New References

53.   Alpert BS, Barfield JA, Taylor WJ: Reappraisal of digitalis in infants with left-to-right shunts and heart failure. J Pediatr 106:66–68, 1985
53a. Baim DS, Colucci WS, Monrad ES, et al: Survival of patients with severe congestive heart failure treated with oral milrinone. J Am Coll Cardiol 7:661–670, 1986
54.   Benotti JR, Lesko LJ, McCue JE, et al: Pharmacokinetics and pharmacodynamics of milrinone in chronic congestive heart failure. Am J Cardiol 56:685–689, 1985
55.   Bostrom PA, Andersson J, Johansson BW, et al: Haemodynamic effects of pre-nalterol and cardiac glycosides in patients with recent myocardial infarction. Eur J Clin Invest 14:175–180, 1984
55a. Bristow MR, Ginsburg R, Umans V, et al: B_1- and B_2-adrenergic receptor subpopulations in nonfailing and failing human ventricular myocardium. Circ Res. In press, 1986
56.   Carlson KJ, DCS Lee, Goroll AH, et al: An analysis of physicians' reasons for prescribing long-term digitalis therapy in outpatients. J Chronic Dis 38:733–739, 1985
57.   Cody RJ, Muller FB, Kubo SH, et al: Identification f the direct vasodilator effect of milrinone with an isolated limb preparation in patients with chronic congestive heart failure. Circulation 73:124–129, 1986
58.   Colucci WS, Wright RF, Braunwald E: New positive inotropic agents in the treatment of congestive heart failure. New Engl J Med 314:290–299, 349–358, 1986
59.   Dawson JR, Thompson DS, Signy M, et al: Acute haemodynamic and metabolic effects of dopexamine, a new dopaminergic receptor agonist, in patients with chronic heart failure. Br Heart J 54:313–320, 1985
60.   Dei Cas L, Bolognesi R, Cucchini F, et al: Hemodynamic effects of ibopamine in patients with idiopathic congestive cardiomyopathy. J Cardiovasc Pharmacol 5:249–253, 1983
61.   Dibianco R, Shabetai R, Silverman BD: Oral amrinone for the treatment of chronic congestive heart failure: Results of a multicenter randomized double-blind and placebo-controlled withdrawal study. J Am Coll Cardiol 4:855–866, 1984
62.   Feldman M, Gwathmey J, Copelas L, et al: Decreased inotropic effect of phosphodiesterase inhibitors in myocardium from patients with end-stage heart failure. Circulation 72:(abs, suppl III):III-404, 1985
63.   Goldberg LI, Rajfer SI: Dopamine receptors: Applications in clinical cardiology. Circulation 72:245–248, 1985
64.   Gomes JAC, Kang PS, El-Sherif N: Effects of digitalis on the human sick sinus node after pharmacologic autonomic blockade. Am J Cardiol 48:783–788, 1981
65.   Gray R, Shah PK, Singh B, et al: Low cardiac output states after open heart surgery. Chest 80:16–22, 1981
65a. Grose R, Strain J, Greenberg M, et al: Systemic and coronary effects of intravenous milrinone and dobutamine in congestive heart failure. J Am Coll Cardiol 7:1107–113, 1986
66.   Hermiller JB, Leithe ME, Magorien RD, et al: Amrinone in severe congestive heart failure: Another look at an intriguing new cardioactive drug. J Pharmacol Exp Ther 228:319–326, 1984
67.   Holmes JR, Kubo SH, Cody RJ, et al: Milrinone in congestive heart failure: Observations on ambulatory ventricular arrhythmias. Am Heart J 110:800–806, 1985
67a. Konstam MA, Cohen SR, Weiland DS, et al: Relative contribution of inotropic and vasodilator effects to amrinone-induced hemodynamic improvement in congestive heart failure. Am J Cardiol 57:242–248, 1986
68.   Lee CO, Abete P, Pecker M, et al: Strophanthidin inotropy: Role of intracellular sodium ion activity and sodium-calcium exchange. J Mol Cell Cardiol 17:1043–1053, 1985
69.   LeJemtel TH, Sonnenblick EH: Should the failing heart be stimulated New Engl J Med 310:1384–1385, 1984
70.   LeJemtel TH, Maskin CS, Mancini D, et al: Systemic and regional hemodynamic effects of captopril and milrinone administered alone and concomitantly in patients with heart failure. Circulation 72:364–369, 1985
71.   Ludmer PL, Wright RF, Arnold MO, et al: Separation of the direct myocardial and vasodilator actions of milrinone administered by an intracoronary infusion technique. Circulation 73:130–137, 1986

72.   Mancini D, LeJemtel T, Sonnenblick E: Intravenous use of amrinone for the treatment of the failing heart. Am J Cardiol 56:8B-15B, 1985

73.   Mancini DM, LeJemtel TH, Factor S, et al: The central and peripheral components of cardiac failure. Am J Med, in press, 1986

74.   Marcus FI; Pharmacokinetic interactions between digoxin and other drugs. J Am Coll Cardiol 5:82A-90A, 1985

75.   Maskin C, Ocken S, Chadwick B, et al: Comparative systemic and renal effects of dopamine and angiotensin-converting enzyme inhibition with enalaprilat in patients with heart failure. Circulation 72:846–852, 1985

76.   Pedersen KE: Digoxin interactions. The influence of quinidine and verapamil on the pharmacokinetics and receptor binding of digitalis glycosides. Acta Med Scand (suppl 697):12–40, 1985

77.   Peters U: Pharmacokinetic review of digitalis glycosides. Eur Heart J 3 (suppl D):65–78, 1982

78.   Podrid P, Lown B, Zielonka J, et al: Effects of acetyl-strophanthidin on left ventricular function and ventricular arrhythmias. Am Heart J 107:882–887, 1984

78a. Rajfer SI, Rossen JD, Douglas F, et al: Effects of long-term therapy with ibopamine on resting hemodynamics and exercise capacity in patients with heart failure. Circulation 73:740–748, 1986

79.   Sinoway LS, Maskin CS, Chadwick B, et al: Long-term therapy with a new cardiotonic agent, WIN 47203: Drug-dependent improvement in cardiac performance and progression of the underlying disease. J Am Coll Cardiol 2:327–331, 1983

80.   Somberg JC, Smith TW: Localization of the neurally mediated arrhythmogenic properties of digitalis. Science 204:321–323, 1979

81.   Unverferth DV, Magorien RD, Altschuld R, et al: The hemodynamic and metabolic advantages gained by a three-day infusion of dobutamine in patients with congestive cardiomyopathy. Am Heart J 106:29–34, 1983

82.   Vik-Mo H, Yasay G, Maroko P, et al: Comparative effects of dobutamine and corwin, a β_1-adrenergic partial agonist, in experimental left ventricular failure. J Cardiovasc Pharmacol 7:784–790, 1985

83.   Wenger TL, Butler VP Jr, Haber E, et al: Treatment of 63 severely digitalis-toxic patients with digoxin specific antibody fragments. J Am Coll Cardiol 5:118A-123A, 1985

84.   Wilmshurst PT, Walker JM, Fry CH, et al: Inotropic and vasodilator effects of amrinone on isolated human tissue. Cardiovasc Res 18:302–309, 1984

Reviews

Colucci WS, Wright RF, Braunwald E: New positive inotropic agents in the treatment of congestive heart failure. New Engl J Med 314:290–299, 349–358, 1986

Mulrow CD, Feussner JR, Velex R: Reevaluation of digitalis efficacy. New light on an old leaf. Ann Intern Med 101:113–117, 1984

L. H. Opie
N. M. Kaplan

6

Diuretic Therapy

By definition a diuretic induces a diuresis of water and solutes. Loss of sodium is essential for the anti-edema effect, and for at least one major component of the antihypertensive effect. The problem is that loss of sodium is inevitably accompanied to some extent by loss of other ions—potassium is most frequently emphasized (Table 6-1). Magnesium and calcium may also be lost especially during a vigorous diuresis, depending on the diuretic used.

When used as antihypertensive agents, diuretics act at least in part by volume and sodium depletion.[21] In addition, diuretics might also be effective by nondiuretic mechanisms[2,28] or at least in doses low enough to avoid the subjective feeling of a diuresis. Here the diuretics may act as vascular dilators, or in a more subtle way by altering the sodium balance. Whatever the exact mechanisms, diuretics given for hypertension are used in lower doses than when a major diuretic effect is required.

Despite the potentially serious side-effects of diuretic therapy when used on a long-term basis, such agents remain very valuable in congestive heart failure (CHF) because of the high ratio of efficacy to really serious side-effects. In other words, **the benefit-risk ratio of diuretics is very high in CHF. In contrast, the risk-benefit ratio of diuretics in the therapy of mild hypertension is increasingly questioned,** especially because of the "wrong-way" blood biochemical changes.[52] Therefore the time-honored role of diuretics as first-line therapy in hypertension is increasingly challenged (see pp 207, 210) with, however, still a prime place for these agents in the therapy of certain groups of hypertensives—the elderly, the obese and blacks, and also for those with renal impairment when loop diuretics are used.

For practical purposes, the three major groups of diuretics are the loop diuretics, the thiazides, and the potassium-retaining diuretics.

LOOP DIURETICS

A particular advantage of loop diuretics (Table 6-2), such as furosemide, is that increasing doses exert an increasing diuresis before the "ceiling" is reached (*high-ceiling diuretics*).

Furosemide

Furosemide (= frusemide; Lasix®) is one of the standard loop diuretics for severe CHF. Furosemide is initial therapy in acute pulmonary edema and in left-sided failure of acute myocardial infarction (AMI). Relief of dyspnea even before diuresis results from venodilation and preload reduction.[6,10] Furosemide is also widely used for maintenance therapy in CHF.

Drugs for the Heart, Second Expanded Edition
Copyright © 1987 by Grune & Stratton, Inc.

ISBN 0-8089-1840-0

111

TABLE 6-1

URINARY ELECTROLYTE COMPOSITION DURING DIURESIS

	Volume (ml/min)	pH	Na+ (mM/l)	K+ (mM/l)	Cl−	HCO₃	Ca²⁺
Control	1	6.0	50	15	60	1	Variable
Thiazides	3	7.4	150	25	150	25	↓
Furosemide	8	6.0	140	10	155	1	↑
Triamterene	3	7.2	130	5	120	15	↓
Amiloride	2	7.2	130	5	110	15	↓

Modified from Mudge GH, in Gilman AG, Goodman LS, Gilman AG (eds): The Pharmacological Basis of Therapeutics, 6th ed. New York, MacMillan Publishing Co, 1980, pp 892–915. With permission.
↓ = decreased; ↑ = increased

Pharmacologic effects and pharmacokinetics.   Loop diuretics including furosemide (Fig. 6-1) inhibit the specific enzymes concerned with the pumping of chloride across the lining cells of the ascending limb of the loop of Henle (Site 2). This site of action is reached intraluminally, after the drug has been excreted by the proximal tubule. The effect of the enzyme inhibition is that chloride, sodium, potassium, and hydrogen ions all remain intraluminally and are lost in the urine with the possible side-effects of hyponatremia, hypochloremia, hypokalemia, and alkalosis. The plasma half-life of furosemide is 1.5 hours; the duration of action is 4–6 hours. Diuresis starts within 10–20 minutes of an IV dose and peaks 1–1.5 hours after an oral dose.[7]

Indications.   Furosemide is frequently the diuretic of choice for severe heart failure for four reasons. First, it is more powerful than the thiazides; second, it is effective (in high doses) in promoting diuresis even in the presence of a low glomerular filtration rate (GFR); third, furosemide promotes venodilatation and preload reduction;[6,10] and fourth, it acts rapidly. Similar reasons make it the initial drug of choice in *acute pulmonary edema.* After initial IV use, oral furosemide is usually continued as standard diuretic therapy, to be replaced by thiazides as the heart failure ameliorates. In *hypertension,* low-dose furosemide can be effective even as monotherapy[35] or combined with other agents such as β-blockers[62] and angiotensin-converting enzyme (ACE) inhibitors. However, if thiazides do not work for hypertension, furosemide probably will not work either unless the problem is a very low GFR. In *severe renal failure,* it is widely believed that furosemide increases the GFR, yet the subject is poorly understood. In *severe hypertension,* IV furosemide is sometimes used, especially if fluid overload is present.

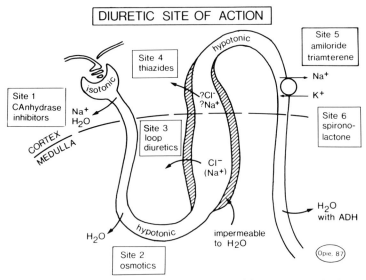

Fig. 6-1.   The six sites of action of diuretic agents. CA = carbonic anhydrase inhibitors.

TABLE 6-2

LOOP DIURETICS: SUMMARY

Drugs	Dose	Duration of Action (hr)	Trade Name® (UK—Europe)	Trade Name® (USA)
1. Furosemide (= frusemide)	20–40 mg (BP); 20–80 mg 1 or 2 × daily (CHF); oral or IV 250–2000 mg (oliguria);* refractory CHF 30–60 mg retard preparation daily	4–5 prolonged over 24 hr	Lasix; Dryptal; Frusetic; Frusid Lasix Retard	Lasix —
2. Bumetanide	0.5–2 mg 1 or 2 × daily oral or IV 5 mg (oliguria); Maintenance: alternate day dosage	4–6	Burinex	Bumex

Modified from Opie LH, Commerford PJ, Swanepoel CR: Diuretic Therapy, in Wenger N, Julian D (eds): Management of Heart Failure. London, Butterworths, 1986, pp 119–142. With permission.

* glomerular filtration rate below 20 ml/min; otherwise such high doses are contraindicated, except in severe refractory congestive heart failure (CHF).

BP = Use for blood pressure lowering; CHF = Use for congestive heart failure.

113

Contraindications. Anuria, although listed as a contraindication, may be treated (as is oliguria) by furosemide in the hope of evoking a diuresis); first exclude dehydration. A history of hypersensitivity to furosemide or sulfonamides. Furosemide (like other sulfonamides) may precipitate or exaggerate lupus erythematosus, photosensitive skin eruptions, or cause blood dyscrasias. Other contraindications include (1) IV use when electrolytes cannot be monitored, (2) AMI in the absence of left ventricular (LV) failure,[34a] (3) when optimal diuresis has already been achieved by other agents, and (4) patent ductus arteriosus in the neonate (see below)

Dose.   *IV furosemide* is usually started as a slow 40 mg injection (give 80 mg slow IV 1 hour later if needed); higher doses are required in elderly patients (surprisingly)[3] and much higher doses in renal failure and severe CHF. *Oral furosemide* also has a wide dose range (20–250 mg/day or even more; 20, 40, and 80 mg tablets in the USA; in Europe also scored 500 mg tablets). A short duration of action (4–5 hours) means that frequent doses are needed when sustained diuresis is required. Once acute relief has been obtained, however, then twice daily dosage reducing to once daily is usually given to rest the kidneys and the patients (at night). When 2 daily doses are required, they should be given in the early morning and mid-afternoon to obviate nocturia and to protect against volume depletion. Because of variable responses, often a brisk initial diuresis with a residual resistant component, the dose regime must be individualized. For *hypertension,* doses are usually lower (20–40 mg 1–2× daily). A retard preparation (Lasix Retard®) available in Europe is given once daily (30–60 mg). In the presence of *oliguria,* as the GFR drops below 20 ml/min, up to 250–2000 mg of furosemide may be required because the site of action in the loop is reached from the lumen only after excretion of furosemide from the proximal tubule (the latter process is reduced as the GFR falls). Similar arguments lead to similar doses of furosemide in *severe refractory heart failure.*[32]

Side-effects.   The risk of *hypokalemia* is greatest with high-dose furosemide, especially when given intravenously, and at the start of myocardial infarction when hypokalemia is in any case common even in the absence of diuretic therapy. Any lowering of plasma potassium can dangerously precipitate arrhythmias in early myocardial infarction.[27] Carefully regulated IV potassium supplements may be required in these circumstances. In acute heart failure too, digitalis toxicity may be precipitated by over-diuresis and hypokalemia. **"Standard oral doses" of furosemide (40–80 mg daily) as used for the chronic therapy of heart failure and hypertension, probably cause less hypokalemia than do some thiazides** (Table 6-1),[12,35,44] although clearly much depends on the doses chosen and the degree of diuresis achieved. The addition of potassium supplements is neither needed nor very effective;[36] addition of potassium-retaining diuretics is probably better.[39,44]

Other side-effects.   In 2580 patients the chief side-effects, in addition to hypokalemia, were hypovolemia and hyperuricemia.[36] Hypovolemia can be lessened by a low starting initial dose (20–40 mg); if it occurs, prerenal azotemia may develop (monitor blood urea).

Despite such fears of hemoconcentration, hemodilution is more likely, as shown by measurements of blood viscosity and hematocrit in patients with acute cardiogenic pulmonary edema treated by IV furosemide.[26] A few patients on high-dose furosemide have developed severe hyperosmolar nonketotic *hyperglycemic states.*[15] *"Atherogenic"* blood lipid changes, similar to those found with thiazides (Table 10-2), have recently been reported for loop diuretics.[65] Occasionally, gout or diabetes may be precipitated; it is not clear whether furosemide causes fewer "metabolic" side-effects than conventional thiazides.

Reversible dose-related *ototoxicity* (electrolyte disturbances of the endolymphatic system) can be avoided by infusing furosemide at rates not greater than 4 mg/min and keeping the oral dose below 1000 mg daily.

In *patent ductus arteriosus,* furosemide inhibits the degradation of prostaglandin E_2, which is a potent dilator of the ductus arteriosus so that the incidence of patent ductus arteriosus is increased.[22]

Drug combinations and interactions.   Additional diuresis may be achieved by a combination of furosemide with hydrochlorothiazide or metolazone. Furosemide-hydrochlorothiazide-amiloride (low-dose Lasix® plus Moduretic®) is a combination which usually avoids the traditional requirement for potassium supplements with furosemide; nonetheless the plasma potassium level requires checking especially in the presence of renal failure.

Captopril appears to enhance the effect of furosemide. In patients with severe heart failure and hyponatremia, combined therapy with furosemide and captopril is able to achieve a brisk sodium loss with correction of the hyponatremia.[17] If treated with captopril alone, the hyponatremia persists.

> Probenecid may interfere with the effects of thiazides or loop diuretics by blocking their secretion into the urine of the proximal tubule.[45,56] Indomethacin and other nonsteroidal anti-inflammatory drugs (NSAIDs) cause loss of response of the kidney to loop diuretics, presumably by interfering with formation of vasodilatory prostaglandins.[49,64] High doses of furosemide may competitively inhibit the excretion of salicylates to predispose to salicylate poisoning with tinnitus. Steroid or ACTH therapy may predispose to hypokalemia. Loop diuretics do not alter blood digoxin levels nor do they interact with warfarin.

LOOP DIURETICS OTHER THAN FUROSEMIDE

Bumetanide

The site of action of bumetanide (Bumex®, Burinex®) and its effects (and side-effects) are very similar to that of furosemide. The onset of diuresis is within 30 minutes, with a peak at 75–90 minutes and a total duration of action of 270 minutes.[4,7] Although it has been claimed that potassium loss may be less than that achieved for a comparable loss of sodium by furosemide,[15] other studies show a powerful potassium losing capacity.[9] Ototoxicity may be less with bumetanide than with furosemide, but renal toxicity more. **The really striking differences between these two agents are the much greater bioavailability and potency of bumetanide** so that smaller (but not less frequent) doses are needed.[7] In practice, as with furosemide, low-dose therapy need not occasion undue concern regarding hypokalemia as a possible side-effect, while higher doses can cause considerable electrolyte disturbances including hypokalemia. Again, as in the case of furosemide, a combined diuretic effect is obtained by addition of a thiazide diuretic.

Dose and clinical uses. In CHF, bumetanide is claimed to be effective in patients with edema resistant to furosemide, but additional studies are required to prove this point. The usual oral dose is 0.5–2 mg (0.5 and 1 mg tablets) with 1 mg bumetanide being equal to 40 mg furosemide;[4] other estimates are that bumetanide is 70× more powerful than furosemide.[7] In renal failure, the comparative potency of bumetanide might be much less than 40.[15] In acute pulmonary edema, a single dose of 1–3 mg can be effective; usually it is given intravenously over 1–2 minutes and the dose can be repeated at 2–3–hourly intervals to a maximum of 10 mg daily. In renal edema, the effects of bumetanide are similar to those of furosemide. In the USA, bumetanide is not approved for hypertension.

> *Side-effects.* These are rather similar to those of furosemide; ototoxicity may be less[15] and renal toxicity more, so that the combination with other potentially nephrotoxic drugs such as aminoglycosides should be avoided. In patients with renal failure, high doses have caused myalgia so that the dose should not exceed 4 mg/day when the GFR is below 5 ml/min.[25] Patients allergic to sulfonamides may also be hypersensitive to bumetanide; however, the package insert suggests that bumetanide might be safe when allergy to furosemide develops. Glucose tolerance may be well preserved.[19]

Summary

Until more careful studies are available on the comparison between bumetanide and furosemide, most clinicians will continue to use the agent they know best, i.e. furosemide unless there is a specific reason for not giving furosemide (allergic reaction, ototoxicity). As furosemide is widely available in generic form, its cost is likely to be less than that of bumetanide. Nonetheless, the use of bumetanide is increasing.

Ethacrynic Acid.   Ethacrynic acid (Edecrin®) closely resembles furosemide in dose (50 mg tablet), duration of diuresis, and side-effects (except for more ototoxicity). Furosemide, with a broader dose-response curve than ethacrynic acid, allows easier definition of the optimal dose for a given patient[45] and is much more widely used.

Piretanide.   This agent is a very new loop diuretic (Arelix®; dose 6–24 mg; available in Europe), and claimed to have little effect on potassium homeostasis despite its potency,[46] and is being promoted for hypertension.

Muzolimine.   This new loop diuretic is being tested in Europe for hypertension and heart failure.

THIAZIDE DIURETICS

Thiazide diuretics (Table 6-3) **remain the most widely used first-line therapy for hypertension,** although increasingly other "first-liners" such as β-blockade, α-blockade, calcium antagonists, and converting enzyme inhibitors are being chosen. Thiazides are also standard therapy for chronic CHF, when edema is modest, either alone or in combination with loop diuretics.

Pharmacologic action and pharmacokinetics.   Thiazide diuretics may act to inhibit the reabsorption of sodium and, with it, chloride in the more distal part of the nephron (Site 3), which allows more sodium to reach the distal tubules where more is exchanged with potassium, particularly in the presence of an activated renin-angiotensin-aldosterone system. Thiazides may also increase the active excretion of potassium in the distal renal tubule.[56]

Thiazides are rapidly absorbed from the gastrointestinal (GI) tract to produce a diuresis within 1–2 hours. Some major differences from the loop diuretics are: (1) the longer duration of action; (2) the different site of action (Fig. 6-1); (3) the relatively low "ceiling" of thiazide diuretics, i.e. the maximal response is reached at a relatively low dosage, and (4) the much decreased capacity of thiazides to work

TABLE 6-3

THIAZIDE DIURETICS: SUMMARY OF PROPERTIES

	Dose	Duration of Action (hr)	Trade Name® (UK—Europe)	Trade Name® (USA)
1. Hydrochlorothiazide	12.5–50 mg (BP); 25–100 mg (CHF)	6–12	Esidrex Hydrosaluric	HydroDIURIL; Esidrix; Thiuretic
2. Hydroflumethazide	25–50 mg (BP); 25–200 mg (CHF)	6–12	Hydrenox	Saluron; Diucardin
3. Chlorthalidone	12.5–50 mg	48–72	Hygroton	Hygroton; Thalitone
4. Metolazone	1–10 mg (BP); 5–20 mg (CHF)	18–25	Metenix; Diulo	Zaroloxyn; Diulo
5. Bendrofluazide = bendroflumethiazide	2.5–5 mg (BP); 10 mg (CHF)	6–12	Aprinox; Centyl; Urizide	Naturetin
6. Polythiazide	1–2 mg (BP)	24–48	Nephril	Renese
7. Chlorothiazide	250–1000 mg	6–12	Saluric	Diuril
8. Cyclothiazide	1–2 mg	6–12	—	Anhydron
9. Trichlormethiazide	1–4 mg	About 24	Fluitran (not in UK)	Metahydrin; Naqua
10. Cyclopenthiazide	0.25 mg	6–12	Navidrex	—
11. Indapamide	2.5 mg (BP)	16–36	Natrilix	Lozol
12. Xipamide	20–40 mg (BP)	6–12	Diurexan	—

Modified from Opie LH, Commerford PJ, Swanepoel CR: Diuretic Therapy, in Wenger N, Julian D (eds): Management of Heart Failure. London, Butterworths, 1986, pp 119–142. With permission.
* = Combination agents.
BP = Use for blood pressure-lowering; CHF = Use for congestive heart failure.
NB: The doses given for antihypertensive therapy are generally *LOWER* than those recommended by the manufacturers. In our view high doses of diuretics are *contraindicated* for hypertension.

in the presence of renal failure (serum creatinine >2.0 mg/dl; GFR below 15–20 ml/min[53]). The fact that thiazides and loop diuretics act at different sites explains the additive effects of these agents.

Dose and indications. In *hypertension,* thiazide doses have generally been too high and high doses continue to be recommended by the manufacturers. Although long-term prospective studies are lacking, indirect evidence suggests a dose of 25 mg hydrochlorothiazide daily[3a,35] or even lower doses, especially in combination therapy.[37] Higher doses are marginally more effective with greater risks of undesirable metabolic and subjective side-effects (Table 6-4: hypokalemia,[23a,23b,35] glucose intolerance, hyperuricemia, and atherogenic lipid changes). In combination with β-blockade, even lower doses (12.5 mg hydrochlorothiazide daily) appear to be effective.[37] **With hydrochlorothiazide, the full antihypertensive effect may take up to 12 weeks**[54] **so that a common error is "*premature step therapy,*" i.e. going on to the next step too soon.** Diuretics may be the initial agent of choice in the elderly, in blacks, and in obese[52a] patients. Chlorthalidone 25–50 mg daily has been used in systolic hypertension in the elderly;[24] the long duration of action and tendency to hypokalemia[23a] may not be advantages. Bendrofluazide 10 mg daily was used in the giant British Trial[41] and compared with propranolol up to 320 mg daily, each had different side-effects with (surprisingly) fatigue and impotence more common in the diuretic group as were arrhythmias (see p 210). A lower dose of bendrofluazide (2.5–5 mg) was however used in Denmark over a 6–year period with fewer metabolic side-effects.[5]

In *CHF,* higher doses are justified (50–100 mg hydrochlorothiazide daily are probably "ceiling" doses), while watching the plasma potassium. In *renal edema,* thiazides are not used if the GFR is low.[53]

Choice of thiazide. It seems to matter little which of the various thiazide preparations are chosen; the majority, including hydrochlorothiazide, have an intermediate duration of action (6–12 hours). However, an ultra-longacting compound such as chlorthalidone (24–72 hours; dose same as hydrochlorothiazide) has the potential disadvantages of nocturia and greater risk of electrolyte disturbances.

Contraindications. Renal edema, hypokalemia, AMI, ventricular arrhythmias, and co-therapy with pro-arrhythmic drugs (see p 81). In hypokalemia (including early AMI), thiazide diuretics may precipitate arrhythmias. Relative contraindications: pregnancy hypertension because of the risk of a decreased blood volume; moreover, thiazides can cross the placental barrier with risk of

TABLE 6-4
SIDE-EFFECTS OF PROLONGED THERAPY
OF MILD HYPERTENSION WITH
HIGH-DOSE THIAZIDE*

Causing withdrawal of therapy
  Impaired glucose tolerance†
  Gout
  Impotence
  Lethargy
  Nausea, dizziness or headache

Blood biochemical changes
  Glucose ↑
  Uric acid ↑
  Urea ↑
  Potassium ↓
  Cholesterol ↑

* Bendroflumethazide 10 mg daily.[41]
† Lower doses of bendroflumethazide (2.5–5.0 mg) have been given over 6 years without any detectable glucose intolerance, uric acid, or cholesterol change and only a minimal fall of potassium.[5]

neonatal jaundice. In renal impairment, the GFR may fall as thiazides decrease the blood volume.

Side-effects.   Besides the increasingly emphasized "wrong way" metabolic side-effects,[52] (p 119), thiazide diuretics rarely cause sulfonamide-type immune side-effects including intrahepatic jaundice, pancreatitis, blood dyscrasias, angiitis, pneumonitis, and interstitial nephritis.

Drug interactions.   Steroids and estrogens (e.g. the contraceptive pill) may cause salt retention to antagonize the action of thiazide diuretics. *Indomethacin* and NSAIDs blunt the response to thiazide diuretics[64] and may worsen CHF.[18] *Captopril or enalapril,* when combined with a potassium-retaining diuretic, may cause hyperkalemia so that this combination should be avoided. Hypokalemia induced by diuretics may predispose to torsades de pointes when there is additional therapy with agents that prolong the QT-interval such as sotalol.[40] The nephrotoxic effects of certain antibiotics such as the aminoglycosides may be potentiated by diuretics. *Probenecid* (for the therapy of gout) may block thiazide effects by interfering with thiazide excretion into the urine. *Lithium* interacts with diuretics by impairing their renal clearance and by possible additive effects of lithium toxicity.

Combination therapy.   Combination with amiloride, triamterene or spironolactone is commonly used in the therapy of hypertension (p 117) and CHF (p 126). For contraindications, see p 122.

OTHER THIAZIDES AND THIAZIDE-LIKE AGENTS

Metolazone—in a Class of its Own?

Metolazone (Zaroloxyn®, Diulo®, Metenix®) belongs to the category of thiazide diuretics. An important additional property is that **metolazone appears to be effective even in patients with reduced renal function,**[11] thus resembling furosemide. The duration of action is up to 24 hours so that a single daily dose is recommended. In combination with furosemide, metolazone may provoke a profound diuresis, with the risk of excessive volume and potassium depletion.[29] Therefore patients should be carefully observed and probably hospitalized when the combination is started especially in elderly patients. Alternately, once-a-day low-dose (2.5 or 5 mg) metolazone may be used instead of 2–3 daily doses of furosemide. If added diuresis is needed, metolazone may be added to furosemide with care, especially in patients with renal as well as cardiac failure. The side-effect profile of metolazone closely resembles that of the ordinary thiazides.

Indapamide

Indapamide (Natrilix®, Lozol®) is a thiazide-like diuretic (albeit with a different molecular structure), which lowers the blood pressure in a dose of 2.5 mg/day, with a terminal half-life of 14–16 hours; in higher doses, a vigorous diuresis can be achieved.[8] Part of the antihypertensive action might be peripheral vasodilation.[31] In hypertension, indapamide can evoke a rapid hypotensive response, more so than the thiazides, so that in elderly patients reduced organ perfusion is a theoretical risk.[54] Although originally thought not to have metabolic side-effects, indapamide 2.5 mg daily has a **similar metabolic side-effect profile to hydrochlorothiazide 50 mg daily,**[31] with particular reference to changes in the serum potassium, serum uric acid, and blood cholesterol (strict comparisons of glucose tolerance were not made). In cardiac edema the drug has little advantage over other well tried diuretics.[38]

Xipamide

This compound, not available in the USA, structurally resembles chlorthalidone and also causes a prolonged diuresis that may be disturbing to elderly patients for whom it is otherwise recommended.[38] Hypokalemia remains a risk. The true place of this agent is not yet known.

MINOR DIURETICS

Carbonic anhydrase inhibitors such as acetazolamide (Diamox®) are weak diuretics. They decrease the secretion of hydrogen ions by the proximal renal tubule (Site 1), with increased loss of bicarbonate and hence of sodium. These agents, seldom used as primary diuretics, have found a place in the therapy of glaucoma because carbonic anhydrase plays a role in the secretion of aqueous humor in the ciliary processes of the eye. In salicylate poisoning, the alkalinizing effect of carbonic anhydrase inhibitors increases the renal excretion of lipid-soluble weak organic acids.[45]

Calcium antagonists have a direct diuretic effect that contributes to the long-term antihypertensive effect.[34,47] For example, nifedipine increases urine volume and sodium excretion[30] and may inhibit aldosterone release by angiotensin.[43] Diuresis explains the tendency to hypokalemia.[47] The diuretic action is quite independent of any change in renal blood flow or glomerular filtration. Thus calcium antagonists may be beneficial in CHF apart from their unloading effects.

METABOLIC SIDE-EFFECTS OF THIAZIDES

Many side-effects of thiazides are similar to those of the loop diuretics: electrolyte disturbances including hypokalemia, hyponatremia, hyperuricemia, the precipitation of gout and diabetes, a decreased blood volume, and alkalosis. "*Atherogenic*" blood lipid changes (Table 10-2) and impotence have recently been described. *Hyponatremia* may sometimes occur in the elderly even with low diuretic doses.

As in the case of loop diuretics, *hypokalemia* is probably an overfeared complication, especially when low doses of thiazides are used.[35] Yet many physicians remain impressed by the average fall in plasma potassium of about 0.7 mM/L, which will lower the K^+ level to below 3.5 mM/L in about one-third of hypertensives with impairment of control of blood pressure.[28a] Hence the frequent choice of potassium-retaining diuretics such as triamterene or amiloride. This choice in turn brings about the alternative but lesser risk that some patients will develop hyperkalemia, especially in the presence of renal impairment or during the concomitant use of potassium supplements or converting enzyme inhibitors.

Arrhythmias.   A recent study highlights the complexity of assessing the relationship between hypokalemia and arrhythmias in patients with mild hypertension treated by diuretics.[42] In a retrospective analysis, only one single fact clearly emerged: in patients chronically treated by bendrofluazide (daily dose: 10 mg), there were more malignant or premalignant arrhythmias. It seemed that diuretic therapy itself rather than a low plasma potassium was associated with arrhythmias; perhaps magnesium depletion played a role. Other trials have also shown the problems of trying to relate *potassium levels* to arrhythmias. In 13 patients with torsades de pointes receiving sotalol,[40] only 6 had potassium values of less than 3.4 mM/L. Correction of diuretic-induced hypokalemia was not linked to a decreased incidence of extrasystoles in patients with uncomplicated systemic hypertension.[50] The problem with some of the above studies may be that the analyses were retrospective. For recent reviews with conflicting conclusions, see references 23a and 49a.

In a prospective trial in patients with mild hypertension and typical effort angina, amiloride 10 mg 2× daily (potassium-retaining) was used as a sole agent in comparison with chlorthalidone 25 mg daily (potassium-losing[58]). Equal control of blood pressure was achieved. The potassium-losing phase brought down plasma K^+ from 4.3 to 3.3 mEq/L and gave a higher incidence of ventricular arrhythmias both during ambulatory monitoring and during programmed stimulation. Plasma magnesium was unchanged throughout. This study proves that **even mild hypokalemia must be avoided in patients with angina pectoris.**

In *AMI*, initial hypokalemia is linked to ventricular arrhythmias including ventricular fibrillation (VF).[16,48] The hypokalemia could be caused both by diuretic therapy and by adrenergic discharge.[59] β-Adrenergic blockade (especially by nonselective agents) appears to inhibit the "stress"-induced hypokalemia with lessening of ventricular arrhythmias.[27] (See p 7.)

Hypomagnesemia,[23b] like hypokalemia, is theoretically blamed for arrhythmias during diuretic therapy, although the facts are few. Even in the case of some digitalis-induced arrhythmias, there is no clear case for a role for hypomagnese-mia. Recently, magnesium infusions have been recommended for patients with early myocardial infarction (see p 78) but many more trials are required. Animal data suggest that hypomagnesemia can be prevented by the addition of a "potassium-retaining" component such as amiloride to the thiazide diuretic.[13,14]

Hypokalemia and Hypomagnesemia: Therapeutic Strategies

Although the arrhythmogenic dangers of thiazide-induced hypokalemia are not convincingly established, common sense says that in patients with a higher risk of arrhythmias, as in ischemic heart disease, heart failure on digitalis, or hypertension with LV hypertrophy, a potassium- and magnesium-retaining diuretic should be part of the therapy unless contraindicated by renal failure or by co-therapy with captopril or enalapril. Such a diuretic may be better than potassium supplementation,[39] especially because the supplements do not avoid hypomagnesemia; yet these issues are not completely resolved. For *heart failure,* a "standard" combination daily therapy might be 1–2 tablets of Moduretic® (hydrochlorothiazide 50 mg, amiloride 5 mg) or 2–4 of Dyazide® (hydrochlorothiazide 25 mg, triamterene 50 mg) or 1–2 tablets of Maxzide® (hydrochlorothiazide 50 mg, triamterene 75 mg). For *hypertension,* the doses are approximately halved, bearing in mind the requirement for the "ideal" thiazide dose of about 25 mg/day as in 1 tablet of Dyazide®. In some countries, a new "mini-Moduretic" (Moduret 25®) with half-strength hydrochlorothiazide (25 mg) and also with amiloride 2.5 mg is now available. K^+-containing supplements such as Slow-K® or K-Lyte® (both with KCl) should not be given unless there is still proven hypokalemia despite the combination therapy. When *captopril or enalapril* is part of the therapy, K supplements must be avoided and *K-retaining diuretics should be replaced by simple hydrochlorothiazide.* It must be stressed that the above proposals are based on extrapolation, albeit reasonable, so that revision may be needed as new data arrive.

When cost is important, a generic thiazide may be cheaper than a potassium-sparing thiazide combination; and when hypokalemia is suspected or detected, oral K-supplementation with a salt substitute is less expensive than KCl supplements.

Diabetogenic Effects

The thiazides are sulfonamide derivatives that explain their potential pancreatic toxicity and provocation of diabetes in a minority of patients. The mechanism may be indirectly via hypokalemia with decreased insulin secretion.[51] Patients with a familial tendency to diabetes may be more prone to the side-effects of thiazide therapy and should be excluded whenever possible.

Urate Excretion

Most diuretics decrease urate excretion with the risk of increasing blood uric acid and causing gout in those predisposed; thus a personal or family history of gout should lead to therapy with non-thiazide diuretics. *Tienilic acid,* in contrast to other thiazides, has a uricosuric effect; unfortunately liver damage has caused withdrawal of this drug. Nevertheless the molecule may serve as a pattern for further agents to come.

"Atherogenic" Changes in Blood Lipids

Thiazides may increase the total blood cholesterol by an average of 15–20 mg/dl,[66] and also the LDL-cholesterol (LDL = low density lipoprotein). Also see Table 10-2. During prolonged thiazide therapy a lipid-lowering diet is advisable.

Prevention of Metabolic Side-Effects

Reduction in the dose of diuretic, restriction of dietary sodium, and additional dietary potassium will reduce the frequency of hypokalemia. Combination thiazide with a K$^+$-retainer usually prevents hypokalemia. Combination therapy of hydrochlorothiazide (about 50 mg daily) with captopril (25–50 mg 2–3× daily) reduces the incidence of hypokalemia and hyperuricemia, and possibly also of hyperglycemia.[66] Combination therapy with hydro-chlorothiazide and conventional K-retaining diuretics is frequently used (see p 122).

POTASSIUM-SPARING DIURETICS

Sodium-potassium exchange in the collecting tubules only accounts for a small part of the sodium re-uptake into the renal cells, so that a powerful diuresis cannot be obtained by distally acting K$^+$-retaining agents acting alone (Table 6-5).

Amiloride and Triamterene

Despite their relatively weak diuretic action (Table 6-1), these agents are frequently used in combination with thiazide diuretics. Advantages are (1) the capacity to retain both potassium and magnesium and (2) an action independent of the activity of aldosterone. **As sole agents they are too weak for diuresis in CHF; they may be antihypertensive in their own right.**[58,61] But the data are incomplete. Side-effects are few; hyperkalemia and acidosis may rarely occur, and then mostly in those with renal disease. In particular the thiazide-related risks of diabetes mellitus and gout have not been reported. There is a suggestion that amiloride may be preferable to triamterene (the latter is excreted by the kidneys with risks of renal casts on standard doses and occasional renal dysfunction[33]). In practice, compounds with triamterene have been widely and extensively used without many detectable risks. For combination with thiazides, see p 122.

Spironolactone

Spironolactone is logical therapy in those few patients who develop heart failure or hypertension in the presence of high mineralocorticoid levels as during prednisone therapy or as part of Conn's syndrome. For others, this agent is **chosen only when diabetes or gout may be present or when there is fear of their precipitation, or when it is important to avoid potassium or magnesium loss and thiazide-combinations are contraindicated.** Spironolactone is a more powerful diuretic than amiloride or triamterene in the presence of hyperaldosteronism, and probably more effective as sole agent in hypertension (strict trials are lacking). One daily dose of spironolactone is adequate for diuresis (25–100 mg); for therapy of Conn's syndrome 100 mg or more 3× daily with meals may be needed (food enhances bioavailability of canrenone). Side-effects include antitestosterone effects such as gynecomastia and impotence, particularly when large doses and long-term treatment are used. Spironolactone may benefit hirsutes in females.

ACE Inhibitors

Because captopril and enalapril ultimately exert an anti-aldosterone effect, they too act as mild potassium-retaining diuretics. Combination therapy with other K$^+$-retainers should be avoided.

TABLE 6-5

POTASSIUM-SPARING DIURETICS (GENERALLY ALSO SPARE MAGNESIUM)

	Dose	Duration of Action	Trade Name® (UK—Europe)	Trade Name® (USA)
1. Spironolactone	25–200 mg	3–5 days	Aldactone	Aldactone
2. Amiloride	2.5–20 mg	4–5 days	Midamor	Midamor
3. Triamterene	25–200 mg	8–12 hr	Dytac	Dyrenium

Modified from Opie LH, Commerford PJ, Swanepoel CR: Diuretic Therapy, in Wenger N, Julian D (eds): Management of Heart Failure. London, Butterworths, 1986, pp 119–142. With permission.

Hyperkalemia—A Specific Risk

The risk of hyperkalemia is also there with most diuretic combinations (see next section). Amiloride, triamterene, and spironolactone may all cause hyperkalemia (serum K^+ equal to or exceeds 5.5 mEq/L) especially in the presence of pre-existing renal disease, diabetes, or in elderly patients during cotherapy with captopril or enalapril, or in patients receiving possible nephrotoxic agents without careful monitoring of the serum K^+. Hyperkalemia is treated by drug withdrawal, infusions of glucose-insulin, and cation exchange resins such as sodium, polystyrene sulfonate, and sometimes dialysis. IV calcium chloride may be required to avoid VF.

COMBINATION DIURETICS

Besides addition of one class of diuretic to another, the fear of hypokalemia has increased the use of K^+-retaining-thiazide combinations (Table 6-6), such as *Dyazide®*, *Moduretic®*, and *Maxzide®*. **When used for hypertension, special attention must be given to the thiazide dose** (25 mg hydrochlorothiazide in Dyazide®; 50 mg in Moduretic® and Maxzide®) where the lower dose may be preferable. On the other hand, amiloride (in Moduretic®) is marginally preferable to triamterene (in Dyazide® and Maxzide®) as judged by renal side-effects.[33] Of interest is the new "mini-Moduretic" (Moduret 25®, 25 mg hydrochlorothiazide, 2.5 mg amiloride) available in Europe. *Maxzide®* (Table 6-6) appears to have few metabolic side-effects especially when given as half-tablet daily (= 25 mg hydrochlorothiazide, 37.5 mg triamterene).[23c] A K^+-retaining furosemide combination (*Frumil®* in Europe) is another reasonable alternative.

Capozide® (Table 6-6). Thiazide diuretics increase renin levels and captopril decreases metabolic side-effects of thiazides. Hence the combination is logical.

TABLE 6-6

SOME COMBINATION DIURETIC AGENTS

		Dose	Trade Name® (UK—Europe)	Trade Name® (USA)
Hydrochlorothiazide +triamterene	25 mg 50 mg	1–2 tablets/day (up to 4 in CHF)	Dyazide	Dyazide
Hydrochlorothiazide +amiloride	50 mg 5 mg	1/2–1 tablet/day (up to 2 in CHF)	Moduretic*	Moduretic
Hydrochlorothiazide +triamterene	50 mg 75 mg	1/2–1 tablet/day (limited clinical experience with higher doses)	—	Maxzide
Spironolactone +hydrochlorothiazide	25 mg 25 mg	1–4 tablets/day	Aldactazide	Aldactazide
Cyclopenthiazide +potassium chloride	0.25 mg 600 mg	1–2 tablets/day	Navidrex K	—
Furosemide +amiloride	40 mg 5 mg	1–2 tablets/day	Frumil	—
Captopril +hydrochlorothiazide	25–50 mg 15–30 mg†	1 tablet 2× day	Capozide	Capozide

Modified from Opie LH, Commerford PJ, Swanepoel CR: Diuretic Therapy, in Wenger N, Julian D (eds): Management of Heart Failure. London, Butterworths, 1986, pp 119–142.

CHF = congestive heart failure

For hypertension, see text—low doses generally preferred and high doses are *contraindicated*.

* available in half-strength in Europe as Moduret® 25 mg.

† lower hydrochlorothiazide content preferred for hypertension.

POTASSIUM SUPPLEMENTS

The routine practice in many centers of giving K^+ supplements with loop diuretics is usually unnecessary (Table 6-1) and leads to extra cost and loss of compliance. Addition of low-dose K^+-retaining diuretics is usually better if really required. Even high doses of furosemide may not automatically require K^+ replacement because such doses are usually given in the presence of renal impairment or severe CHF when renal potassium handling may be abnormal. Clearly potassium levels need periodic checking during therapy with all diuretics. *To avoid hypokalemia*, low-dose diuretics are preferred. A high-potassium, low-salt diet is advised and can be simply and cheaply achieved by the use of salt substitutes. Sometimes, despite all reasonable care, problematic hypokalemia develops especially after prolonged diuretic therapy or in the presence of diarrhea or alkalosis. Then potassium supplements may become necessary.

Potassium chloride (KCl) in liquid form is theoretically best because (1) co-administration of chloride is required to correct fully K^+-deficiency in hypokalemic hypochloremic alkalosis;[57] (2) slow-release tablets may cause GI ulceration (see next section) which liquid KCl does not.[50a] The dose is variable. About 20 mEq daily are required to avoid K^+-depletion and 40–100 mEq to treat K^+-depletion. Absorption is rapid and bioavailability good. To help avoid the frequent GI irritation, liquid KCl needs dilution in water or another liquid and titration against the patient's acceptability. KCl may also be given in some effervescent preparations (next section). *Slow-release potassium chloride* wax-matrix tablets (Slow-K®, each with 8 mEq or 600 mg KCl; Klotrix® and K-Tab® each contain 10 mEq KCl; Kaon-CL®, 6.7 or 10 mEq KCl) although widely used and well tolerated, should not be given (according to the package insert in the USA) unless liquid or effervescent potassium preparations are not tolerated. The chloride salt, although able to correct co-existing chloride deficiency, carries the risk of GI ulceration or bleeding, especially when GI motility is impaired as in elderly or immobile or diabetic patients or in the presence of scleroderma, esophageal stricture, massive left atrial enlargement, or co-therapy with anticholinergic drugs including disopyramide. To avoid esophageal ulceration, tablets should be taken with the patient upright or sitting, and with a meal or beverage, and anticholinergic therapy should be avoided. *Microencapsulated* KCl (Micro-K®, 8 mEq KCl or 10 mEq KCl) may reduce GI ulceration to only 1 per 100,000 patient years, but the package insert still carries the same warning as for wax-matrix tablets. High doses of Micro-K® cause GI ulcers especially during anticholinergic therapy.[50a]

Effervescent preparations lessen the risk of GI ulceration and those with KCl include Klorvess® (20 mEq), K-Lor® (20 mEq KCl per packet), K-Lyte/Cl® (25 mEq per tablet), and K-Lyte/Cl 50® (50 mEq tablet). K-Lyte® contains potassium bicarbonate and citrate, 25 mEq. GI intolerance frequently limits the use of these agents that are best given with liquid meals and in relatively small doses. *Potassium gluconate* (with citrate), Bi-K® 20 mEq, or Twin K® tends to minimize the GI irritative effects of the effervescent preparations but lacks chloride.

K^+ Supplements—Summary

The simplest is a high-potassium low-sodium diet achieved by salt substitutes. When drug supplements become essential, KCl is preferred. The best preparation will be one well tolerated by the patient and inexpensive. "No comprehensive adequately controlled studies of the relative efficacy of the various KCl preparations in clinical settings are available."[57]

SPECIAL DIURETIC PROBLEMS

Over-Diuresis

During therapy of *edematous states*, over-vigorous diuresis may so reduce venous pressure and ventricular filling so that the cardiac output drops and tissues become underperfused. The renin-angiotensin axis is further activated. Probably many patients are protected against the extremely effective potent diuretics by poor compliance. Over-diuresis is most frequently seen during hospital admissions when a rigid policy of regular administration of diuretics is carried out.

Fixed diuretic regimes are largely unsatisfactory in edematous patients. Often intelligent patients can manage their therapy well by tailoring a flexible diuretic schedule to their own needs, using a simple bathroom scale, knowing how to recognize pedal edema and the time course of maximal effect of their diuretic often allows a patient to adjust his own diuretic dose and administration schedule to fit in with daily activities.

Patients who may experience *adverse effects* due to over-diuresis include (1) those with mild chronic heart failure overtreated with potent diuretics; (2) patients requiring a high filling pressure particularly those with a "restrictive" pathophysiology as in restrictive cardiomyopathy or hypertrophic cardiomyopathy; and (3) early phase AMI,[20] when the problem of excessive diuresis is most commonly encountered when using potent IV diuretics for acute heart failure. It may be necessary cautiously to administer a *"fluid challenge"* with saline solution or a colloid preparation while checking the patient's cardiovascular status. If the resting heart rate falls, renal function improves, and blood pressure stabilizes, the ventricular filling pressure has been inadequate.[67]

Diuretic Resistance

Repetitive diuretic administration leads to a levelling off of the effect, because (in the face of a shrunken intravascular volume) the part of the tubular system not affected reacts by reabsorbing more sodium. Additional mechanisms are an abnormally low cardiac output in patients with heart failure; prominent activation of the angiotensin-renin axis; or an electrolyte-induced resistance (Fig. 6-2; Table 6-7). Apparent resistance can also develop (see p 118) when there is concomitant therapy with indomethacin or other NSAIDs (exception: sulindac;[64,69]) or probenecid. The thiazide diuretics (exception: metolazone) will not work well if the GFR is below 15–20 ml/min.[53] When potassium depletion is severe, diuretics will not work well for complex reasons.

Is there compliance with dietary salt restriction? Is complete bed rest required? Is the optimal agent being used, avoiding thiazide diuretics (except

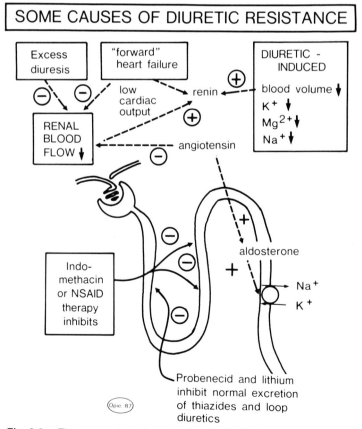

Fig. 6-2.   The causes of resistance to diuretics (for further details see text).

TABLE 6-7
SOME CAUSES OF APPARENT RESISTANCE TO DIURETICS IN THERAPY OF CARDIAC FAILURE

1. *Incorrect use of diuretic agent*
   — combination of 2 thiazides or 2 loop diuretics instead of 1 of each type
   — use of thiazides when GFR is low* (exception: metolazone)
   — excessive diuretic dose (see 2 and 3)
   — poor compliance, especially caused by multiple tablets of oral K^+ supplements

2. *Electrolyte volume imbalance*
   — hyponatremia, hypokalemia, hypovolumia
   — hypomagnesemia may need correction to correct hypokalemia

3. *Poor renal perfusion diuretic-induced hypovolemia*
   — cardiac output too low
   — excess hypotension (unloading agents)

4. *Excess circulating catecholamines*
   (frequent in severe congestive heart failure; causes vasoconstriction and limits renal blood flow)
   — correct by increased inotropic support if possible, or by appropriate unloading agents

5. *Activation of renin-angiotension-aldosterone system*
   (frequent in severe congestive heart failure)
   — correct by angiotensin-converting enzyme inhibition (captopril, enalapril)

6. *Interfering drugs*
   — indomethacin and other non-steroidal anti-inflammatories inhibit diuresis (prostaglandins inhibit action of vasopressin)
   — probenecid and lithium inhibit tubular excretion of thiazides and loop diuretics

* GFR = glomerular filtration rate below 15–20 ml/min.

metolazone) when the GFR is low? Is the optimal dose being used? Are there interfering drugs or severe electrolyte or volume imbalances that can be remedied? Has the general cardiovascular status been made optimal by judicious use of unloading or inotropic drugs? **To achieve ideal metabolic-hormonal status, captopril or enalapril may have to be added to thiazide or loop diuretics, or metolazone combined with loop diuretics. In out-patients, compliance and dietary salt restriction must be carefully checked, while all unnecessary drugs are eliminated. Sometimes fewer drugs work better than more (here the prime sinners are K supplements, requiring many daily tablets frequently not taken).**

Renal Failure

In patients with mild chronic renal failure, treated without success with high-dose furosemide (up to 480–500 mg/day), the addition of hydrochlorothiazide 25–50 mg 2× daily may produce a marked diuresis, so that the combination may be effective when either agent singly fails.[68] Metolazone and furosemide may likewise be combined (see section on metolazone) especially when the GFR is really low. Whether the latter combination is truly more powerful than hydrochlorothiazide-furosemide (as some anecdotal observations suggest), remains to be rigorously tested.[23]

Hyponatremia

In patients severely ill with CHF, a hyponatremic state may develop from water retention. Recent studies point to (1) the "inappropriate release" of arginine vasopressin—antidiuretic hormone;[55,60] and (2) increased activity of angiotensin II.[18]

Adverse Drug Interactions

Indomethacin and other NSAIDs may cause serious deterioration of cardiovascular status in some patients with severe heart failure[18] because the vasoconstrictor response to angiotensin may evoke the release of vasodilatory prostaglandins to exert a compensatory effect on the circulation. Most NSAIDs impair thiazide control of blood pressure (exception: *sulindac* = Clinoril®).[69] *Probenecid* and *lithium* decrease the normal renal excretion of thiazide and loop diuretics, so that the diuretic effect is decreased.

LESS COMMON USES OF DIURETICS

Less common indications are: (1) hypernatremia when not due to fluid depletion; (2) IV furosemide in malignant or premalignant hypertension especially if there is associated CHF and fluid retention; (3) high-dose furosemide for acute or chronic renal failure when it is thought that diuresis may be initiated; (4) in hypercalcemia, high-dose loop diuretics increase urinary excretion of calcium; IV furosemide is used in the emergency treatment of severe hypercalcemia; (5) thiazides for the nephrogenic form of diabetes insipidus—the mechanism of action is not clear but there is a diminution in "free water" clearance; and (6) thiazide diuretics decrease the urinary calcium output through a mechanism that is not well understood, so that they are used in idiopathic hypercalciuria to decrease the formation of renal stones (in contrast, loop diuretics increase urinary excretion of calcium). **The inhibitory effect of thiazides on urinary calcium loss may explain why these agents may increase bone mineralization,**[63] hence suggesting a possible *new therapeutic use for thiazides in osteoporosis.* The latter benefit is another argument for first-line (low-dose) diuretic therapy in elderly hypertensives.

An additional use, entirely unrelated, is in mania when *lithium* therapy is insufficient (thiazides sensitize to lithium effects).

STEP-CARE THERAPY OF CHF

In *mild to moderate CHF,* the usual "step-care" diuretic therapy is (1) dietary sodium restriction and the use of thiazide diuretics; (2) increasing doses of thiazides to the "ceiling" which is rapidly reached, and monitoring plasma potassium (and sometimes magnesium); (3) low-dose furosemide; and (4) high-dose furosemide or other loop diuretics.

For *severe CHF,* when congestion and edema are prominent symptoms, initial therapy is usually with furosemide, especially when renal perfusion may be impaired. Complete bed rest helps to promote an early diuresis.[1] The dose of furosemide required may be very high (500–1500 mg daily). Digitalis is introduced when diuresis by itself seems inadequate—probably at the stage of low-dose furosemide unless there is atrial fibrillation in which case digitalis will be introduced earlier. In the United States and in Germany, however, digitalis is still generally introduced at an earlier stage, sometimes even as the primary agent. (For use of digitalis in heart failure, see p 94).

Load-reducing agents are added at variable stages. The current tendency is to add such agents sooner rather than later, because in CHF diuretic action may be inhibited by poor renal perfusion and renin formation, the low GFR, and an increased renal interstitial pressure and lessened sodium reabsorption. The problem with load-reducers is, in general, the frequent development of tolerance—a possible problem also with digitalis (see p 94) so that these agents in turn are now frequently being replaced by ACE inhibitors.

ACE inhibitors are increasingly used in heart failure (see p 156), especially in preference to high-dose diuretics or other vasodilators. Relatively little tolerance has been found with *captopril,* which is an 'indirect' diuretic by its ultimate anti-aldosterone effect. Unfortunately the use of all ACE inhibitors may be limited by hypotension (use low initial dose). Neutropenia or renal damage are possible yet rare risks, seldom expected at captopril doses used for CHF (12.5–50 mg 2–3× daily after an initial dose of 6.25 mg). *Enalapril* is now also increasingly used for CHF (dose: 10–20 mg, 1–2× daily after an initial dose of 2.5 mg).

Special problems. In those unusual patients who have heart failure and severe restriction of the GFR (such as 15–20 ml/min), high doses of furosemide alone or combined with metolazone are used. In patients with borderline diabetes or mild diabetes or increasing glucose intolerance or gout, neither thiazides nor furosemide can be used with impunity; now spironolactone becomes the agent of choice yet it is unfortunately only of low diuretic potency. Therefore captopril or enalapril is a reasonable alternative.

SUMMARY

Diuretics are powerful therapeutic agents with the potential for major and serious side-effects. Thus the risk-benefit ratio in the therapy of mild hypertension is increasingly questioned except in three groups of patients: the elderly, black patients and the obese. Patients with renal impairment also require a diuretic (loop or metolazone). For most hypertensives, low-dose thiazide diuretic, probably with a potassium-retaining component (amiloride or triamterene) might be the answer. The risk-benefit ratio of diuretics is high in the therapy of heart failure, and their use remains standard.

Yet not all patients require vigorous diuresis; rather each patient needs careful clinical evaluation with a specific cardiological diagnosis so that surgically correctable defects are appropriately handled. Thereafter a thiazide diuretic (for mild heart failure) or a loop diuretic (for severe heart failure) may be chosen. With intermediate severities of failure, increasing doses of thiazide or metolazone may be used before switching to a loop diuretic such as furosemide. We stress that automatic addition of oral potassium supplements is not ideal practice. Rather, the combination of a loop diuretic plus low-dose thiazide plus potassium-retaining diuretic is reasonable, except in the presence of renal failure when loop diuretics with metolazone seem better.

The next step is variable. High-dose furosemide used to be the next choice and can still be used; the dangers of volume depletion, electrolyte imbalance, and activation of the renin-angiotensin axis are very real. Therefore additional therapy with captopril or enalapril seems preferable unless limited by side-effects such as hypotension. Potassium-retaining diuretics (amiloride, triamterene, spironolactone) must be avoided with ACE inhibitors, as should oral potassium supplements, unless there is still proven hypokalemia.

ACKNOWLEDGMENT

This Chapter was reviewed with the kind assistance of P.J. Commerford, C.R. Swanepoel, and W.P. Leary.

REFERENCES

1. Abildgaard U, Aldershvile J, Ring-Larsen H, et al: Bed rest and increased diuretic treatment in chronic congestive heart failure. Eur Heart J 6:1040–1046, 1985
2. Acchiardo SR, Skoutakis VA: Clinical efficacy, safety, and pharmacokinetics of indapamide in renal impairment. Am Heart J 106:237–244, 1983
3. Andreasen F, Hansen U, Husted SE: The influence of age on renal and extrarenal effects of furosemide. Br J Clin Pharmacol 18:65–74, 1984
3a. Beermann B, Groschinsky-Grind M: Antihypertensive effect of various doses of hydrochlorothiazide and its relation to the plasma level of the drug. Eur J Clin Pharmacol 13:195–201, 1978
4. Asbury MJ, Gatenby PBB, O'Sullivan S, et al: Bumetanide: Potent new "loop" diuretic. Br Med J 1:211–213, 1972
5. Berglund G, Andersson O: Beta-blockers or diuretics in hypertension A six year follow-up of blood pressure and metabolic side-effects. Lancet i:744–747, 1981
6. Biddle TL, Yu PN: Effect of furosemide on hemodynamics and lung water in acute pulmonary edema secondary to myocardial infarction. Am J Cardiol 43:86–90, 1979
7. Brater DC, Chennavasin P, Day B, et al: Bumetanide and furosemide. Clin Pharmacol Ther 34:207–213, 1983
8. Caruso FS, Szabadi RR, Vukovich RA: Pharmacokinetics and clinical pharmacology of indapamide. Am Heart J 106:212–220, 1983
9. Carriere S, Dandavino R: Bumetanide, a new loop diuretic. Clin Pharmacol Ther 20:424–438, 1976
10. Chatterjee K, Parmley WW: Vasodilator therapy for acute myocardial infarction and chronic congestive heart failure. J Am Coll Cardiol 1:133–153, 1983
11. Dargie HJ, Allison MEM, Kennedy AC, et al: High dosage metolazone in chronic renal failure. Br Med J 4:196–198, 1972
12. Davidov ME, McNight JE, Osborne JL: A cross-over comparison between chlorthalidone and furosemide in essential hypertension. Curr Ther Res 25:1–9, 1979
13. Devane J, Ryan MP: The effects of amiloride and triamterene on urinary magnesium excretion in conscious saline loaded rats. Br J Pharmacol 72:285–289, 1981

14. Devane J, Ryan MP: Evidence for a magnesium-sparing action by amiloride during renal clearance studies in rats. Br J Pharmacol 79:891–896, 1983

15. Drug and Therapeutics Bulletin: Choice of a powerful diuretic. Drug Ther Bull 17:47–48, 1979

16. Dyckner T, Helmers C, Lundman T, et al: Initial serum potassium level in relation to early complications and prognosis in patients with acute myocardial infarction. Acta Med Scand 197:207–210, 1975

17. Dzau VJ, Hollenberg NK: Renal response to captopril in severe heart failure: Role of furosemide in natriuresis and reversal of hyponatremia. Ann Intern Med 100:777–782, 1984

18. Dzau VJ, Packer M, Lilly LS, et al: Prostaglandins in severe congestive heart failure. Relation to activation of the renin-angiotensin system and hyponatremia. New Engl J Med 310:347–352, 1984

19. Flamenbaum W, Friedman R: Pharmacology, therapeutic efficacy and adverse effects of bumetanide, a new "loop" diuretic. Pharmacotherapy 2:213–222, 1982

20. Forrester JS, Diamond G, Chatterjee K, et al: Medical therapy of acute myocardial infarction by application of haemodynamic subsets. New Engl J Med 295:1356–1362, 1404–1413, 1976

21. Freis ED: How diuretics lower blood pressure. Am Heart J 106:185–187, 1983

22. Green TP, Thompson TR, Johnson DE, et al: Furosemide promotes patent ductus arteriosus in premature infants with respiratory distress syndrome. New Engl J Med 308:743–748, 1983

23. Greenberg A, Walia R, Puschett JB: Combined effect of bumetanide and metolazone in normal volunteers. Abstract. First International Conference on Diuretics, 1984, p 36

23a. Helfant RH: Hypokalemia and arrhythmias. Am J Med 80 (suppl 4A):13–22, 1986

23b. Hollifield JW: Thiazide treatment of hypertension. Effects of thiazide diuretics on serum potassium, magnesium, and ventricular ectopy. Am J Med 80 (suppl 4A):8–12, 1986

23c. Hollenberg NK, Bannon JA: The PACT Study: Post-marketing surveillance in 47,465 patients treated with Maxzide (triamterene/ hydrochlorothiazide). An interim report. Am J Med 80 (suppl 4A):30–36, 1986

24. Hulley SB, Furberg CD, Gurland B, et al: Systolic hypertension in the elderly program (SHEP): Antihypertensive efficacy of chlorthalidone. Am J Cardiol 56:913–920, 1985

25. Huston G: Diuretics, in Hamer J (ed): Drugs for Heart Disease. London, Chapman and Hall, 1979, pp 513–547

26. Jahnsen T, Skovborg F, Hansen F, et al: Variations in blood viscosity in patients with acute cardiogenic pulmonary oedema treated with frusemide. Scand J Clin Lab Invest 43:297–300, 1983

27. Johansson BW, Dziamski R: Malignant arrhythmias in acute myocardial infarction. Relationship to serum potassium and effect of selective and non-selective β-blockade. Drugs 28 (suppl 1):77–85, 1984

28. Jones B, Nanra RS: Double-blind trial of antihypertensive effect of chlorothiazide in severe renal failure. Lancet ii:1258–1260, 1979

28a. Kaplan NM, Carnegie A, Raskin P, et al: Potassium supplementation in hypertensive patients with diuretic-induced hypokalemia. New Engl J Med 312:746–749, 1985

29. Kehoe WA, Guslielmo BJ: Excessive potassium depletion with metolazone and furosemide. Clin Pharmac 2:304–305, 1983

30. Klutsch K, Schmidt P, Grosswendt J: Der Einfluss von BAYa1040 auf die nierenfunktion des hypertonikers. Arzneim-Forschung (Drug Res) 22:377–380, 1972

31. Kreeft JH, Langlois S, Ogilvie RI: Comparative trial of indapamide and hydrochlorothiazide in essential hypertension with forearm plethysmography. J Cardiovasc Pharmacol 6:622–626, 1984

32. Kuchar DL, O'Rourke MF: High dose furosemide in refractory cardiac failure. Eur Heart J 6:954–958, 1985

33. Lancet review: Triamterene and the kidney. Lancet i:424, 1986

34. Landmark K: Antihypertensive and metabolic effects of long-term therapy with nifedipine slow-release tablets. J Cardiovasc Pharmacol 7:12–17, 1985

34a. Larsen FF, Mogensen L: Influence of prophylactic furosemide on arrhythmias in acute myocardial infarction—a controlled study. Eur Heart J 7:210–216, 1986

35. Licht JH, Haley RJ, Pugh B, et al: Diuretic regimens in essential hypertension. A comparison of hypokalemic effects, BP control, and cost. Arch Int Med 143:1694–1699, 1983

36. Lowe J, Gray J, Henry DA, et al: Adverse reactions to frusemide in hospital inpatients. Br Med J 2:360–362, 1979

37. MacGregor GA, Banks RA, Markandu ND, et al: Lack of effect of β-blocker on flat dose response to thiazide in hypertension: Efficacy of low-dose thiazide combined with β-blocker. Br Med J 286:1535–1538, 1983

38. Maclean D, Tudhope GR: Modern diuretic treatment. Br Med J 286:1419–1422, 1983

39. Maronde RF, Milgrom M, Vlachakis ND, et al: Response of thiazide-induced hypokalemia to amiloride. JAMA 249:237–241, 1983

40. McKibbin JK, Pocock WA, Barlow JB, et al: Sotalol, hypokalaemia, syncope, and torsade de pointes. Br Heart J 51:157–162, 1984

41. Medical Research Council Working Party on Mild to Moderate Hypertension: Adverse reactions to bendrofluazide and propranolol for the treatment of mild hypertension. Lancet ii:539–543, 1981

42. Medical Research Council Working Party on Mild to Moderate Hypertension: Ventricular extrasystoles during thiazide treatment: substudy of MRC mild hypertension trial. Br Med J 287:1249–1253, 1983

43. Millar JA, McLean K, Reid JL: Calcium antagonists decrease adrenal and vascular responsiveness to angiotensin II in normal man. Clin Sci 61:65S-68S, 1981

44. Morgan DB, Davidson C: Hypokalemia and diuretics: an analysis of publications. Br Med J 280:905–908, 1980

45. Mudge GH: Diuretics and other agents employed in the mobilization of edema fluid, in Gilman AG, Goodman LS, Gilman AG (eds): The Pharmacological Basis of Therapeutics, 6th ed. New York, MacMillan Publishing Co, 1980, pp 892–915

46. Muller FO, Meyer BH, de Waal A, et al: Potassium balance in piretanide and digoxin treatment. Clin Pharmacol Ther 31:339–342, 1982

47. Murphy MB, Scriven AJI, Dollery CT: Role of nifedipine in treatment of hypertension. Br Med J 287:257–259, 1983

48. Nordrehaug JE, von der Lippe G: Hypokalaemia and ventricular fibrillation in acute myocardial infarction. Br Heart J 50:525–529, 1983

49. Oliw E, Kover G, Larsson C, et al: Reduction by indomethacin of furosemide effects in the rabbit. Eur J Pharmacol 38:95–100, 1976

49a. Papademetriou V: Diuretics, hypokalemia, and cardiac arrhythmias: A critical analysis. Am Heart J 111:1217–1224, 1986

50. Papademetriou V, Fletcher R, Khatri I, et al: Diuretic-induced hypokalemia in uncomplicated systemic hypertension: Effect of plasma potassium correction on cardiac arrhythmias. Am J Cardiol 52:1017–1022, 1983

50a. Patterson DJ, Weinstein GS, Jeffries GH: Endoscopic comparison of solid and liquid potassium chloride supplements. Lancet ii:1077–1078, 1983

51. Perez-Stable E, Caralis PV: Thiazide-induced disturbances in carbohydrate, lipid and potassium metabolism. Am Heart J 106:245–251, 1983

52. Perry HM: Some wrong-way chemical changes during antihypertensive treatment: Comparison of indapamide and related agents. Am Heart J 106:251–257, 1983

52a. Raison J, Achimastos A, Asmar R, et al: Extracellular and interstitial fluid volume in obesity with and without associated systemic hypertension. Am J Cardiol 57:223–226, 1986

53. Reubi FC, Cottier PT: Effects of reduced glomerular filtration rate on responsiveness to chlorothiazide and mercurial diuretics. Circulation 23:200–210, 1961

54. Reyes AJ, Leary WP: Indapamide: A review. S Afr Med J 64 (suppl):1–5, 1983

55. Riegger GAJ, Liebau G, Kochsiek K: Antidiuretic hormone in congestive heart failure. Am J Med 72:49–52, 1982

56. Smith TW, Braunwald E: The management of heart failure, in Braunwald E (ed): Heart Disease, 2nd ed. Philadelphia, Saunders, 1984, pp 527–534

57. Stanaszek WF, Romankiewicz JA: Current approaches to management of potassium deficiency. Drug Intell Clin Pharm 19:176–183, 1985

58. Stewart DE, Ikram H, Espiner EA, et al: Arrhythmogenic potential of diuretic induced hypokalaemia in patients with mild hypertension and ischaemic heart disease. Br Heart J 54:290–297, 1985

59. Struthers AD, Whitesmith R, Reid JL: Prior thiazide diuretic treatment increases adrenaline-induced hypokalaemia. Lancet i:1358–1361, 1983

60. Szatalowicz VL, Arnold PE, Chaimovitz C, et al: Radioimmunoassay of plasma arginine vasopressin in hyponatremic patients with congestive heart failure. New Engl J Med 305:263–266, 1981

61. Thomas JP, Thompson WH: Comparison of thiazides and amiloride in treatment of moderate hypertension. Br Med J 286:2015–2018, 1983

62. Van der Elst E, Dombey SL, Lawrence J: Controlled comparison of the effects of furosemide and hydrochlorothiazide added to propranolol in the treatment of hypertension. Am Heart J 102:734–740, 1981

63. Wasnich RD, Benfante RJ, Yano K, et al: Thiazide effect on the mineral content of bone. New Engl J Med 309:344–347, 1983

64. Webster J: Interactions of NSAIDs with diuretics and β-blockers. Mechanism and clinical implications. Drugs 30:32–41, 1985

65. Weidmann P, Uehlinger DE, Gerber A: Antihypertensive treatment and serum lipoproteins. J Hypertens 3:297–306, 1985

66. Weinberger MH: Influence of an angiotensin converting enzyme inhibitor on diuretic-induced metabolic effects in hypertension. Hypertension 5 (suppl III):132–138, 1983

67. Williams ES, Fisch C: Treatment of Cardiac Failure, in Rosen MR, Hoffman BF (eds): Cardiac Therapy. Boston, Martinus Nijhoff, 1983, pp 453–479

68.   Wollam GL, Tarazi RC, Bravo EL, et al: Diuretic potency of combined hydroch-
       lorothiazide and furosemide therapy in patients with azotemia. Am J Med 72:929–
       938, 1982
69.   Wong DG, Spence JD, Lamki L, et al: Effect of non-steroidal anti-inflammatory drugs
       on control of hypertension by beta-blockers and diuretics. Lancet i:997–1001, 1986

Reviews

Lant A: Diuretics. Clinical Pharmacology and Therapeutic Use (Part I). Drugs 29:57–87,
   1985
Lant A: Diuretics. Clinical Pharmacology and Therapeutic Use (Part II). Drugs 29:162–
   188, 1985

L. H. Opie
K. Chatterjee
D. C. Harrison

7

Vasodilating Drugs

PRINCIPLES

Vasodilation, once a specialized procedure, is now common place in cardiac therapy as the peripheral circulation has become one of the prime sites of action. There are two major classifications for vasodilators. Clinically most important is the vascular bed involved: nitrates are predominantly venodilators, hydralazine and the calcium antagonists predominantly arteriolar dilators, whereas nitroprusside, prazosin, and the new angiotensin-converting enzyme (ACE) inhibitors are mixed agents. Reduction of the preload is chiefly required in "backward" congestive heart failure (CHF) or in acute pulmonary edema, whereas reduction of the afterload is required in "forward" CHF or in other low output states (not resulting from obstructive valvular disease), or in systemic hypertension. Arteriolar dilators may also act regionally and more specifically on certain vascular beds such as in Raynaud's syndrome (calcium antagonists), extracranial vessels (verapamil for migraine), cerebral vessels (nimodipine for subarachnoid hemorrhage), pulmonary circulation (nitrates, calcium antagonists, hydralazine), and the renal circulation (dopamine-like agents). Second, vasodilators may be classified according to the mechanism of action (Table 7-1) that is now reasonably well understood except for the "direct" agents such as hydralazine.

Neurohumoral Effects of Severe Heart Failure

Increased activity of the autonomic nervous system and elevation of circulating norepinephrine (NE) as one of the compensating mechanisms for heart failure gained widespread acceptance in the 1960s. The next concept was that excessive vasoconstriction by a similar mechanism aggravated heart failure to become a new site for action of therapeutic agents. The third concept was that enhanced activity of the renin-angiotensin system, another result of excess adrenergic activity, made a further contribution to the increased peripheral vascular resistance and to fluid retention by stimulation of the secretion of aldosterone (*renin-angiotensin-aldosterone activation*). Fourth, angiotensin may stimulate the release of vasopressin which contributes to abnormal volume regulation and hyponatremia in severe CHF.[12a]

Similar compensating mechanisms and their physiologic excess may occur even in mild forms of heart failure. These hypotheses suggest that there is an "afterload mismatch" between the level of vascular resistance and the heart's ability to deliver enough blood to meet the body's demands, especially during exertion, because the systolic wall stresses are too high for depressed contractility. Today, vasodilators are widely used as adjuvants in the therapy of heart failure (Table 7-2).

Drugs for the Heart, Second Expanded Edition
Copyright © 1987 by Grune & Stratton, Inc.

TABLE 7-1

CLASSIFICATION OF VASODILATORS

Category	Proposed Mechanism	Examples
Nitrate-like agents	Stimulate guanylate cyclase with formation of cyclic GMP	Nitrates Nitroprusside
Direct vasodilators	Unknown	Hydralazine Diazoxide Minoxidil
α_1-antagonists	Inhibition of α_1 mediated calcium ingress	Prazosin Labetalol (Indoramin)*
α_1-α_2-antagonists	Inhibition of α_1-α_2 mediated calcium ingress	Phentolamine Phenoxybenzamine
Calcium antagonists	Inhibit calcium ingress	Nifedipine Verapamil Diltiazem New dihydropyridines*
Angiotensin-converting enzyme inhibitors	Decrease formation of vaso-constrictory angiotensin II, inhibit secretion of aldosterone	Captopril Enalapril Ramipril*
β_2-agonists	Inhibit formation of cyclic AMP to decrease myosin light chain kinase activity in vessel wall	Isoproterenol Dobutamine Salbutamol-albuterol
Dopamine agonists	Inhibition of release of NE from terminal neurons	Dopamine (Ibopamine, Dopexamine)*
Central α_2 agonists	Central inhibition of adrenergic outflow	Clonidine Methyldopa
Under development	Serotonin antagonism Prostacyclin-like agents Atrial natriuretic peptide	(Ketanserin)* — —

Compiled by LH Opie
* Not in the USA

TABLE 7-2

VASODILATORS: ROUTE OF ADMINISTRATION AND MAJOR SITE OF ACTION

Agent	Vascular Bed
Intravenous Only	
Nitroprusside	Balanced arteriolar and venous
Dobutamine	Arteriolar
Dopamine	Arteriolar and renal
IV and Oral	
Nitrates	Venous > arteriolar
Labetalol	Arteriolar (also β-blocking)
Diazoxide	Arteriolar
Verapamil	Arteriolar (negative inotropic effect)
Hydralazine	Arteriolar
Furosemide	Venous (diuretic chiefly)
Sublingual	
Nitrates	Venous > arteriolar
Nifedipine	Arteriolar including pulmonary
Captopril	Arteriolar > venous
Oral	
Nitrates	Venous > arteriolar
α_1 Antagonists	Venous + arteriolar
ACE inhibitors	Arteriolar > venous
Calcium antagonists	Arteriolar
Direct dilators	Arteriolar
β-Agonists	Arteriolar >> venous

Compiled by LH Opie

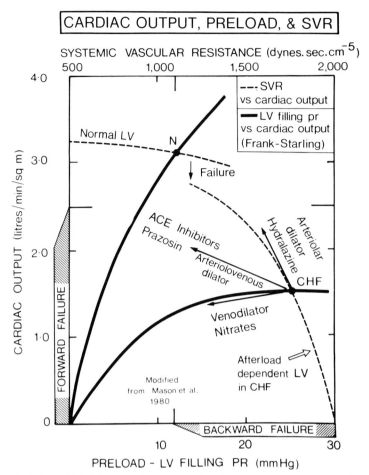

Fig. 7-1. A high left ventricular (LV) end-diastolic pressure causes congestive symptoms, i.e. dyspnea. A low cardiac output causes symptoms of forward failure, i.e. fatigue. Two basic therapies are vasodilators reducing the LV end-diastolic pressure; and agents increasing contractile activity of the heart such as digitalis. In normal heart (point N), cardiac output (CO) is principally regulated by changes in preload; alterations in impedance are of minor importance. In contrast, in congestive heart failure (CHF), CO is principally regulated by changes in impedance ("afterload-dependent"); alterations in preload are of minor importance. In CHF, the pure arteriodilator, hydralazine, raises lowered CO markedly with mild decline of elevated left ventricular end-diastolic pressure (LVEDP); the angiotensin-converting enzyme inhibitors and prazosin act on both venous and arterial systems to raise the lowered CO and to decrease elevated LVEDP; and the pure venodilator, sublingual nitroglycerin, decreases elevated LVEDP markedly with little or no improvement of lowered CO. (Modified from Mason DT, Awan NA, Joye JA, et al: Treatment of acute and chronic congestive heart failure by vasodilator afterload reduction. Arch Intern Med 140: 1577–1581, 1980. With permission).

Preload Reduction

The preload is the left ventricular (LV) filling pressure, raised in left heart failure (Fig. 7-1). It is measured indirectly by insertion of a Swan-Ganz flotation catheter via the right heart into the pulmonary capillary bed to obtain the "wedge" pressure. Normally as the preload increases so also does the peak LV systolic pressure, and the cardiac output rises (ascending limb of the Frank-Starling curve, Fig. 7-2). But in diseased hearts the increase in cardiac output is much less than normal, and the output may even fall as the filling pressure rises (the controversial descending limb of the curve, Fig. 7-2). However, the optimal

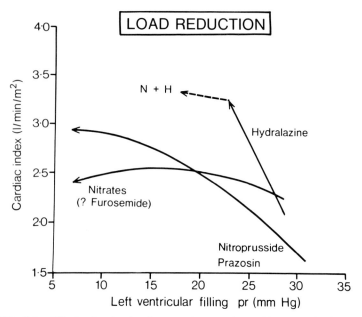

Fig. 7-2. Effects of oral unloading agents on patients with congestive heart failure. Prazosin reduces both preload and afterload with an increased cardiac index. Hydralazine has a more impressive inotropic effect (by afterload reduction and directly); however reduction of filling pressure requires added nitrates. Nitrates decrease the filling pressure without increasing the cardiac index, unless there is added arteriolar dilation. Nitroprusside has a "balanced" effect decreasing preload and afterload. N + H = nitrates + hydralazine.

filling pressure for the diseased heart is higher than normal so that excess reduction of the preload should be avoided. Clinically, the major drugs reducing the preload in CHF are furosemide with its combined diuretic-vasodilator effect (see pp 112 and 126) and nitrates that dilate the systemic veins to reduce the venous return and the filling pressure on the left heart (Table 7-3).

Afterload Reduction

In strict terms, the aim of arteriolar vasodilation therapy is to reduce the aortic impedance (aortic pressure divided by the aortic flow at the same instant). In heart failure, the emphasis is put upon the reduction of the peripheral vascular resistance—this is not the same as blood pressure reduction, because a compensatory increase in the cardiac output tends to maintain the arterial pressure. According to the LaPlace law, the tension on the walls of a thin-walled sphere equals the intraluminal pressure times the radius. Wall tension is one of the major determinants of the myocardial oxygen uptake. Afterload reduction hence implies a decrease in the myocardial oxygen uptake. In contrast, positive inotropes such as digitalis increase the work of the heart and the oxygen uptake unless they reduce the heart size, which will reduce wall tension and tend to reduce oxygen uptake.

Thus, as in ischemic heart disease, one of the aims in chronic heart failure is to improve the myocardial oxygen balance. In CHF, the tension on the LV wall rises as the LV end-diastolic pressure increases and the cavity dilates; this process predisposes to subendocardial ischemia which, in turn, may perpetrate myocardial failure even in the absence of ischemic cardiomyopathy.[28]

Hypertension

In systemic hypertension, a raised peripheral vascular resistance is an important perpetuating and/or initiating mechanism, so that arteriolar vasodilation is an increasingly popular mode of action of antihypertensive agents.

TABLE 7-3   THE PRINCIPLE HEMODYNAMIC EFFECTS OF NONPARENTERAL VASODILATORS IN CHRONIC HEART FAILURE

Vasodilator	Heart Rate	Blood Pressure	Cardiac Output	Systemic Vascular Resistance	Right Atrial Pressure	Pulmonary Venous Pressure	Pulmonary Vascular Resistance
Nitrates	0/↑	Slight ↓	0/↓	0/ (high dose ↓)	↓↓	↓↓	↓
Hydralazine Endralazine	0/↑	0/↓	↑↑	↓↓	0	0/↓	0/↓
Minoxidil	0/↑	0/↓	↑↑	↓↓	0	0/↓	0/↓
Prazosin Trimazosin	0/↓	↓	↑	↓↓	↓↓	↓↓	↓
Captopril Enalapril	0/↓	↓	↑	↓↓	↓	↓	0/↓
Nifedipine Felodipine	0/↑	↓	↑	↓	0/↓	0/↓	↓
Diltiazem	↓/↓↓	↓	0/↑	↓	0/↓	0/↓	0/↓
Pirbuterol	0/↑	0/↓	↑	↓	↓	↓	0/↓
Salbutamol	0/↑	0/↓	↑	↓	0/↓	0/↓	0/↓

Modified from Chatterjee K: Vasodilators, in Weatherall DJ, Ledingham JCG (eds): Oxford Textbook of Medicine. Oxford, Oxford University Press, 1986 (in press). With permission.

0 = no effect
↑ = moderate increase; ↑↑ = marked increase
↓ = moderate decrease; ↓↓ = marked decrease.

Originally only hydralazine was available for prolonged oral therapy; its use was limited by side-effects such as reflex tachycardia and fluid retention, so that it was seen largely as a third-line agent, after diuretics and β-blockers. **Now the advent of a new generation of vasodilators with relatively few side-effects, including the calcium antagonists and ACE inhibitors, means that vasodilation is increasingly seen as a possible second or even first-line therapy.**

NITRATE-LIKE VASODILATORS

Nitroprusside*

IV nitroprusside (Nitride®) remains the reference vasodilator for severe low output left-sided heart failure because it acts rapidly and has a balanced effect, dilating both arterioles and veins. Nitroprusside seems particularly useful for increasing LV stroke work in severe refractory heart failure caused by mitral or aortic incompetence. Hemodynamic and clinical improvement are also observed in patients with severe pump failure complicating acute myocardial infarction (AMI), in heart failure after cardiac surgery, and in patients with acute exacerbation of chronic heart failure. Because of the increased stroke volume there may be considerable hemodynamic improvement without much hypotension; but, in general, some hypotension accompanies and may limit the therapeutic effect of nitroprusside.

Pharmacokinetics. With infusion of nitroprusside the hemodynamic response (direct vasodilation) starts within minutes and stops equally quickly. Nitroprusside given intravenously is converted to cyanmethemoglobin and free cyanide in the red cells; the free cyanide is then converted to thiocyanate in the liver, and is cleared by the kidneys (half-life 7 days).

Dose. An initial infusion of 10 μg/min is increased by 10 μg/min every 10 minutes up to 40–75 μg/min with a top dose of 300 μg/min.

Precautions. The infusion rate needs careful titration against the blood pressure, which must be continously monitored to avoid excess hypotension. Nitroprusside must not be abruptly withdrawn because of the danger of rebound hypertension. Extravasation must be avoided. The solution in normal saline (avoid alkaline solutions) must be freshly made and then shielded from light during infusion; it should be discarded when 4 hours old, or before if discolored. Cyanide may accumulate with prolonged high doses of nitroprusside to produce a lactic acidosis. Toxicity can be avoided by monitoring blood lactate and blood thiocyanate (toxic level 100 μg/mL). But in lactic acidosis due to poor tissue perfusion nitroprusside may be beneficial.

Indications. (1) For hemodynamic improvement in selected patients with myocardial infarction and LV failure; (2) severe CHF with regurgitant valve disease; (3) in hypertensive crises associated with LV failure; (4) in dissecting aneurysm; and (5) postoperative coronary bypass surgery, when patients frequently have reactive hypertension as they are removed from hypothermia, so that nitroprussides or nitrates are routinely given by most cardiovascular surgical units for 24 hours provided that hypotension is no problem.

Contraindications. Pre-existing hypotension (systolic < 90 mmHg, diastolic < 60 mmHg). All vasodilators are contraindicated in severe obstructive valvular heart disease (aortic or mitral or pulmonic stenosis). In patients with ventricular septal defect, nitroprusside can cause a disproportionate increase in pulmonary vascular resistance with increased left-to-right shunt.

Side-effects. Overvigorous treatment may cause an excessive drop in LV end-diastolic pressure, severe hypotension, and myocardial ischemia. Fatigue, nausea, vomiting, and disorientation tend to arise especially when treatment continues for more than 48 hours. In patients with renal failure, thiocyanate accumulates with high dose infusions and may produce hypothyroidism after prolonged therapy. In chronic cor pulmonale, hypoxia may develop (increased ventilation-perfusion mismatch with pulmonary vasodilation).

Combination with other agents. Nitroprusside may be combined with inotropic agents such as dopamine and dobutamine (Fig. 7-3) and with digitalis to optimize the hemodynamic benefit. Maintaining an adequate ventricular filling pressure is essential with these combined therapies and invasive monitoring is required.

---

*For references, see previous edition.

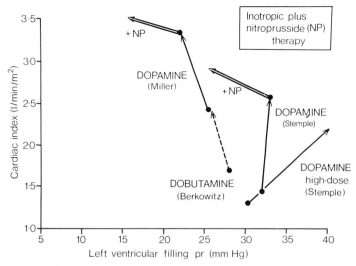

Fig. 7-3. Combined inotropic and vasodilator therapy with dopamine or dobutamine plus nitroprusside. Only vasodilator therapy decreases left ventricular filling pressure; inotropic therapy increases cardiac index.

Nitroprusside—Summary

Nitroprusside, the prototype IV vasodilator, has balanced venous and arteriolar effects. It is a powerful agent that requires invasive monitoring to avoid excess reduction of preload or hypotension which can develop very rapidly. When no longer required, nitroprusside must be tapered and not abruptly reduced. The use of sublingual nifedipine for acute afterload reduction and the efficacy of nitrates and furosemide for preload reduction, have tended to decrease the indications for nitroprusside that must be much more carefully monitored than the other agents because of its very rapid onset and cessation of activity. Nonetheless, nitroprusside is still the vasodilator of choice in many acute emergency situations.

Nitrates*

Nitrates are now used in the therapy of both acute LV failure and chronic heart failure. Their major effect is venous rather than arteriolar dilation, thus being most suited to patients with raised pulmonary wedge pressure and clinical features of pulmonary congestion. A newly described effect is pulmonary arteriolar dilation, thereby easing the work of the right ventricle during exercise. They are not suited for the therapy of hypertension uncomplicated by CHF.

Dose. Sublingual nitrates (0.8–2.4 mg every 5–10 minutes) or isosorbide dinitrate (10 mg sublingually or orally) are becoming popular in the management of acute pulmonary edema; they induce a "pharmacologic phlebotomy". In chronic CHF, the dose of isosorbide dinitrate is 10 mg sublingually every 4 hours or 80 mg 4× daily. Doses for other preparations are given in Table 2-1.

Indications. (1) In acute pulmonary edema, sublingual nitrates are usually given with IV furosemide; (2) severe chronic CHF, used as sole vasodilators or in combination with other agents such as hydralazine (see summary) or ACE inhibitors; (3) in ischemic heart disease associated with CHF, nitrates may also have a direct coronary vasodilating effect; hence nitrates are the agents of choice in the presence of both angina and heart failure; (4) postoperative hypertension, where nitrates are as effective as nitroprusside; (5) in occasional patients with precapillary pulmonary hypertension, nitrates give hemodynamic and clinical benefit with however unpredictable effects.

---

*For references, see Chapter 2.

Side-effects of nitrates.   Headaches, a troublesome feature of vasodilator therapy for hypertension and angina, may be less common in heart failure. For other side-effects, see Table 2-2.

Vascular tolerance.   Whether high-dose nitrates used in the treatment of CHF cause clinically significant tolerance, as in the therapy of angina pectoris, is controversial. When nitrates first work and then seem not to, a "nitrate-free" interval (first reducing and then stopping the dose) provides a test.

Nitrates—Summary

In CHF, nitrates are used for preload reduction. They are especially of benefit when given sublingually in acute pulmonary edema. Although nitrate tolerance may be a problem during prolonged therapy, isosorbide dinitrate 40 mg 4× daily combined with hydralazine 300 mg daily has been shown to produce unequivocal long-term benefits in patients with severe heart failure in a double-blind, randomized trial.[11a]

DIRECT ACTING VASODILATORS

Hydralazine

Hydralazine (Apresoline®), a drug that has been in and out of favor over the years and firmly in favor at the time of the first edition of this book (1980), now once again seems to be on the wane. The introduction of other vasodilators such as nifedipine has limited the use of hydralazine in hypertension. Nonetheless, hydralazine is still widely used as a third-line agent in hypertension and the agent of choice in some obstetrical patients with pre-eclampsia. The observation that tolerance occurs during prolonged hydralazine therapy of CHF[8] has further limited its use. Thus after 9 months of therapy of CHF, tolerance to hydralazine was a specific tachyphylaxis with a maintained response to nitroprusside. Despite these caveats, combined vasodilator treatment of CHF with two drugs (hydralazine and nitrates), both thought to induce tolerance, has achieved long-term benefit.[11a]

Pharmacologic effects.   Hydralazine is predominantly an arteriolar dilator and may also have some indirect positive inotropic effect.[6] It causes a marked increase in cardiac output with little or no decrease in pulmonary wedge or right atrial pressures (Fig. 7-2). In healthy subjects, the arteriolar vasodilation causes a reflex tachycardia, but in CHF hydralazine causes little change in the heart rate, perhaps because the failure dampens reflex arcs.[1] Hydralazine is particularly effective in patients with mitral regurgitation. It increases forward stroke volume and decreases regurgitant volume.[2]

Pharmacokinetics.   Hydralazine is rapidly absorbed from the gut (peak concentration 1–2 hours). The plasma half-life is 2–8 hours but the hypotensive effect is long-lasting, possibly because hydralazine is taken up avidly by the arterial wall. It is metabolized via acetylation in the liver with subsequent excretion in the urine. In severe renal failure, the dosage should be reduced. Patients with fast acetylation rates need a dose about 25 percent higher than those with slow rates. The lupus syndrome is more likely to develop in a slow acetylator.

Dose and indications.   In *chronic LV failure*, oral hydralazine (50–75 mg every 6 hours, top dose 800 mg/day) is effective for at least 4–6 weeks when added to digoxin and diuretics.[4] Long term benefit is doubtful, unless combined with nitrates.[8,11a] With high doses the risk of lupus must be weighed against possible benefits.

In *severe aortic regurgitation*, oral hydralazine 150–200 mg only every 12 hours gave moderately well sustained effects over 12 hours with a low incidence of acute side-effects; this regime should improve patient compliance and can also be tested in severe heart failure of other etiologies.[22]

In *severe mitral regurgitation*, acute hydralazine (0.3 mg/kg IV, maximum 20 mg over 5 minutes) increases forward stroke volume and reduces regurgitation.[5] The oral dose is 50–100 mg 4× daily.

In *dilated cardiomyopathy*, IV hydralazine (5 mg doses every 5 minutes, 10–60 mg) acts by a reduction of the elevated LV wall stress, with little or no inotropic effect.[26]

In *hypertensive emergencies* (Table 11-5), an infusion of 20–40 mg takes about 20 minutes to act. Compensatory tachycardia (blunted in patients with chronic heart failure) contraindicates hydralazine in acute hypertension with pre-existing angina.

In *mild to moderate hypertension*, the usual dose is 50–75 mg 6- or 8-hourly, but two divided doses a day are equally effective.

In *heart failure following cardiac surgery*, hydralazine (test dose 2.5–5.0 mg IV, up to 7.5 mg every 4–6 hours) generally gives improvement within 8 hours.[10]

In *pregnancy with pre-eclampsia*, IV hydralazine 40 mg can be infused by itself or with diazepam 40 mg (both in 500 mL) to keep the blood pressure below 150/100 mmHg. Hydralazine is said to improve uterine blood flow, but data are scant. *Dihydralazine* (Nepresol®) is frequently used as 6.25–12.5 mg IV slowly or infused at 0.1 mg/min to a total of 25 mg.

In *precapillary pulmonary hypertension*, hydralazine may decrease pulmonary vascular resistance; however, without hemodynamic monitoring, hydralazine therapy should not be initiated as severe side-effects may also occur.

In *dilated cardiomyopathy*, hydralazine therapy leads to a regression of myocardial cellular hypertrophy,[28] perhaps because of the dominant unloading effect.

In contrast, in experimental *myocardial hypertrophy of hypertension*, hydralazine can bring down the pressure without causing regression of the hypertrophy, presumably because of the partial inotropic effect or the reflex stimulation of the adrenergic nervous system.

The *intramuscular* use of dihydralazine or hydralazine is still unfortunately frequent but must be avoided because variable rates of absorption may cause unpredictable hypotension with dangerous end-organ underperfusion.

Side-effects.   Side-effects include fluid retention (renin release) that may necessitate diuretic therapy. In hypertension, the direct inotropic effect and the tachycardia limit the usefulness of hydralazine in patients with angina pectoris not on β-blockade. In contrast, in CHF, reflex tachycardia is unusual, perhaps because reflex arcs are blunted. The lupus syndrome is rare with doses below 200 mg a day or with total doses below 100g. Patients on higher doses or prolonged therapy should be checked for antinuclear factors. Headache, nausea, and abdominal pain are not unusual at the start of therapy. Postural hypotension is occasionally seen in patients with congestive failure. Polyneuropathy (usually responsive to pyridoxin) and drug fever are rare side-effects.

Combination with other agents.   In hypertension, hydralazine is best combined with β-blockade (to avoid headache, tachycardia, angina) and diuretics (to avoid fluid retention). In heart failure, long-term combination with isosorbide dinitrate beneficially improves mortality.[11a] Hydralazine should normally not be combined with captopril (possibility of enhanced immune effects).

Hydralazine—Summary

Hydralazine is now used less in the therapy of CHF but retains popularity in hypertension as a third-line agent, although gradually being displaced by calcium antagonists such as nifedipine. Hydralazine-isosorbide dinitrate is well documented vasodilator therapy for CHF.

Diazoxide

Diazoxide is now only occasionally used as the IV preparation in hypertensive crises, and even there its use is being replaced by IV labetalol or sublingual nifedipine. An IV bolus of 300 mg acts too quickly; smaller doses are preferable (initial bolus 150 mg followed by boluses of 100–150 mg every 5 minutes) and controlled infusions (5 mg/kg at 15 mg/min) are safest. It is difficult to control the hypotensive effect that may be excessive. Chronic oral treatment may cause diabetes mellitus, fluid retention and the vasodilator effect is not sustained so that diazoxide is not suited for chronic afterload reduction.

Minoxidil

Minoxidil (Loniten®) is another direct acting arteriolar vasodilator with serious side-effects, seldom used except in the therapy of *resistant hypertension* where there are now so many other agents that are effective that the risk of frequent hirsuties or rare pericardial disease seems not worthwhile, although minoxidil can be more effective than hydralazine.[20] In CHF, controlled studies failed to demonstrate any improvement in maximum oxygen consumption and exercise tolerance, despite increased cardiac output in monoxidil-treated patients.[15] Furthermore, almost all patients developed edema and required increased diuretics. Thus, minoxidil has little value in the management of chronic CHF. The oral dose is up to 40 mg/day, there is renal excretion without hepatic metabolism, and the biologic half-life is 1–4 days. Concomitant β-blockade is required to reduce tachycardia and diuretics are required to avoid fluid retention when minoxidil is used for hypertension.

α-RECEPTOR ANTAGONISTS

Two types of α-receptors have been defined—the presynaptic α_2-receptors and the postsynaptic or vascular α_1-receptors. Sustained α_1 blockade may lead to tolerance, especially with prazosin.[7,13,21] This tolerance may in part depend on the complexity of the feedback loops whereby unimpaired α_2-receptor stimulation inhibits the release of NE from the terminal adrenergic neurons. Now the major use of these agents is against hypertension and not chronic heart failure. Postsynaptic α_2-receptors, recently described, may permit vasoconstriction via a process inhibited by calcium antagonists; no specific α_2-receptor blockers are yet available for clinical use.

Prazosin

Prazosin (Minipress®; Hypovase® in UK) antagonizes vascular α_1-receptors and is an established agent for hypertension. Although also used for the therapy of refractory heart failure, tachyphylaxis is a major problem.[10a,11a,23a] Prazosin dilates both peripheral arterial and venous systems, thus acting as an "oral nitroprusside" to decrease the blood pressure, to reduce the preload, and to increase the cardiac output. The venous effects may account for first-dose syncope, unless a low dose is used. Arteriolar dilation should cause a reflex tachycardia, yet for some reason the heart rate rises little in hypertension or in CHF, so for a given fall of blood pressure prazosin produces less increase in the cardiac output than does nitroprusside so that a negative inotropic effect has been suspected.[24]

Pharmacokinetics. Prazosin has to be given orally and is well absorbed. The plasma half-life is 3–4 hours, yet the antihypertensive effect is prolonged. Although 3× daily doses are conventional, 2× daily doses suffice. Prazosin can be used in renal failure because renal blood flow is not altered and the drug is chiefly excreted in the feces. Substantial first-pass liver metabolism indicates the need for caution in patients with liver disease.

Dose. The initial dose should be low and taken at night (2 mg for heart failure, 0.5 or 1 mg for hypertension) then 2× daily (previously 3× daily was recommended). As the dose is worked up to a maximum of 20 mg/day, 1 mg then 2 mg then 5 mg tablets 2× daily is convenient. There is no evidence that 30 mg daily gives a better response than 20 mg. Sharp increases in the dose may cause syncope.

Side-effects. *First-dose syncope* may be due to decreased preload and is especially likely when there is no LV failure or during co-therapy with nitrates or potent diuretics. Chronic postural dizziness is a less frequent side-effect. *Tachyphylaxis*, whereby increasing doses are required to produce the same effect, may develop in the treatment of both heart failure and hypertension. Tachyphylaxis is a specific phenomenon and should be distinguished from tolerance, a nonspecific resistance to therapy with all vasodilators; and from transient attenuation to the effect of prazosin, most evident in the therapy of hypertension. In some studies, prazosin has been clinically beneficial over 2–3 months of therapy for CHF. Yet a recent double-blind placebo-controlled study showed no effect of prazosin over six months when given to patients with CHF (Class III disability, already receiving digitalis and diuretics[7]). Several recent double-blind studies confirm that prazosin is not effective in the long-term therapy of CHF.[10a,11a,23a] If the clinical response appears inadequate or blunted, there are several practical approaches such as changing to captopril or enalapril (because prazosin can activate the angiotensin-renin system[3]), giving prazosin intermittently or in alternation with other vasodilators. Diuretic doses may need reduction if the LV filling pressure becomes too low. Conversely, weight gain and edema may call for more diuretics.

Tolerance has now also been described in the therapy of hypertension[21] and may explain why upward adjustment of the dose of prazosin is so frequently needed.

Nonspecific side-effects include drowsiness, lack of energy, nasal congestion, depression, and occasional retrograde ejaculation. Tachycardia is usually not common but in some patients can be troublesome. Positive antinuclear factors may develop without clinical lupus.

Combination with other agents.   In hypertension, prazosin may be combined with β-blockers or with centrally acting agents such as methyldopa and clonidine. Fluid and sodium retention may necessitate the addition of diuretics. Prazosin is sometimes used together with other vasodilators such as hydralazine, nifedipine, and verapamil. There may be an added interaction between prazosin and calcium antagonists so that excess or added hypotension results.[18,25] In patients with angina and ischemic heart disease, both nitrates and prazosin may cause syncope so that combinations require care; prazosin plus β-blockade or verapamil may be better therapy. In CHF, prazosin in combination with the ACE inhibitors can produce better hemodynamic and clinical effects at the risk of enhanced hypotension.

Prazosin—Summary

Prazosin is widely used in the therapy of hypertension, both in combination with diuretics/β-blockade or as monotherapy. During chronic therapy the dose may have to be increased, possibly the result of tachyphylaxis. In CHF, prazosin is one of the agents that can be used acutely but the long-term effect is similar to that of placebo.

Labetalol

This β-antagonist agent (Trandate®, Normodyne®) (see p 14) with added α-antagonist activity is a vasodilatory β-blocker well-documented in the use of hypertension. It acts much more rapidly than pure β-blockade in the therapy of acute hypertension (Table 11-5), even though the α-antagonist activity is much less than the β-antagonist activity. There is not enough α-antagonism for the management of intense α-adrenergic activity as in some patients with pheochromocytoma or clonidine-withdrawal. Because the α-blocking activity of labetalol is limited to the vascular α_1-receptors, some of its effects and side-effects must be similar to those of prazosin. The dominant β-blocking effect in the chronic therapy of hypertension may be due at least in part to tolerance to the blockade of α_1 vascular receptors. Labetalol has not been well studied in angina pectoris, apart from effort angina combined with hypertension, where 200 mg 2× daily was as effective as atenolol 100 mg daily; the higher heart rates with labetalol could be an advantage especially in elderly patients.[19]

Indoramin

This α_1-blocking agent (Baratol® in UK; Wydora® in Germany; not in the USA) finds its chief application as an adjuvant in the therapy of hypertension (oral dose 25–50 mg 2× daily). Arguments favoring α_1-blockade over β-blockade for hypertension (see p 208) can also be applied to indoramin which seems to have a different spectrum of side-effects[26a] from prazosin with more prominent sedation, dizziness and dry mouth and less first dose syncope. These potential differences, however, are not well documented. Compared with β-blockade, advantages include absence of adverse hemodynamic effects of indoramin, and no change of blood lipid profile.

Phentolamine

Phentolamine specifically blocks both α_1 and α_2-adrenoceptors, especially the α_2-receptors. Release of NE from the terminal neurons could account for the tachycardia and inotropic effect. In low output LV failure, large IV doses are required (10–20 μg/kg/min) for continuous vasodilation at high expense. Phentolamine is now used only in hypertensive crises when there is excess sympathetic α-stimulation as in pheochromocytoma, clonidine-withdrawal, excess use of sympathomimetic agents, or when breakdown of NE by monoamine oxidase is inhibited.

Phenoxybenzamine

Phenoxybenzamine is a powerful α-blocking agent with a slow mode of action but with long-lasting effects and used chiefly in the management of pheochromocytoma. The IV dose is 15–40 mg given slowly or up to 100 mg. The solution should be freshly diluted and clear.

CALCIUM ANTAGONISTS

The peripheral unloading effect may offset a direct negative inotropic effect, especially in the case of nifedipine and felodipine (see pp 44 and 47). These vasodilator properties are of established benefit in the therapy of angina pectoris and hypertension.

In *CHF*, the calcium antagonists are not generally used because of the potential negative inotropic effect. Nevertheless, in less severe heart failure, nifedipine works as an afterload reducer[12] and may be combined with nitro-glycerin.[21a] One-third of patients may deteriorate in response to nifedipine, presumably because the negative inotropic effect is not adequately controlled by peripheral vasodilation.[14] Limited data suggest that the initial vasodilator effect is sustained during long-term therapy. Verapamil is generally not well tolerated by patients with overt heart failure. Experience with diltiazem is also limited. The new calcium antagonist, *felodipine*,[27] appears to be a potent vaso-dilator and improves cardiac function significantly, even in the presence of severe heart failure; further experience will be required to establish its value. *Presently calcium antagonists should be considered chiefly in patients with mild to moderate heart failure associated with angina or hypertension.*

> In patients with *hypertrophic cardiomyopathy*, verapamil may improve diastolic function (see p 40), whereas nifedipine therapy runs the risk of increasing the LV outflow tract gradient.[11]
>
> In *precapillary pulmonary hypertension*, calcium antagonists may sometimes decrease pulmonary artery pressure and pulmonary vascular resistance; how-ever, an adverse response such as systemic hypotension and decreased cardiac output might also occur so that careful hemodynamic monitoring is required.

In *hypertension*, calcium antagonists may be of special benefit in elderly or black hypertensives. Nifedipine is increasingly seen as a desirable agent either in addition to diuretics/β-blockade or even as monotherapy. However, the use of nifedipine is limited by the short half-life requiring $3\times$ daily dosage and the side-effects of flushing and headache. It is likely that slow-release preparations (Adalat Retard®, not in the USA) or longer acting agents of a similar structure such as nitrendipine or felodipine will soon be used widely in systemic hyper-tension. Extensive recent testing has also shown the benefit of verapamil and diltiazem in hypertension. Verapamil is likely to be the first calcium antagonist approved for use in hypertension in the USA.

In *severe hypertension* where urgent reduction of blood pressure is re-quired, sublingual nifedipine is usually rapidly effective and safe (see p 44); Table 11-5). When, however, there is danger of end-organ under-perfusion such as in patients with a history of cerebral or myocardial ischemia or overt renal failure, then the safety of such acute blood pressure reduction is not established and there is possible danger of precipitation of stroke or myocar-dial infarction. Therefore in such patients controlled IV administration of other agents such as labetalol is usually preferred. IV verapamil (5 mg), although not usually used in severe hypertension, was found to be effective many years ago.

OTHER VASODILATORS

Adrenergic blockers. *Guanethedine* blocks postganglion sympathetic but not parasympathetic transmission and causes hypotension that is mainly postural. The initial dose is 10–20 mg/day; usual dose 0–75 mg/day, up to 400 mg/day. Onset of action is 2–3 days. Hypertensive crises used to be managed with 10–20 mg given intramuscularly or slowly intravenously.

Clonidine stimulates the central α_2-receptors to inhibit the peripheral release of NE and could theoretically be useful in CHF besides its established use in hypertension.

Trimethaphan.   Trimethaphan blocks both sympathetic and parasympathetic ganglionic transmission and is largely used for controlling surgical hypertension and in the management of *aortic dissection* (infusion starts at 3 mg/min) because of the rapidity of onset and cessation of action.

Furosemide (= frusemide).   Furosemide (Lasix®), when injected intravenously in standard doses, can rapidly improve the acute pulmonary edema (in patients with AMI, even before there is an increase in urinary output[2]). The probable mechanism of this early effect is venodilation. In chronic CHF, LV function may transiently deteriorate as plasma renin activity increases following IV furosemide[16] to limit the early benefit. (For dose, see p 114.)

Phosphodiesterase inhibitors.   The phosphodiesterase inhibitors *amrinone* and *milrinone* (see p 106) act in CHF largely by peripheral vasodilation although also having a direct inotropic effect. Acutely, both these agents work well; during prolonged therapy efficacy seems to fall and side-effects arise.

VASODILATORS UNDER DEVELOPMENT

β-Adrenergic Agonists

The β-agonists act on the vascular receptors to cause peripheral vasodilation. Their direct cardiac effect makes them unsuitable for use in hypertension. Dobutamine and dopamine (see pp 101 and 104) may owe part of their beneficial effect in heart failure to β-mediated vasodilation. Conversely, the peripheral vasoconstriction found with some β-blocking agents may also be explained by unopposed peripheral α-adrenergic activity. The following β-agonists are under assessment:

Salbutamol (= **albuterol** in the USA; Ventolin®; Proventil®) is a selective β-agonist chiefly used as a bronchodilator. (Its use as a vasodilator is investigational in the USA). It improves indices of contractility when infused (0.5 μg/min/kg) into patients with congestive cardiomyopathy who have already received digitalis and diuretics.[9] Thus it is potentially useful especially in patients with CHF and obstructive lung disease. In patients with myocardial infarction and severe LV failure, IV salbutamol may improve cardiac output, although the heart rate rises only slightly.

Pirbuterol (available in Europe) is also a β_2-agonist and, to a lesser extent, a partial β-blocker. It usually increases cardiac output and decreases pulmonary wedge pressure in patients with chronic heart failure. However, there may be ventricular arrhythmias and a rapid attentuation of clinical response.

Xamoterol (Corwin®, soon to be available in Europe) is another combined β-stimulator-blocker with predominant stimulant properties. Xamoterol is, however, β_1-specific, thus being a "pure" inotropic agent and not a vasodilator.

Other New Vasodilators

Dopamine receptor stimulators (see p 105) are now becoming available in oral form and may have the special advantage of prominent renal vasodilation and little or no effect on the heart rate.

Atrial natriuretic peptide (= atrial natriuretic factor: ANP or ANF) has very recently been isolated. This is the peptide that is secreted by the cardiac atria in response to volume distension. Thus it is the natural hypovolemic agent, acting on the renal vasculature, to cause a powerful vasodilation and diuresis. Thereby the polyuria frequently associated with paroxysmal supraventricular tachycardia (PSVT) can be explained. ANP acts on vascular cells to produce vasodilatory cyclic GMP.[17] *Human ANP* has been synthesized and tested in man, with the expected natriuretic and diuretic qualities. ANP is now being tested in acute heart failure and in certain forms of hypertension. In chronic heart failure, an added potential benefit of ANP is decreased secretion of aldosterone.

DIFFERING EFFECTS OF VASODILATORS
IN HYPERTENSION AND HEART FAILURE

All vasodilators decrease vascular resistance in both conditions. In *heart failure*, cardiac output increases because the ventricle is afterload-dependent (Fig. 7-1). When the initial filling pressure is high and the patient lies on the flat portion of the ventricular function curve (Fig. 7-1)), decreased preload due to venodilation does not cause any appreciable reduction or increase in stroke volume (nitrate effect, Fig. 7-2). In contrast, when the ventricular function curve moves upwards and to the left, stroke volume and cardiac output rise (prazosin, nitroprusside, hydralazine; Fig. 7-2). The common denominator to these agents is their effect in reducing systemic vascular resistance. In heart failure, the higher the systemic vascular resistance, the greater is the increase in cardiac output achieved by peripheral arteriolar vasodilation.

In *hypertension*, when the LV filling pressure is normal and the patient is on the steep portion of the function curve, a dominant venodilator effect as with nitrates may not increase but rather may decrease the stroke volume. When a predominant arteriolar vasodilator is used, the reduction in aortic impedance causes little change in the cardiac output (Fig. 7-1), because the ventricle is not afterload-dependent. In response to vasodilation, self-adjusting circulatory reflexes allow only enough tachycardia to compensate for the peripheral vasodilation. Sometimes, as with hydralazine, tachycardia may be excessive suggesting that hydralazine has a direct effect on the heart. In contrast, the same vasodilators usually do not produce any change in heart rate in patients with heart failure, presumably due to blunted baroreceptor activity and a concomitant increase in pulse pressure.

VASODILATOR VERSUS INOTROPIC THERAPY
IN HEART FAILURE

The "step-care" of CHF, starting with sodium restriction and diuretics, is considered elsewhere (see p 126). Thereafter vasodilators and inotropic agents may be considered; they improve cardiac function and systemic hemodynamics acting by different mechanisms. Vasodilators decrease resistance to LV ejection and also, frequently, the LV filling pressure and diastolic volume. Thus myocardial oxygen consumption generally tends to decrease which should benefit patients with heart failure due to coronary artery disease. Vasodilators may, however, cause hypotension to enhance myocardial ischemia by decreasing the diastolic perfusion pressure. Inotropic agents, in contrast, improve cardiac function by increasing myocardial contractility that undesirably enhances myocardial oxygen requirements. **These two differing physiological principles, afterload reduction and increased contractility, may be combined to provide better hemodynamic benefits and fewer side-effects** (see "Inodilators," Table 5-8). Both these principles act completely differently from the basic first principle in CHF: diuretic therapy. Inotropic agents are particularly worth considering in (1) patients who are hypotensive (systolic blood pressure <90 mmHg) and (2) patients who remain in refractory heart failure despite vasodilator therapy.

In other circumstances, vasodilators may be preferable to inotropic agents. It is reasonable to try vasodilator/diuretic therapy instead of digitalis/diuretics in selected patients with CHF, such as those in whom digoxin is contraindicated (renal failure), those prone to digoxin toxicity, or when digoxin no longer seems to work. Likewise, patients with ventricular arrhythmias or ischemic heart disease may also respond better to vasodilators than to inotropic therapy. Vasodilators may also be considered when large doses of diuretics (furosemide > 160 mg daily) are required. In other patients, combined inotropic-vasodilation therapy may be tried empirically (see p 101).

Choice of Vasodilator

As ACE inhibitors provide some advantages over other vasodilators, these agents should be considered initially (Chapter 8). Their superiority to prazosin is particularly well documented.[10a,11a,23a] Patients who develop hypotension may benefit from other vasodilators such as a combination of an arteriolar dilator (hydralazine) and a venodilator (nitrates) with documented long-term benefit,[11a] or may require inotropic support. A reasonable short-term alternate therapy is prazosin, which acutely benefits many patients with heart failure, especially if overdiuresis is avoided. During continued prazosin therapy, tolerance may require interrupted prazosin therapy or usually a switch to ACE inhibitors. Intermittent nocturnal nitrates may improve nocturnal dyspnea. Intermittent dobutamine or a sustained 3-day dobutamine infusion may produce considerable improvement in interval exercise tolerance (see p 102). It needs to be emphasized that **there is accumulating evidence that vasodilator therapy improves the prognosis of patients with chronic heart failure.** Thus the Veterans Administration Heart Failure Trial showed that hydralazine 300 mg with isosorbide dinitrate 160 mg (total daily doses) reduced mortality by 23 percent over 2 years in patients with mild to moderate heart failure; prazosin 5 mg 3× daily had no effect.[11a]

End-Stage Heart Failure

Special management may be required in this condition, when the myocardium is largely destroyed and, in addition, the number of β-adrenoceptor sites falls, probably as a result of prolonged excessive and increasing adrenergic stimulation as the CHF intensifies, so that the receptors become "downgraded." To restore the number of binding sites, circulating catecholamines must be diminished as can theoretically be achieved by vasodilator therapy (especially ACE inhibition, see p 159), while sympathomimetic stimulation is avoided. Recently, low-dose β-antagonists have been used to up-regulate the β-receptors and in an attempt to improve CHF. Logically, mixed β-agonists-antagonists may be novel and desirable therapy (see p 104). **In general, vasodilator therapy earlier in the course of CHF could be an advantage in avoiding end-stage heart failure, although there are no firm data to support this proposal.**

CONCLUSIONS

Vasodilation is now an integral part of the therapy of hypertension and CHF. In hypertension, the benefits of arteriolar dilators are relatively easily measured by the blood pressure, although there may be added advantages in the reduction of myocardial hypertrophy (not, however, achieved by hydralazine). In the case of CHF, vasodilation is now established add-on therapy in patients already digitalized and treated by diuretics. Until the factors regulating exercise tolerance in CHF are better understood, the agent of choice is to some extent a pragmatic procedure. Nonetheless, ACE inhibition (Chapter 8) seems likely better to counter the overall metabolic-hormonal abnormalities in severe heart failure, whereas nitrates seem likely better to reduce pulmonary congestion, and afterload reducers such as hydralazine or nifedipine or ACE inhibitors may be best to improve renal blood flow. Which agent is likely best to improve skeletal muscle perfusion during exercise is still unknown, although ACE inhibitors are promising. Such guidelines, although useful, should not obscure the frequent requirement for a flexible, pragmatic approach to the individual patient.[23]

REFERENCES

References from Previous Edition

For details see previous edition of Opie et al: Drugs for the Heart, American Edition. Orlando, Florida, Grune and Stratton, 1984, pp 129–151

1. Chatterjee K, Massie B, Rubin S, et al: Am J Med 65:134–145, 1978
2. Chatterjee K, Parmley WW: J Am Coll Cardiol 1:133–153, 1983
3. Colucci WS: Ann Intern Med 97:67–77, 1982
4. Fitchett DM, Marin JA, Oakley CM, et al: Am J Cardiol 44:303–309, 1979
5. Greenberg BH, Massie BM, Brundage BH, et al: Circulation 58:273–279, 1978

6.   Khatri I, Uemara N, Notargiacomo A, et al: Am J Cardiol 40:38–42, 1977
7.   Markham RV, Corbett JR, Gilmore A, et al: Am J Cardiol 51:1346–1352, 1983
8.   Packer M, Meller J, Medina N, et al: New Engl J Med 306:57–62, 1982
9.   Sharma B, Goodwin JF: Circulation 58:449–460, 1978
10.   Sladen RN, Rosenthal MH: J Thorac Cardiovasc Surg 78:195–202, 1979

New References

10a. Bayliss J, Canepa-Anson R, Norell MS, et al: Vasodilatation with captopril and prazosin in chronic heart failure: Double-blind study at rest and on exercise. Br Heart J 55:265–273, 1986
11.   Betocchi S, Cannon RO, Watson RM, et al: Effects of sublingual nifedipine on hemodynamics and systolic and diastolic function in patients with hypertrophic cardiomyopathy. Circulation 72:1001–1007, 1985
11a. Cohn JN, Archibald DG, Ziesche S, et al: Effect of vasodilator therapy on mortality in chronic congestive heart failure. Results of a Veterans Administration Cooperative Study. New Engl J Med 314:1547–1552, 1986
12.   Colucci WS, Fifer MA, Lorell BH, et al: Calcium channel blockers in congestive heart failure: Theoretic considerations and clinical experience. Am J Med 78 (suppl 2B):9–17, 1985
12a. Creager MA, Faxon DP, Cutler SS, et al: Contribution of vasopressin to vasoconstriction in patients with congestive heart failure: Comparison with the renin-angiotensin system and the sympathetic nervous system. J Am Coll Cardiol 7:758–765, 1986
13.   Elkayam U, Lejemtel TH, Mathur M, et al: Marked early attenuation of hemodynamic effects of oral prazosin therapy in chronic congestive heart failure. Am J Cardiol 44:540–545, 1979
14.   Elkayam U, Weber L, Torkan B, et al: Acute hemodynamic effect of oral nifedipine in severe chronic congestive heart failure. Am J Cardiol 52:1041–1045, 1983
15.   Franciosa JA, Jordan RA, Wilen MM, et al: Minoxidil in patients with chronic left heart failure: Contrasting hemodynamic and clinical effects in a controlled trial. Circulation 70:63–68, 1984
16.   Francis GS, Siegel RM, Goldsmith SR, et al: Acute vasoconstrictor response to intravenous furosemide in patients with chronic congestive heart failure. Ann Intern Med 10:1–6, 1985
17.   Garcia R, Thibault M, Cantin M, et al: Effect of a purified atrial natriuretic factor on rat and rabbit vascular strips and vascular beds. Am J Physiol 247:R34–R39, 1984
18.   Jee LD, Opie LH: Acute hypotensive response to nifedipine added to prazosin in treatment of hypertension. Br Med J 287:1514–1516, 1983
19.   Jee LD, Opie LH: Double-blind trial comparing labetalol with atenolol in therapy of hypertension with effort angina. Am J Cardiol 56:551–554, 1985
20.   Johnson BF, Black HR, Beckner R, et al: A comparison of minoxidil and hydralazine in non-azotemic hypertensives. J Hypertens 1:103–107, 1983
21.   Khatri IM, Levinson P, Notargiacomo A, et al: Initial and long-term effects of prazosin on sympathetic vasopressor responses in essential hypertension. Am J Cardiol 55:1015–1018, 1985
21a. Kubo SH, Fox SC, Prida XE, et al: Combined hemodynamic effects of nifedipine and nitroglycerin in congestive heart failure. Am Heart J 110:1032–1034, 1985
22.   McKay CR, Nana M, Kawanishi DT: Importance of internal controls, statistical methods, and side-effects in short-term trials of vasodilators: A study of hydralazine kinetics in patients with aortic regurgitation. Circulation 72:865–872, 1985
23.   Packer M: Conceptual dilemmas in the classification of vasodilator drugs for severe chronic heart failure. Advocacy of a pragmatic approach to the selection of a therapeutic agent. Am J Med 76:3–13, 1984
23a. Packer M, Medina N, Yushak M: Comparative hemodynamic and clinical effects of long-term treatment with prazosin and captopril for severe chronic congestive heart failure secondary to coronary artery disease or idiopathic dilated cardiomyopathy. Am J Cardiol 57:1323–1327, 1986
24.   Packer M, Meller J, Gorlin R, et al: Differences in hemodynamic effects of nitroprusside and prazosin in severe chronic congestive heart failure. Evidence for a direct negative inotropic effect of prazosin. Am J Cardiol 44:310–317, 1979
25.   Pasanisi F, Elliott HL, Meredith PA, et al: Combined alpha-adrenoceptor antagonism and calcium channel blockade in normal subjects. Clin Pharmacol Ther 36:716–723, 1984
26.   Smucker ML, Sanford CF, Lipscomb KM: Effects of hydralazine on pressure-volume and stress-volume relations in congestive heart failure secondary to idiopathic dilated cardiomyopathy. Am J Cardiol 56:690–695, 1985
26a. Stannard M, Cohen M, Marrott PK, et al: Antihypertensive therapy with indoramin: Risk-benefit profile in clinical practice. J Cardiovasc Pharmacol 8 (suppl 2):S48–S52, 1986
27.   Timmis AD, Jewitt DE: Studies with felodipine in congestive heart failure. Drugs 29 (suppl 2):66–75, 1985

28.   Unverferth DV, Mehegan JP, Magorien RD, et al: Regression of myocardial cellular hypertrophy with vasodilator therapy in chronic congestive heart failure associated with idiopathic dilated cardiomyopathy. Am J Cardiol 51:1392 1398, 1983

Review

Remme WJ: Congestive heart failure—Pathophysiology and medical treatment. J Cardiovasc Pharmacol 8 (suppl 1):S36–S52, 1986

K. Chatterjee
L. H. Opie

8

Angiotensin-Converting Enzyme Inhibitors

Angiotensin converting enzyme (ACE) inhibitors (= CEI) act on the angiotensin-renin-aldosterone system by inhibition of the ACE. The ACE inhibitors, captopril and enalapril (and many others will soon appear), act as mixed arteriolar and venous vasodilators. Besides beneficial hemodynamic effects in congestive heart failure (CHF) and hypertension, they also powerfully alter the underlying neurohumoral events that exaggerate the severity of heart failure. Theoretically, ACE inhibitors should benefit most when CHF is accompanied by high-plasma renin activity, or when hypertension is caused by a high-renin state as in renal artery stenosis. Yet these agents frequently benefit ordinary essential hypertension and mild degrees of CHF. As angiotensin inhibitors do not alter glucose tolerance, blood uric acid, or cholesterol levels and as these agents seldom cause subjective side-effects, their use in hypertension is rapidly increasing. In CHF, angiotensin inhibitors are increasingly seen as the vasodilators of choice because of their added neurohumoral benefit, and are therefore being used earlier and earlier. The "permissive" role of angiotensin in the release of norepinephrine (NE) from the terminal adrenergic neurons and elsewhere (Fig. 8-1) leads to the proposal that angiotensin inhibitors may be tested in various other "hyperadrenergic" states such as acute myocardial infarction (AMI) and some ventricular arrhythmias.

The Principle

Angiotensin II is the vasoconstrictive hormone that increases the tension of the smooth muscles of the vascular bed via stimulation of the angiotensin receptors. Angiotensin also enhances vascular tone by several indirect mechanisms. First, angiotensin potentiates the activity of the sympathetic nervous system (Fig. 8-1) and enhances synthesis and release of NE. Second, angiotensin is a secretagogue for aldosterone from the adrenal glands. Aldosterone, in turn, can increase the systemic vascular resistance directly by its effect on vascular smooth muscle, and also indirectly by increasing the water and sodium content of the vascular wall to promote stiffness. Third, angiotensin may mediate the release of vasopressin, particularly in patients with severe CHF. Vasopressin, in turn, may contribute to abnormal volume regulation frequently observed in severe heart failure. Vasopressin may also be a direct vasoconstrictor.

Drugs for the Heart, Second Expanded Edition
Copyright © 1987 by Grune & Stratton, Inc.

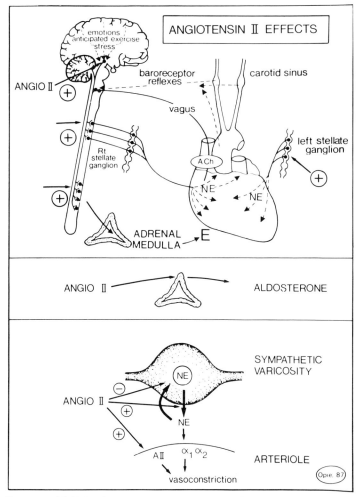

Fig. 8-1. Multiple sites of action of angiotensin II (= angio II), including central adrenergic activation, facilitation of ganglionic transmission, release of aldosterone from the adrenal medulla, release of norepinephrine (NE) from terminal sympathetic varicosities with inhibition of re-uptake and direct stimulation of vascular angiotensin II receptors. The major net effect is powerful vasoconstriction. (Modified from Opie LH: The Heart: Physiology, Metabolism, Pharmacology and Therapy. Orlando and London, Grune and Stratton, 1984. With permission).

Possible Sites of Angiotensin Inhibition

Angiotensin II is an octapeptide, and its formation from its precursor, decapeptide, angiotensin I, requires the converting enzyme (Fig. 8-2). Renin is the rate-limiting enzyme required to form angiotensin I from the substrate angiotensinogen, which comes from the liver (Fig. 8-3). The synthesis of angiotensin II can be prevented by blunting the action of the converting enzyme by the ACE inhibitors. The synthesis of both angiotensin I and II can be prevented by blocking the formation of renin, normally synthesized and released by the juxtaglomerular cells of the kidney, by the experimental renin-inhibiting peptide, H-142. Finally, angiotensin II can undergo competitive antagonism at its receptor sites by the IV investigational agent, saralasin.

Bradykinin

Another function of the converting enzyme is to degrade the potent vasodilator kinin peptide (bradykinin) to inactive metabolites (Fig. 8-2). ACE inhibition therefore increases bradykinin to contribute to peripheral vasodilation by stimulating the synthesis and release of vasodilator prostaglandins. This sequence explains why indomethacin attenuates the effects of the ACE inhibitor, captopril.[47]

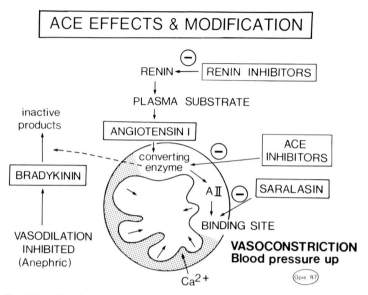

Fig. 8-2. Site of action of angiotensin-converting enzyme (ACE) and its modifiers. ACE is found especially in the pulmonary vascular bed. ACE inhibitors reduce formation of angiotensin II (AII), and also decrease breakdown of the vasodilator, bradykinin. The latter mechanism is thought to account for an effect of captopril detected even in anephric patients. Saralasin is a receptor antagonist which, by interacting with the same vascular binding site as an angiotensin II, causes vasodilation. Saralasin is not in clinical use. Anti-renin agents are under development. (Modified from Opie LH: The Heart: Physiology, Metabolism, Pharmacology and Therapy. Orlando and London, Grune and Stratton, 1984).

CAPTOPRIL

Captopril (Capoten®; Lopril® in France; Lopirin® in Germany; Captopril® in Japan), the first widely available ACE inhibitor, was originally seen to be an agent with significant and serious side-effects such as loss of taste, renal impairment, and neutropenia. Now it is recognized that these are rather rare side-effects and can be avoided largely by reducing the daily dose and by the appropriate monitoring. The result is that captopril is now widely used both for CHF and hypertension. Captopril impairs neither intellectual nor sexual function, nor causes fatigue, so that it compares very favorably with other antihypertensives such as methyldopa and propranolol by preserving the "quality of life."[10]

Pharmacokinetics. After absorption from the stomach, captopril is metabolized by the liver and kidney with an elimination half-life of approximately 6–8 hours. A dose of 20 mg given orally to normal volunteers blocks the pressor response to exogenous angiotensin I within 15 minutes and for over 2 hours.[16] In hypertension its biological half-life is long enough to allow 2× daily dosage.

Dose and indications. Captopril has an average daily dose of 25–50 mg orally given 2× daily (instead of much higher 3× daily doses previously prescribed). For maximum bioavailability, captopril should be taken on an empty stomach. Yet food has little influence on the overall antihypertensive effect.[36] In *hypertension*, although 2× daily doses are conventional, a single daily dose of 50–100 mg may be used with dietary salt restriction.[35] The risk of excess hypotension is highest in patients with high renin states (renal artery stenosis, pre-existing vigorous diuretic therapy or severe sodium restriction) when the

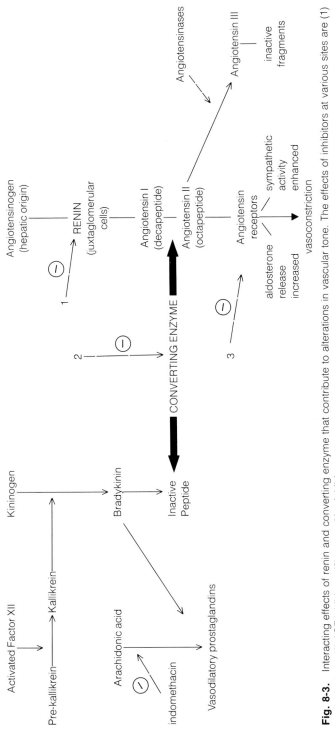

Fig. 8-3. Interacting effects of renin and converting enzyme that contribute to alterations in vascular tone. The effects of inhibitors at various sites are (1) renin blockers, (2) ACE inhibitors, (3) competitive inhibitors.

151

initial dose should be low (6.25–12.5 mg). When given sublingually, 25 mg captopril (chewed) may relieve severe hypertension,[42] but renal contraindications must first be excluded.

In *CHF*, the usual dose is 75–450 mg daily in three divided doses; 2× daily therapy seems logical but undocumented. Lower doses need more evaluation especially in view of the risk of proteinuria with doses exceeding 150 mg/day. Captopril may cause excessive hypotension especially in vigorously diuresed patients so that a *test dose* of 6.25 mg is required (if given sublingually the safety can be assessed within 1 hour). Studies with an investigational IV form of captopril show that high plasma levels may be required for an optimal effect in CHF.[34]

In *renal disease*, when not contraindicated (next section), the dose is reduced. (For use in diabetic nephropathy, see p 159).

In *rheumatoid arthritis*, captopril appears to work by virtue of the sulfhydryl (SH) group.[21]

Contraindications.   Bilateral renal artery stenosis; renal artery stenosis in a single kidney; immune-based renal disease; severe renal failure (serum creatinine > 1.6 mg/dL or > 150 μmol/L). Pre-existing neutropenia. Systemic hypotension. *Relative contraindications:* co-administration of other drugs likely to alter immune function such as procainamide, tocainide, hydralazine, probenecid and possibly acebutolol; mild renal impairment.

Side-effects.   In general, the side-effects are seldom serious provided that the total daily dose is 150 mg daily or less.[17] Side-effects caused less withdrawal than equivalent antihypertensive doses of methyldopa or propranolol.[10] In principle, there are two types of side-effects: (1) those common to all ACE inhibitors whereby hypotension may cause renal failure in the presence of pre-existing renal impairment and (2) immune-based side-effects probably specific to captopril, such as taste disturbances, skin rashes, and (in a subgroup of patients) neutropenia.

Neutropenia (< 1000/mm^3) may occur with captopril, extremely rarely in hypertensive patients with normal renal function (1/8600 according to the package insert), more commonly (1/500) with pre-existing impaired renal function with a serum creatinine of 1.6 mg/dL or more and as a serious risk (4/100) in patients with both collagen vascular disease and renal impairment. In CHF, neutropenia is a risk especially in the presence of impaired renal function or during co-therapy with procainamide. With neutropenia, there may also be thrombocytopenia or even pancytopenia. Logically co-therapy with other drugs altering the immune response (see contraindications) should be avoided. When captopril is discontinued, recovery from neutropenia is usual except when there is associated serious disease such as severe renal or heart failure or collagen vascular disease.

Proteinuria occurs in about 1 percent of patients receiving captopril especially in the presence of pre-existing renal disease or high doses of captopril (> 150 mg/day[22]). There appears to be a double mechanism for renal damage induced by captopril (Fig. 8-4): first, an altered immune response, and second, excess hypotension, as shared with enalapril.[4] Paradoxically, captopril may be used in the therapy of diabetic nephropathy with proteinuria.[10]

Other side-effects include hypotension (frequent in the treatment of CHF), impaired taste (2–7 percent), skin rashes (4–10 percent), sometimes with eosinophilia, and rarely (1/100 to 1/1000) serious angioedema. Hepatic damage is also very rare. Renal failure in patients with CHF may be exacerbated by captopril. Cough and wheeze occur occasionally.[38]

Pretreatment precautions.   Because the immune-based side-effects are largely found in patients with collagen vascular disease or receiving other drugs likely to alter the immune response, it is advised that **all patients should have pre-captopril renal evaluation, tests for antinuclear antibodies, a full blood count and a screen of all other medications (check for K$^+$-retaining diuretics).** Bilateral renal artery stenosis should be excluded as far as possible.

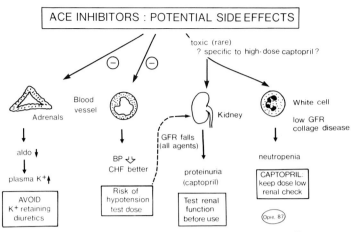

Fig. 8-4.   Potential side-effects of converting enzyme inhibitors. For precaution, see text.

Patients with renal impairment caused by collagen disease or patients receiving immunosuppressives or immune system modifiers such as steroids and hydralazine should be excluded, as also patients with a history of hematological disease or pretreatment depression of neutrophils or platelets. Pretreatment hypotension excludes therapy.

Precautions at the start of therapy.   First-dose hypotension may occur especially in patients with high-renin states including those over-diuresed or on very severe salt restriction or with severe hyponatremia or with renal artery stenosis. Hypotension is a common risk in patients with CHF. Hypotension may be avoided by: (1) an *initial test dose* with captopril (6.25 mg in heart failure, 6.25–12.5 mg in patients with hypertension or high-renin states) and (2) a decrease of diuretic therapy with attention to volume repletion in CHF. In all cases, therapy should be started under close medical supervision (**emphasized in the package insert**). A sublingual test dose of captopril may be tried in out-patient practice when the patient does not require hospital admission.

Precautions during treatment.   Regular monitoring of neutrophil counts is required in patients with pre-existing renal impairment (pretreatment, 2 weekly counts for 3 months). Captopril should normally not be given to patients with collagen vascular disease. In hypertensive patients without renal impairment, patients are warned to report any sore throats. In patients with pre-existing renal disease, renal function requires repetitive monitoring; dipsticks on the first morning urine may be sufficient. The risk of renal damage from captopril may be reduced by keeping total daily doses below 150 mg/day.[22]

Drug interactions.   The most common drug interaction is excess hypotension in over-diuresed patients. Co-therapy with other drugs altering the immune status (procainamide, hydralazine, acebutolol, probenecid) may predispose to neutropenia. Indomethacin and nonsteroidal anti-inflammatories may decrease the antihypertensive effect of captopril. K^+-retaining diuretics can cause excess hyperkalemia.

Combination therapy.   Captopril is frequently combined with a diuretic in the therapy of hypertension, and β-blocker or calcium antagonist combinations are also in use (see pp 157–158). In CHF, combination with digoxin and diuretics is standard, and combination with other vasodilators is being explored. Captopril should not normally be combined with potassium-retaining diuretics (Moduretic®, Dyazide®, Maxzide®, spironolactone, triamterene, amiloride) for fear of excess hyperkalemia.

ENALAPRIL

Enalapril (Vasotec® in the USA; Innovace® in the UK; Xanef®, Renitec® or Pres® in Europe; Renivace® in Japan) is now available throughout the world. In many ways enalapril is similar to captopril with, however: (1) a longer half-life, (2) a slower onset of effect because of the requirement of hydrolysis of the pro-drug to the active form, enalaprilat, in the liver so that the therapeutic effect depends on hepatic metabolism, and (3) the absence of the SH group from the structure, thus theoretically lessening or removing the risk of immune-based side-effects. On the other hand, captopril has been in use for several years longer than enalapril with more accumulated clinical experience (Table 8-1).

Pharmacokinetics.   About 60 percent of the oral dose is absorbed[40] with no influence of meals. Enalapril is de-esterified in the liver to the active form, enalaprilat which, however, is poorly absorbed when given orally. The time to the peak serum concentration is about 2 hours for enalapril and about 5 hours for enalaprilat[37] with some delay in CHF. Excretion is 95 percent renal as enalapril or enalaprilat (hence the lower doses in renal failure). The elimination half-life of enalaprilat is about 4–5 hours in hypertension and 7–8 hours in CHF.[37] Following multiple doses, the effective elimination half-life of enalaprilat is 11 hours (package insert). One oral 10 mg dose of enalapril yields sufficient enalaprilat to cause significant ACE inhibition for 19 hours.[40] The peak hypotensive response to enalapril occurs about 4–6 hours after the oral dose both in hypertensives and in CHF[37] that may account for the marked depression of renal function which may occur at that time.[4] Peak effects on cardiac index and other hemodynamic parameters occur earlier, after about 1–2 hours and are sustained for at least 12 hours.[13] In severe liver disease, the dose may have to be increased.

TABLE 8-1

CAPTOPRIL VERSUS ENALAPRIL

	Captopril	Enalapril
Active principle	captopril	enalaprilat
Pharmacokinetics	no liver metabolism	liver metabolism required
Liver disease	little/no effect on pharmacokinetics	delayed formation of enalaprilat; delayed clearance of enalaprilat in severe CHF*
Speed of onset	within 1 hr	slower
Oral dose	25–75 mg 2× daily (3× usual in CHF)	10–20 mg 2× daily or once daily
Sublingual dose	25 mg (in severe hypertension)	—
Duration of action	6–12 hr	12–24 hr
Sulfhydryl groups	present	absent
Immune-based side-effects	rare but present (taste, skin, white cells)	probably absent or very low incidence
Angioedema	rare but present risk	emphasized in package insert but uncommon
Drug-induced renal damage	high-dose proteinuria	creatinine clearance may fall in CHF
Diabetic nephropathy	may benefit	not known
Possible adverse drug interactions	Procainamide, hydralazine, acebutolol, immunosuppressives	not known
Hypotensive risk in CHF	present	present
Clinical experience	many years	recent

Table compiled by LH Opie; CHF = congestive heart failure

Dose.   In hypertension, the dose is 2.5–20 mg as 1 or 2 daily doses.[2,5,14] A low initial dose (2.5 mg) is a wise precaution especially when enalapril is added to a diuretic or the patient is salt-depleted,[45] or in the elderly. In CHF (not yet approved in the USA), enalapril is started under close supervision in hospital with an initial dose of 2.5 mg (risk of hypotension and renal failure) and a usual maintenance dose 10–20 mg 2× daily.[9,13] An IV form of enalaprilat is under investigation.[25] In renal failure (glomerular filtration rate [GFR] below 30 ml/min), the dose of enalapril must be reduced.

Contraindications.   Bilateral renal artery stenosis, renal artery stenosis in a single kidney; severe renal failure (see captopril, p 4); systemic hypotension.

Side-effects.   The major potential side-effects are renal (Fig. 8-4), probably mediated by hypotension and especially found in patients with severe CHF or underlying renal disease including renal artery stenosis. As in the case of captopril, administration of enalapril especially to high-renin patients may lead to an excessive hypotensive response with oliguria and/or azotemia. In animals, very high doses of enalapril may cause renal tubular damage, probably the result of excess prolonged hypotension. Rarely has neutropenia been reported and the relationship to enalapril not proven. Taste disturbances have not occurred and enalapril can be safe when captopril has induced a skin rash.[28] **Angioedema is a risk highlighted in the package insert** (0.2 percent of patients) and may cause fatal laryngeal edema. Unexplained cough and wheeze are not yet well documented.[38]

Precautions.   As in the case of captopril, (1) the major risk is excess hypotension (use low initial dose); and (2) pretreatment evaluation of renal function and of drug co-therapy is essential. In hypertensives, bilateral renal artery stenosis or stenosis in a single kidney should be excluded. It is presumed that enalapril, without the SH group found in captopril, may not develop the same immune-based toxic effects and regular monitoring of the neutrophil count or proteinuria does not seem essential. Until this question is fully settled, it is commonsense to keep the dose of enalapril low (for example 10 mg 2× daily). If ACE inhibition is required for patients with collagen vascular disease or during co-therapy with other drugs altering the immune status, enalapril seems preferable to captopril; yet the white cell count would still need periodic monitoring (package insert).

Drug interactions.   As in the case of captopril, enalapril should not normally be combined with potassium-retaining diuretics unless hypokalemia is documented.

ACE INHIBITORS FOR HYPERTENSION

Mechanism of Antihypertensive Action

In hypertension, increased activity of the renin-angiotensin-aldosterone system is most obvious in cases of unilateral renal artery stenosis when the decreased perfusion pressure to the renal arteries results in increased release of renin from the juxtaglomerular apparatus. However, the renin-angiotensin system also helps to maintain blood pressure both in normal people and in essential hypertension. Therefore, although ACE inhibition leads to the most dramatic falls of blood pressure in the presence of an underlying renal mechanism, ACE inhibition may also be an effective antihypertensive therapy in mild to moderate hypertension, probably acting by indirect adrenergic modulation (Fig. 8-1).

ACE inhibitors appear to lower blood pressure by four mechanisms. They inhibit the normal conversion of angiotensin I to the powerful vasoconstrictor angiotensin II. Second, they reduce the secretion of aldosterone to induce a natriuresis. Third, the inactivation of vasodilatory bradykinins is reduced. Fourth, specific renal vasodilation may enhance natriuresis.

Clinical Use in Hypertension

When it is important to avoid intellectual or sexual impairment and to maintain well-being, captopril will increasingly be chosen over adrenergic inhibitors such as methyldopa or propranolol.[10] Enalapril likewise carries fewer side-effects than atenolol or hydrochlorothiazide.[19]

In *renovascular hypertension* where circulating renin is high and a critical part of the mechanism, ACE inhibition is logical first-line therapy. Captopril was first shown to be effective. Enalapril 10–40 mg daily is sufficiently effective to obviate the need for surgery in most patients.[20] The GFR falls acutely[4] to recover in cases of unilateral but not bilateral disease. The proposed mechanism of the renal damage is that ACE inhibition opens up intrarenal shunts to bypass the glomeruli and to reduce the filtration fraction.[4] This potential effect on renal function is variable and may be absent.[20] The mechanism is quite different from the immune-based renal toxicity sometimes caused by captopril and manifest in some of the early high-dose captopril studies. The acute hypotensive effects both of captopril and enalapril may cause hypotension-mediated renal damage. Whether low-dose captopril regimes fully avoid the immune-based renal problems is not known, but possible. Logically, either of the ACE inhibitors should be started in low doses in patients with renovascular hypertension and given only with great care (if at all) when there is pre-existing bilateral renal artery disease or unilateral disease in a solitary kidney or when renal failure complicates renal artery stenosis.

In *acute severe hypertension*, sublingual (chewed) captopril rapidly brings down the blood pressure,[42] but it is not clear how bilateral renal artery stenosis can be excluded quickly enough to make the great speed of action of captopril an important point. Furthermore, the safety of such sudden falls of blood pressure in the presence of possible renal impairment (always a risk in severe hypertension) has not been evaluated. Because enalapril has a slower mode of action than captopril, it should be tested in such patients.

In *hypertension unresponsive to conventional therapy*, renal artery stenosis must be considered and ACE inhibition may be especially effective (precaution: bilateral disease).

In *diabetic hypertensives*, captopril may be better than β-blockade because of the potential benefit of captopril against nephropathy[41] and because blood sugar regulation is unaltered.

In *mild to moderate hypertension*, either captopril or enalapril can be used as monotherapy even in low-renin patients,[46] or in combination with thiazide diuretics,[44] β-blockers or calcium antagonists. High-dose captopril and enalapril are equipotent.[44] About 50–75 percent of mild to moderate hypertensives respond to monotherapy with ACE inhibition,[18] which is as effective as β-blockade or hydrochlorothiazide with fewer adverse subjective or metabolic or hypovolemic effects.[2,10,19] Combination captopril or enalapril with a thiazide diuretic achieves an additive antihypertensive effect while decreasing the thiazide-induced hypokalemia (see p 122).

ACE INHIBITORS FOR CHF

Rationale. In patients with heart failure associated with decreased cardiac output, systemic vascular resistance is usually elevated. The vasoconstriction partly results from activation of the renin-angiotensin- aldosterone system. Plasma renin activity is elevated in many patients with heart failure and there is some correlation between the severity of heart failure and plasma renin activity. The principle reasons for use of ACE inhibitors in patients with heart failure are to reduce the systemic vascular resistance and to counteract the secondary neurohumoral changes found in severe heart failure. Thus ACE inhibition decreases the elevated levels of plasma catecholamines found in CHF[26] unless there is excess hypotension.

Effects. In the therapy of severe CHF, *captopril* (25–100 mg 3× daily after lower initial doses) is one of the only two vasodilators to show sustained benefit during double-blind randomized trials,[6] the other being high-dose isosorbide dinitrate (see p 28). Because of the rapid onset of action of captopril, reactive hypotension may be a problem so that a test dose of 6.25 mg is usually given first, while vigorous diuretic doses are avoided and the circulating volume maintained. *Enalapril* (5 mg 2× daily after test dose of 2.5 mg, range 2.5–20 mg 2× daily; not yet approved in the USA) is likely to be equally effective because its efficacy over 3 months has been shown in a double-blind randomized trial.[39] Enalapril also improved exercise tolerance over the same period in a randomized but non-blinded study.[9] Because of the slow onset of action, reactive hypotension may be less of a problem with enalapril than with captopril, yet first-dose reactions can occur with doses as low as 2.5 mg,[13] and prolonged action may be a problem. **Hypotension with either agent carries with it the risk of renal failure and angina.**[13] Patients with pre-existing hyponatremia may be at greatest risk of hypotension[32] presumably because they also have the highest renin secretion. In CHF with severe liver dysfunction, captopril would appear to be preferable to enalapril because of the requirement of the latter for activation by the liver. Patients with CHF may constitute a high risk group for serious *ventricular arrhythmias* (risk factors: myocardial disease, therapy with digoxin and thiazide diuretics; excess circulating catecholamines). ACE inhibitors, by relieving heart failure and decreasing circulating NE levels[13] can be expected to have an antiarrhythmic effect;[7] specific studies are required.

Selection of Patients with CHF for ACE Inhibitor Therapy.   ACE inhibitors should be considered in patients with CHF who remain symptomatic despite diuretics and digitalis therapy. An important unanswered question is whether ACE inhibitors can be used instead of digitalis. Mostly the efficacy of these agents has been shown in patients not responding well to diuretics and digitalis. Certain conditions are particularly suitable for ACE inhibitor therapy: (1) hypertension or relative hypertension and CHF; (2) angina plus CHF when ACE inhibitors may improve coronary blood flow; (3) CHF with an elevated plasma renin activity; however, as with hypertension, captopril also works when the renin level is normal.[26] Plasma sodium concentrations of 130 mEq/L or less are more frequently associated with increased plasma renin activity, and may warn of a brisk response to captopril.[32] In patients with high plasma renin levels, captopril may be less effective than anticipated because of persistent pulmonary vasoconstriction.[30]

Precautions.   (1) *Hypotension* may occur in many patients with CHF with pre-existing normal or low blood pressures treated by ACE inhibitors. Transient hypotension has the risk of precipitating arrhythmias or prerenal azotemia. Hypotension may be avoided by decreasing the diuretic dose, maintaining circulating blood volume and by low initial doses. Otherwise, therapy of CHF with ACE inhibition is relatively straightforward, provided that the precautions outlined under captopril are followed. Readjustment of the diuretic or ACE inhibitor dose may be required. (2) *Hyperkalemia* is a risk in patients treated by potassium-retaining diuretics or with excess potassium supplements. (3) *Aortic stenosis* is a contraindication to all vasodilator therapy. (4) *Renal failure* is also a contraindication, because of the risk of prolonged deterioration in renal function following excess hypotension.

ACE INHIBITORS : COMBINATION THERAPY

ACE Inhibitors plus Diuretics

Captopril or enalapril may be combined with other antihypertensive or antifailure regimes. In *hypertension*, captopril may be combined with thiazide diuretics[2] to enhance its hypotensive effects, but with some diuretic-related loss of "quality of life".[10] Combination captopril-hydrochlorothiazide (Capozide®) is now available in several countries (Table 6-6). During co-therapy with hydrochlorothiazide 50 mg, it matters little whether the captopril daily dose is 37.5 or 150 mg daily.[43] Enalapril 20 mg once daily, combined with only 12.5 mg hydrochlorothiazide, gives as good an antihypertensive effect as with more diuretics.[11] In severe hypertension, combination with loop diuretics gives added benefit. Pretherapy renal disease should always be excluded. The combination with thiazide diuretics is thought to be synergistic, because diuretics increase renin, the effects of which are antagonised by ACE inhibitors.[5] ACE inhibitors also tend to decrease the metabolic and hypovolemic side-effects of diuretic therapy.[2] When combined with potassium-retaining thiazide diuretics (Dyazide®, Moduretic®, Maxzide®) and especially spironolactone,[39] there is a *risk of hyperkalemia* because captopril/enalapril decreases aldosterone secretion.

In *CHF*, additive effects of ACE inhibitors on the preload may lead to syncope or hypotension so that the diuretic dose may need to be decreased or omitted for several days before starting captopril/enalapril therapy. Thereafter the diuretic dose usually needs upward adjustment,[13] but may require downward adjustment.[9] Although captopril/enalapril may have severe side-effects when the serum sodium is low (high aldosterone levels retain sodium that stimulates vasopressin secretion), captopril/enalapril may also be most effective in such patients.

ACE Inhibitors plus Other Vasodilators

ACE inhibition may act more dominantly on the arteriolar than on the venous circulation. In the case of captopril, during chronic therapy, captopril acts as a dominant arteriolar dilator in about two-thirds of patients and a dominant pulmonary arterial dilator in about one-third of patients.[30] Because the exercise capacity is closely related to right rather than to left ventricular (LV) performance, the predominant systemic vasodilation caused by captopril may not cause an optimal hemodynamic situation in some patients.[33] Accordingly, therapy with nitrates rather than captopril may give a better response in some patients.[33] Hyponatremic patients are more likely to experience systemic vasodilation with captopril and therefore more likely to experience symptomatic hypotension.[32] Milrinone, added to captopril, may increase the stroke volume without enhancing the hypotensive effect of captopril[23]

As different vasodilators have different supplementary qualities, each patient has to be individualized on a pragmatic basis. A patient with prominent pulmonary congestion may respond better to nitrates, whereas captopril is more logical to promote diuresis or correct hyponatremia. Combination of captopril with other vasodilators such as nitrates, nifedipine or hydralazine should be undertaken with care (added risk of hypotension). The combination hydralazine-captopril may have an added risk of altered immune system function, so that careful monitoring of neutrophils is mandatory.

ACE Inhibitors plus β-Blockade

This combination has been widely used in hypertension, although logically not the combination of choice because both agents have in common an ultimate antirenin effect. Thus the overall antihypertensive response to captopril-β-blockade is less than additive. Although not reported, the possibility of an added immune-based interaction between captopril and acebutolol warrants consideration.

ACE Inhibitors plus Calcium Antagonists

This combination, now increasingly used in the therapy of hypertension, appears to be logical, because of the two different modalities of attack, first the renin-angiotensin system and second the increased peripheral vascular resistance found especially in moderate and severe hypertension. Furthermore, both types of agents should be free of central nervous side-effects.

NEUROHUMORAL EFFECTS IN CHF : ACE INHIBITORS VERSUS OTHER VASODILATORS

Aldosterone Secretion

As expected, ACE inhibitors, such as captopril or enalapril, decrease aldosterone levels due to decreased production of angiotensin II. In some patients with chronic heart failure, prazosin may cause a small increase in aldosterone level.[26] An increased aldosterone level appears to be due to increased plasma renin activity.

Fluid Retention and Hyponatremia

Sodium and water retention occurs not infrequently in response to classical vasodilators. In contrast, during maintenance therapy with captopril or enalapril, the dose of diuretics needs to be reduced in many patients. Hyponatremia is frequently corrected with ACE inhibitors, whereas hyponatremia may persist with other vasodilators, despite similar hemodynamic improvement. Hyponatremia in CHF reflects excess angiotensin II and carries a bad prognosis.

Adrenergic Activity

Captopril and enalapril usually decrease plasma NE levels, particularly after chronic therapy. Plasma NE levels either remain unchanged or may even increase with prazosin or hydralazine. Thus, heightened sympathetic activity, observed in patients with heart failure, tends to lessen following therapy with ACE inhibitors, but remains unchanged with prazosin[26] and may increase with hydralazine.[15]

Drug Tolerance

In approximately 70 percent of patients, some tolerance develops in response to continued hydralazine or prazosin therapy[3] especially in high-renin patients.[26] In contrast, tolerance to the effects of captopril is less common (25–30 percent). Hydralazine or prazosin appear to activate the renin-angiotensin-aldosterone system, at least in some patients. ACE inhibitors, however, decrease angiotensin II and aldosterone levels and, therefore, their potential mechanism for tolerance is obviated.[26]

Exercise Tolerance

Both captopril and enalapril improve exercise tolerance. For other arterial vasodilators, the evidence is less convincing.[1,3,7] Sometimes venous dilators such as nitrates may be best (see p 158).

Patient Survival in CHF

Captopril was markedly better than hydralazine in a small number of patients randomized for one year of therapy.[24]

RENAL IMPAIRMENT

ACE inhibitors may have a specific renal vasodilatory effect.[1a]

In severe CHF and impaired creatinine clearance, ACE inhibitors (especially captopril) may maintain renal function (renal vasodilator effect) and yet there is risk of exaggeration of the renal defect.[31]

In *diabetic nephropathy*, captopril (37.5 mg 3× daily) improved proteinuria without changing serum creatinine possibly by reduction of intrarenal hypertension.[41]

In *early renal failure* of hypertension, ACE inhibitors are being tested for a possible beneficial reduction of intrarenal hypertension.[8]

In *ischemic renal failure*, ACE inhibitors should theoretically relieve angiotensin-induced vasoconstriction.[27]

NEW ACE AND RENIN INHIBITORS

A large number of ACE inhibitors are under investigation including (1) *lisinopril*, a long-acting once-daily lysine derivative of enalapril which requires no prior hepatic activation; (2) *ramipril*, also long-acting and hypotensive in a 5–10 mg dose once daily,[12] but like enalapril a pro-drug; (3) *zofenopril*, 5×

more potent than captopril, longer-acting and with the SH-group complexed to a ring structure; (4) *fosenopril,* under development for hypertension; and (5) *perindopril*, which is claimed to have α-inhibitory qualities. Specific *renin-inhibition* can be achieved by a modified analog of human angiotensinogen with specific renin-inhibition and therefore acting on the renin-angiotensin-aldosterone axis at a different site from the ACE inhibitors (Site 1, Fig. 8-3).

SUMMARY

ACE inhibitors have a radically different and new site of therapeutic attack, the renin-angiotensin axis. Initially used only in refractory cases of hypertension and CHF, they are now employed earlier and earlier in those conditions especially with the emergence of much safer new low-dose regimes for captopril, and the development of structurally different compounds such as enalapril, lisinopril, and ramipril. The major side-effect of ACE inhibitors is excess hypotension. The major contraindications are pre-existing hypotension or severe renal impairment (exception: captopril for diabetic nephropathy) or collagen vascular disease (in the case of captopril). The major danger is renal impairment, especially when hypotension occurs in the presence of pre-existing renal damage as in severe heart failure or renal artery stenosis (particularly when bilateral). A major advantage of ACE inhibitors is that they favorably modify the basic neurohumoral abnormalities in CHF, thus representing a distinct advance over traditional vasodilators. In mild to moderate hypertension, the major advantage of ACE inhibitors is the absence of side-effects such as fatigue or mental or sexual impairment or exercise limitation, so that a feeling of well-being is usual.

REFERENCES

1. Agnosti PG, De Cesare N, Doria E, et al: Afterload reduction: A comparison of captopril and nifedipine in dilated cardiomyopathy. Br Heart J 55:391–399, 1986
1a. Ando K, Fujita T, Ito Y, et al: The role of renal hemodynamics in the antihypertensive effect of captopril. Am Heart J 111:347–352, 1986
2. Bauer JH, Jones LB: Comparative studies: Enalapril versus hydrochlorothiazide as first-step therapy for the treatment of primary hypertension. Am J Kidney Dis 4:55–62, 1984
3. Bayliss J, Canepa-Anson R, Norell MS, et al: Vasodilatation with captopril and prazosin in chronic heart failure: Double-blind study at rest and on exercise. Br Heart J 55:265–273, 1986
4. Bender W, La France N, Walker WG: Mechanism of deterioration in renal function in patients with renovascular hypertension treated with enalapril. Hypertension 6 (suppl I):I-193–I-197, 1984
5. Bergstrand R, Herlitz H, Johansson S, et al: Effective dose range of enalapril in mild to moderate essential hypertension. Br J Clin Pharmacol 19:605–611, 1985
6. Captopril Multicenter Research Group: A placebo-controlled trial of captopril in refractory chronic congestive heart failure. J Am Coll Cardiol 2:755–763, 1983
7. Cleland JGF, Dargie HJ, Ball SG, et al: Effects of enalapril in heart failure: A double blind study of effects on exercise performance, renal function, hormones, and metabolic state. Br Heart J 54:305–312, 1985
8. Cooper WD, Doyle GD, Donohoe J, et al: Enalapril in the treatment of hypertension associated with impaired renal function. J Hypertens 3 (suppl 3):S471–S474, 1985
9. Creager MA, Massie BM, Faxon DP, et al: Acute and long-term effects of enalapril on the cardiovascular response to exercise tolerance in patients with congestive heart failure. J Am Coll Cardiol 6:163–170, 1985
10. Croog SH, Levine S, Testa MA, et al: The effects of antihypertensive therapy on the quality of life. New Engl J Med 314:1657–1664, 1986
11. Dahlof B, Andren L, Eggertsen R, et al: Potentiation of the antihypertensive effect of enalapril by randomized addition of different doses of hydrochlorothiazide. J Hypertens 3 (suppl 3):S483–S486, 1985
12. de Leeuw PW, Lugtenburg PL, van Houten H, et al: Preliminary experiences with HOE 498, a novel long-acting converting enzyme inhibitor, in hypertensive patients. J Cardiovasc Pharmacol 7:1161–1165, 1985
13. DiCarlo L, Chatterjee K, Parmley WW, et al: Enalapril: A new angiotensin-converting enzyme inhibitor in chronic heart failure: Acute and chronic hemodynamic evaluations. J Am Coll Cardiol 2:865–871, 1983
14. Dunn FG, Oigman W, Ventura HO, et al: Enalapril improves systemic and renal

hemodynamics and allows regression of left ventricular mass in essential hypertension. Am J Cardiol 53:105–108, 1984

15. Elkayam U, Roth A, Hsueh W, et al: Neurohumoral consequences of vasodilator therapy with hydralazine and nifedipine in severe congestive heart failure. Am Heart J 111:1130–1138, 1986

16. Ferguson RK, Turini GA, Brunner HR, et al: A specific orally active inhibitor of angiotensin-converting enzyme in man. Lancet i:775–778, 1977

17. Frohlich ED, Cooper RA, Lewis EJ: Review of the overall experience of captopril in hypertension. Arch Intern Med 144:1441–1444, 1984

18. Gavras H, Biollaz J, Waeber B, et al: Antihypertensive effect of the new oral angiotensin converting enzyme inhibitor "MK-421". Lancet ii:543–549, 1981

19. Helgeland A, Strommen R, Hagelund CH, et al: Enalapril, atenolol and hydrochlorothiazide in mild to moderate hypertension. Lancet i:872–875, 1986

20. Hodsman GP, Brown JJ, Cumming AMM, et al: Enalapril (MK421) in the treatment of hypertension with renal artery stenosis. J Hypertens 1 (suppl 1):109–117, 1983

21. Jaffe IA: Adverse effects profile of sulfhydryl compounds in man. Am J Med 80:471–476, 1986

22. Jenkins AC, Dreslinski GR, Tadros SS, et al: Captopril in hypertension: Seven years later. J Cardiovasc Pharmacol 7:S96–S101, 1985

23. LeJemtel TH, Maskin CS, Mancini D, et al: Systemic and regional hemodynamic effects of captopril and milrinone administered alone and concomitantly in patients with heart failure. Circulation 72:364–369, 1985

24. Lilly L, Dzau VJ, Williams GH, et al: Captopril vs hydralazine in advanced congestive heart failure: Comparison of one year survival. Circulation 72 (suppl III):III-408, 1985

25. Maskin CS, Ocken S, Chadwick B, et al: Comparative systemic and renal effects of dopamine and angiotensin-converting enzyme inhibition with enalaprilat in patients with heart failure. Circulation 72:846–852, 1985

26. Mettauer B, Rouleau J-L, Bichet D, et al: Differential long-term intrarenal and neurohumoral effects of captopril and prazosin in patients with chronic congestive heart failure: Importance of initial plasma renin activity. Circulation 73:492–502, 1986

27. Myers BD, Moran SM: Hemodynamically mediated acute renal failure. New Engl J Med 314:97–105, 1986

28. Navis GJ, De Jong PE, Kallenberg CGM, et al: Absence of cross-reactivity between captopril and enalapril. Lancet i:1017, 1984

29. Packer M: Mechanisms of nitrate action in patients with severe left ventricular failure: Conceptual problems with the theory of venosequestration. Am Heart J 110:259–264, 1985

30. Packer M, Lee WH, Medina N, et al: Hemodynamic and clinical significance of the pulmonary vascular response to long-term captopril therapy in patients with severe chronic heart failure. J Am Coll Cardiol 6:635–645, 1985

31. Packer M, Lee WH, Medina N, et al: Comparative effects of two converting-enzyme inhibitors on renal function in patients with severe chronic heart failure: A prospective randomized clinical trial. J Am Coll Cardiol 7:70A, 1986

32. Packer M, Medina N, Yushak M: Relation between serum sodium concentration and the hemodynamic and clinical responses to converting enzyme inhibition with captopril in severe heart failure. J Am Coll Cardiol 3:1035–1043, 1984

33. Packer M, Medina N, Yushak M, et al: Comparative effects of captopril and isosorbide dinitrate on pulmonary arteriolar resistance and right ventricular function in patients with severe left ventricular failure: Results of a randomized crossover study. Am Heart J 109:1293–1299, 1985

34. Rademaker M, Shaw TRD, Williams BC, et al: Intravenous captopril treatment in patients with severe cardiac failure. Br Heart J 55:187–190, 1986

35. Reyes AJ, Leary WP, Acosta-Barrios TN: Once-daily administration of captopril and hypotensive effect. J Cardiovasc Pharmacol 7:S16–S19, 1985

36. Salvetti A, Pedrinelli R, Magagna A, et al: Influence of food on acute and chronic effects of captopril in essential hypertensive patients. J Cardiovasc Pharmacol 7:S25–S29, 1985

37. Schwartz JB, Taylor A, Abernethy D, et al: Pharmacokinetics and pharmacodynamics of enalapril in patients with congestive heart failure and patients with hypertension. J Cardiovasc Pharmacol 7:767–776, 1985

38. Semple PF, Herd GW: Cough and wheeze caused by inhibitors of angiotensin-converting enzyme. New Engl J Med 314:61, 1986

39. Sharpe DN, Murphy J, Coxon R, et al: Enalapril in patients with chronic heart failure: A placebo-controlled, randomized, double-blind study. Circulation 70:271–278, 1984

40. Sweet CS, Ulm EH: Enalapril. New Drugs Ann: Cardiovasc Drugs 2:1–17, 1984

41. Taguma Y, Kitamoto Y, Futaki G, et al: Effect of captopril on heavy proteinuria in azotemic diabetics. New Engl J Med 313:1617–1620, 1985

42. Tschollar W, Belz GG: Sublingual captopril in hypertensive crises. Lancet ii:34–35, 1985

43. Veterans Administration Cooperative Study Group on Antihypertensive Agents: Low-

dose captopril for the treatment of mild to moderate hypertension. Arch Intern Med 144:1947–1953, 1984

44. Vlasses PH, Conner DP, Rotmensch HH, et al: Double-blind comparison of captopril and enalapril in mild to moderate hypertension. J Am Coll Cardiol 7:651–660, 1986
45. Webster J, Newnham DM, Petrie JC: Initial dose of enalapril in hypertension. Br Med J 290:1623–1624, 1985
46. Wilkins LH, Dustan HP, Walker JF, et al: Enalapril in low-renin essential hypertension. Clin Pharmacol Ther 34:297–302, 1983
47. Witzgall H, Hirsch F, Scherer B: Acute hemodynamic and hormonal effects of captopril are diminished by indomethacin. Clin Sci 62:611–615, 1982

Reviews

Edwards CRW, Padfield PL: Angiotensin-converting enzyme inhibitors: Past, present and bright future. Lancet i:30–34, 1985
Gomez HJ, Cirillo VJ, Irvin JD: Enalapril: A review of human pharmacology. Drugs 30 (suppl 1):13–24, 1985
Riley LJ, Vlasses PH, Ferguson RK: Clinical pharmacology and therapeutic applications of the new oral converting enzyme inhibitor, enalapril. Am Heart J 109:1085–1089, 1985
Robertson JIS: Circulatory basis for the use of angiotensin converting enzyme inhibitors in hypertension and cardiac failure. J Cardiovasc Pharmacol 8 (suppl 1):S2–S8, 1986
Romankiewicz JA, Brogden RN, Heal RC, et al: Captopril: An update review of its pharmacologic properties and therapeutic efficacy in congestive heart failure. Drugs 25:6–40, 1983

L. H. Opie
B. J. Gersh

9

Antithrombotic Agents: Platelet Inhibitors, Anticoagulants, and Fibrinolytics

MECHANISMS OF THROMBOSIS

To form a thrombus, the three steps are (1) exposure of the circulating blood to a thrombogenic surface, such as a damaged vascular endothelium; (2) a sequence of platelet-related events, involving first platelet adhesion, then platelet aggregation and release of agents further promoting aggregation and causing vasoconstriction; and (3) activation of the clotting mechanism with an important role for thrombin in the formation of fibrin. Once formed, the clot may be broken down by plasmin-stimulated fibrinolysis. Current antithrombotic medications include those inhibiting platelets (antiplatelet agents), anticoagulants and fibrinolytics.

Two types of clot may form—the *white thrombus* that is predominantly composed of platelets and tends to form when blood flows rapidly as in arteries, whereas the *red thrombus* is rich in red cells and thrombus and tends to form where blood flow is stagnant as in veins. Inhibitors of platelet function are more likely to inhibit the white thrombus, whereas the anticoagulants, heparin and warfarin, are agents active against venous but not arterial thrombosis.

The above sequence relates to the three main types of agents considered in this chapter. First, platelet inhibitors may be expected to act on arterial thrombi and to help prevent their consequences such as transient ischemic attacks (TIAs) and myocardial infarction. Second, anticoagulants may be expected to benefit thromboembolism derived from veins such as those in the legs, or from a dilated left atrium. Third, fibrinolytics will be most useful in clinical syndromes of acute arterial thrombosis and occlusion, typified by acute myocardial infarction (AMI), but also including peripheral arterial thrombosis.

In addition to their potential for acting against arterial thrombosis, it may be predicted that platelet inhibitors should also protect against other proposed consequences of platelet malfunction such as excessive vasoconstriction and, possibly, atherogenesis because platelets release powerful vasoconstricting agents, such as serotonin and platelets, which may play a role in stimulating growth of the arterial intima, thereby promoting atheroma.

The processes of platelet adhesion and aggregation are intimately involved with the pathways of prostaglandin synthesis which has two chief end-products with opposing effects: thromboxane A_2 is pro-aggregatory and vasoconstrictive, whereas prostacyclin is anti-aggregatory and vasodilator.

Drugs for the Heart, Second Expanded Edition
Copyright © 1987 by Grune & Stratton, Inc.

163

Platelet Adhesion

This is the first of the three steps in the development of an arterial throm-bus, typically occurring in relation to a damaged arterial endothelium at the site of an atherosclerotic plaque or on an artificial surface, such as a prosthetic heart valve, or on the arteriovenous shunt used for renal dialysis. Microfibrils of collagen from the deeper layers of the vessel wall become exposed as a result of endothelial injury, and appear to promote platelet adhesion. It is also pro-posed that platelets may adhere to normal or nearly normal arteries by a process involving the Willebrand factor; the subsequent release of platelet-derived growth factor and the ensuing smooth muscle intimal proliferation constitute one hypothetical sequence of events in early atherogenesis. Platelet adhesion to the vessel wall is not affected by thromboxane A_2 or by prostacy-clin or by agents modifying their production, but rather by another antiplatelet agent, dipyridamole. The latter effect is, however, of unproven clinical value.

Platelet Aggregation and Release Phenomena

The critical but not yet fully explained event causing aggregation of platelets is a rise in intracellular platelet calcium by two mediators, adenosine diphosphate (ADP) and thromboxane A_2. The ADP is derived from platelets or tissue injury (Fig. 9-1) and thromboxane A_2 is synthesized by the prostaglandin pathway. An enhanced platelet calcium has several consequences, including (1) activation of the pathways breaking down the platelet phospholipids even-tually to form thromboxane (Fig. 9-2) and (2) activation of platelet actin and myosin present to cause contraction and promote platelet aggregation. Plate-let activation also involves membrane alterations to allow platelets to stick to each other. Not only does calcium promote the formation of thromboxane A_2, but once thromboxane A_2 is formed, it enhances intraplatelet calcium by an unknown mechanism, possibly acting to inhibit the formation of cyclic AMP. Conversely, prostacyclin, formed from the vessel wall, acts to decrease platelet calcium by promotion of the formation of cyclic AMP within platelets, and cyclic AMP in turn decreases platelet calcium (in platelets, as in vascular smooth

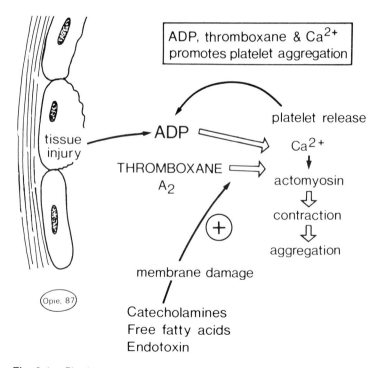

Fig. 9-1.   Platelet aggregation depends on a combination of endothelial tis-sue injury with release of adenosine diphosphate (ADP), thromboxane A_2 and an increase in platelet calcium (Ca^{2+}).

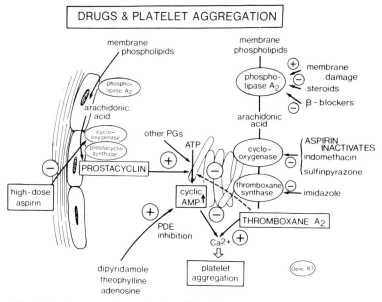

Fig. 9-2. Agents active on platelets. The critical event in platelet aggregation is an increase of platelet calcium that can be inhibited by prostacyclin (PGI_2), and promoted by thromboxane A_2. Most clinically used inhibitors act on cyclo-oxygenase. Aspirin inactivates cyclo-oxygenase and in high doses inhibits prostacyclin formation.

muscle, cyclic AMP decreases cytosolic calcium). As cytosolic calcium rises, the platelet contracts and at the same time releases ADP from the platelet-dense granules into the extracellular space; such ADP acts on the membrane receptors of adjacent platelets to release intracellular calcium in those platelets, thereby promoting the whole process of platelet aggregation by a self-perpetuating mechanism. Platelet aggregation may be further enhanced by circulating catecholamines and free fatty acids, as may be elevated as part of the "stress" reaction.

Activation of Clotting Mechanisms

The intrinsic coagulation pathway involves the ultimate generation of thrombin during activation of the platelet membrane. The extrinsic coagulation pathway involves thromboplastin generated by the vessel wall, which is then converts prothrombin to thrombin. Prothrombin is one of several vitamin-K-dependent clotting factors; the oral anticoagulants such as warfarin are vitamin-K-antagonists. Thrombin from either source enhances platelet membrane activation further to promote platelet aggregation and to convert fibrinogen to fibrin, which adheres to platelet surfaces to stabilize and fix the arterial thrombus. Fibrinolytic mechanisms, involving the conversion of plasminogen to plasmin, act to limit the size of the clot and eventually to dissolve it at least in part.

Platelets and Vascular Contraction

During and after platelet aggregation, platelets release 5–hydroxytryptamine (serotonin) and other potentially important products such as platelet factor 4 and β-thromboglobulin that may help in the formation of the hemostatic plug. Serotonin normally causes vasodilation in the presence of an intact vascular endothelium. In contrast, when the endothelium is damaged, serotonin causes vasoconstriction[86] that may promote vascular stasis and thrombosis. Hence platelets are suspected of a role in vasoconstrictive diseases such as coronary spasm or Raynaud's disease. This vasoconstrictive effect of platelets may be aided by leukotrienes.

Leukotrienes are newly described prostaglandin-like agents released from white cells and tissue macrophages to act as powerful vasoconstrictors. Because they are prostaglandin derivatives and also eventually derived from arachidonic acid, aspirin and other inhibitors of cyclo-oxygenase may act by leukotriene inhibition. Such concepts are still being explored.

PROSTAGLANDINS AND THEIR ROLE
IN PLATELET FUNCTION

Synthesis of Prostaglandins and Cyclo-Oxygenase Inhibitors

Prostaglandins are compounds with a long-chain cyclical structure, eventually derived from the unsaturated fatty acid, arachidonic acid, which in turn is formed from the phospholipids of the cell membranes. The name prostaglandin is derived from the parent compound, prostanoic acid, first isolated from prostatic tissue by von Euler (the Swedish Nobel Prizewinner). Now it seems that prostaglandins have widespread effects throughout the body, but only minimal effects on prostatic function. Membrane phospholipids, especially in the vascular wall or the platelets, are converted to arachidonic acid under the influence of the enzyme phospholipase A_2 (Fig. 9-2). Next to be formed are the cyclic endoperoxides (enzyme: cyclo-oxygenase) that in turn become converted to either prostacyclin (enzyme: prostacyclin synthetase) or to thromboxane A_2 (enzyme: thromboxane synthetase). Each of these enzymatic steps is potentially subject to therapeutic inhibition by different inhibitors of platelet function (Fig. 9-2).

Prostacyclin (PGI_2) is the major prostaglandin formed in the vessel walls, with vasodilator and antithrombotic properties, acting chiefly by inhibition of platelet aggregation. Prostacyclin is synthesized from arachidonic acid in the endothelial wall by a pathway involving cyclo-oxygenase and potentially inhibited by aspirin. PGI_2 is very rapidly broken down to become 6-keto-$PGF_{1\alpha}$ and also 6-keto-PGE_1. The generation of prostacyclin is probably a physiologic mechanism indirectly to protect the vessel wall by its inhibitory effect on platelet aggregation. Therapeutically, the very short half-life of prostacyclin makes it unsuitable for use in conditions such as unstable angina, and presently prostacyclin analogs are under evaluation.

Thromboxane A_2 promotes platelet aggregation, acts as a vasoconstrictor, and may ultimately play a role in the promotion of vascular disease. Thromboxane A_2, like prostacyclin, is also eventually formed from arachidonic acid by a sequential pathway that can be blocked at several sites, including the cyclo-oxygenase step inhibited by aspirin. Selective inhibition of thromboxane synthetase is clearly more specific and now made possible by new experimental agents (Table 9-1). Thus prostacyclin and thromboxane A_2 potentially have opposing effects, as also shown experimentally in coronary artery stenosis.[73]

Cyclo-Oxygenase Inhibitors

Cyclo-oxygenase plays a crucial role in the synthesis of the endoperoxides that are the precursors to both (1) vasodilatory anti-aggregatory prostaglandins of which the prototype is prostacyclin and (2) the vasoconstrictor pro-aggregatory prostaglandins of which the prototype is thromboxane A_2. Thus inhibitors of this enzyme have both potential harmful and beneficial effects. The wide variety of ultimate effects of cyclo-oxygenase inhibitors that may be dose-related, including vasodilation and vasoconstriction, explain the apparently contradictory or only mildly beneficial results of numerous therapeutic trials of these agents in the postinfarct stage. Of these agents, the one with clearest therapeutic benefit is aspirin.

PLATELET INHIBITION BY ASPIRIN

The major mechanism whereby aspirin acts is by inactivation of cyclo-oxygenase especially in platelets and also in vascular endothelium (Fig. 9-1); other mechanisms of action may also operate.[32,44] **Aspirin irreversibly acetylates cyclo-oxygenase, and activity is not restored until new platelets are formed.** Platelets, being very primitive cells, cannot synthesize new proteins so

TABLE 9-1   PLATELET-INHIBITOR AGENTS UNDER INVESTIGATION

Agent	Mechanism	Comment
Indomethacin (reference drug)	Cyclo-oxygenase inhibition Anti-inflammatory	Vasoconstrictive; many drug interactions
Dazoxiben; UK-38485; AH-23848; OKY-046	Thromboxane Synthetase inhibition	Short duration of action usually limits use
BM-13179 and others	Thromboxane receptor antagonism	Promising in limitation of experimental ischemia
β-Blockers	"Membrane stabilization"	High-dose propranolol
Ca^{2+} antagonists	Ca^{2+} required for platelet aggregation	Nifedipine; modest effects in clinical doses
α-Blockers	Ca^{2+} inhibition	Nicergoline and others being tested
Ketanserin	Serotonin antagonist	Modest clinical benefit
Pentoxifylline	PDE-inhibitor	Chiefly hemorrheologic
Ticlopidine	Cyclo-oxygenase inhibitor other specific effects	Clinically promising
Clofibrate	Chiefly hypolipidemic	Little used
Prostacyclin analogs	Promote effects of prostacyclin	Not yet in clinical use
Nafazatrom	Stimulates prostacylin release and inhibits its breakdown	Free radical scavenger; tested in myocardial ischemia[74]

that aspirin removes all the platelet cyclo-oxygenase activity for the lifespan of the platelet.[92] Thereby aspirin stops the production of the pro-aggregatory thromboxane A_2 and eventually acts as an antithrombotic agents.[54] On the other hand, aspirin also has important non-platelet effects and in the vascular endothelium likewise inactivates cyclo-oxygenase that could diminish formation of anti-aggregatory prostacyclin. The difference is that vascular cyclo-oxygenase can be resynthesized within hours. Theoretically, aspirin has both antithrombotic and prothrombotic effects. Since the former effect seems to predominate, the net result is that platelet inhibition may be achieved by both low and high-dose aspirin.

Differential Selective Inactivation of Cyclo-Oxygenase in Platelets and in Vascular Endothelium

Theoretically, aspirin should inhibit production of platelet thromboxane more than that of vascular prostacyclin. Many studies have tried to translate this attractive theory into reality, using as end-points platelet aggregation and the generation of thromboxane versus that of prostacyclin. Normal doses of aspirin (325–650 mg) powerfully inhibit platelet aggregation for 4–7 days.[58] Clear-cut selective inhibition of thromboxane A_2 has not been obtained even with aspirin doses down to 20–40 mg daily, in comparison with 325 mg daily.[58,92] However, with the ultra-low dose of aspirin (20 mg), vascular endothelium more readily synthesizes prostacyclin than do the platelets make thromboxane.

Aspirin Kinetics

Aspirin undergoes substantial presystemic hydrolysis to form salicylic acid, which is only a weak inactivator of cyclo-oxygenase with however a longer half-life of 2–3 hours versus 15–20 minutes for aspirin.[67] Because the concentration of the parent compound is highest in the splanchnic circulation, the platelets circulating in that region will be exposed to a higher dose of aspirin than those in the systemic vascular bed. This difference may explain why ultra-low doses of aspirin (20 mg) could have a greater platelet inhibitory than vascular inhibitory effect.[66]

Clinical Indications for Aspirin

(1) Unstable angina. Two trials have shown benefit: 325 mg daily in men[49] and 1300 mg daily both in men and women.[11] Aspirin is started within 2–8 days of hospitalization and continued for up to 2 years. In men the lower dose should be used for compliance, but in women it is the higher dose that has the documented effect (heparin is added in the acute phase, see p 176). (2) Theatened stroke. In TIAs, aspirin 1300 mg daily (650 mg 2× daily or 325 mg 4× daily) had a men-only benefit with stroke and death as end-points.[12,22] When considering the occurrence of TIAs as an end-point, women also seem to benefit.[7,22] (3) Postinfarction. There is no evidence that aspirin 1–2 g daily prevents the recurrence of myocardial infarction[56] unless the many trials are grouped together;[43] this is a procedure with some statistical reserve, yet the Food and Drug Administration (FDA) has recently approved aspirin for postinfarct protection.[21]

Less firm indications for aspirin are: (1) postcoronary bypass surgery. In two relatively small series, aspirin 975 mg daily prevented graft occlusion,[10] as did "low-dose" aspirin, 100 mg daily,[52] and in both cases it was essential to start aspirin as early as possible after the operation (the combination aspirin-dipyridamole is usually preferred, see p 171); (2) artificial heart valves, to prevent emboli[16] although warfarin is superior to aspirin alone (see p 177); (3) arteriovenous shunts, aspirin 160 mg daily decreases thrombosis;[33] there are reservations and problems;[51] (4) prevention of pregnancy-induced hypertension, aspirin, 60 mg daily, may benefit;[89] (5) following balloon dilation percutaneous transluminal coronary angioplasty (PTCA) aspirin is widely used for reasons similar to bypass surgery without proof of efficacy in this setting.

Side-effects.   In the normal therapeutic doses usually used in unstable angina, minor gastrointestinal (GI) side-effects occur in about half the patients and may be dose-limiting in about 10–20 percent (dyspepsia, nausea, vomiting). GI bleeding may occur in about 7 percent, with frank melena only in about 1 percent of patients per year and hematemesis in about 0.1 percent per year. Uncommonly, gout may be aggravated (mechanism: impaired urate secretion). GI side-effects may be reduced by *buffered* (Bufferin® 324 mg) or *enteric-coated aspirin* (Cosprin® 325–650 mg, Easprin® 975 mg)[59] or by Alka-Selzer® (with however 567 mg sodium per tablet) or by dose-reduction or by intermittent therapy—(in the UK, Disprin® contains 300 mg aspirin, 90 mg calcium carbonate).

Side effects of high-dose aspirin.   A truly high dose of aspirin (4000 mg/day) can aggravate angina in patients with Prinzmetal's variant angina, possibly by promotion of coronary artery spasm;[61] this dose also increases fibrinolytic activity[63] and GI side-effects are much more likely. Clinically, however, similar high doses have been used in rheumatoid arthritis for an average period of 10 years without any increase in angina, sudden death or stroke; rather, there was a reduction of myocardial infarction in men.[50]

Contraindications.   Aspirin intolerance, hemophilia, history of GI bleeds or of peptic ulcer or other potential sources of GI or genito-urinary bleeding. Congestive heart failure (CHF) is a contraindication to Alka-Selzer® (sodium content). Renal failure or stones; hepatic cirrhosis.[20] *Relative contraindications* include potentially dangerous drug interactions (next section), dyspepsia, iron deficiency anemia, gout, and the possibility of enhanced peri-operative bleeding[85] unless the dose is 20 mg daily.[92] Retinal hemorrhages are not a contraindication to low-dose aspirin.

Precautions.   Besides checking for contraindications and drug interactions, patients chronically receiving aspirin should have their hemoglobin checked periodically in case of occult GI bleeding. Blood sugar and urate may need periodic checks (next section).

Drug interactions.   Generally, nonsteroidal anti-inflammatory drugs (NSAIDs) attenuate the efficacy of antihypertensive therapy by complex mechanisms;[90] aspirin appears not to share this interaction. Aspirin may decrease the urinary excretion of uric acid, the levels of which need monitoring in patients also receiving thiazides or in patients with a family history of gout.[30] Aspirin may interfere with the uricosuric effect of sulfinpyrazone and probenecid and reduce the natriuretic effect of spironolactone. Aspirin may rarely precipitate gout, so there is a potential indirect interaction with thiazides. The risk of aspirin-induced GI bleeding is increased by alcohol, corticosteroid therapy, and NSAIDs. Enteric-coated preparations may have their efficacy reduced by antacids by altering the pH of the stomach. Phenobarbital decreases aspirin efficacy by hepatic enzyme induction. Hypoglycemia: the effect of oral hypoglycemic agents and insulin might be enhanced. Aspirin, especially in high doses, may exaggerate a bleeding tendency and anticoagulant-induced bleeding[63] that may explain why disopyramide-warfarin causes less bleeding than aspirin-warfarin in patients with bypass surgery.[15] (For the combination dipyridamole-aspirin, see p 171).

High Versus Low-Dose Aspirin

The proven benefit of conventional doses such as 325–1300 mg daily in unstable angina or after bypass surgery suggests that the prostacyclin-thromboxane "balance" theory with the presumed superior inhibition of thromboxane formation by low-dose aspirin may not be correct. It seems as if in clinical terms doses of 300–1300 mg should be regarded as proven doses, doses below those as "low-dose", doses down to 20 mg as "ultra-low-dose", and "high-dose" as those above 1300 mg.

Aspirin Dose, Men Versus Women

A greater benefit of aspirin (1300 mg daily) in men than in women was shown in a Canadian trial on threatened stroke;[12] a similar dose was however equally effective in men and women with unstable angina.[11] These differences are not easily explicable.

"Prophylactic" Aspirin

Many patients are being prescribed aspirin, usually in low doses, on the unproven supposition that thromboembolic events may be diminished, that coronary atherogenesis may be inhibited,[6] and that thrombosis and myocardial infarction can be prevented. When aspirin is given in this "prophylactic" and as yet unproven way, it would make sense to give no more than one baby (= Junior = childrens) aspirin, containing about 80 mg every day or even every second or third day. Even this dose may be too high for truly prophylactic indications.[44]

Aspirin—Summary

Aspirin is now of proven value in unstable angina to prevent myocardial infarction and in TIAs to prevent strokes (men only) and recurrent attacks. In postinfarct patients, its protective effects are recognized by the FDA although the statistics involve trial combinations. Aspirin is also used (but is usually combined with dipyridamole) for the prevention of thromboembolism following bypass surgery, and in selected patients with artificial heart valves or arteriovenous shunts. The optimal dose remains unsure, but most trials showing beneficial outcome have used 300–1300 mg daily and higher doses do not seem warranted. For postinfarct prophylaxis, 325 mg daily is recommended by the FDA. Some experimental evidence suggests that in normals even ultra-low dose aspirin (20 mg daily) may preferentially inhibit thromboxane A_2 formation. In the absence of clinical proof of efficacy of such ultra-low doses, conventional doses will continue to be used with, however, a dose reduction in patients intolerant to aspirin.

PLATELET INHIBITION BY SULFINPYRAZONE

Sulfinpyrazone (Anturane®) also inhibits cyclo-oxygenase and has similar ultimate effects to those of aspirin, decreasing the production of the prostanoids, prostacyclin, and thromboxane A_2. The mechanism of action on the cyclo-oxygenase is different from aspirin in that sulfinpyrazone competitively and reversibly inhibits the enzyme whereas aspirin inactivates, so that sulfinpyrazone is a much weaker inhibitor.[67] Sulfinpyrazone also limits platelet adhesion to collagen, an action not shared by aspirin. The critical questions are (1) whether sulfinpyrazone, which is more expensive and needs multiple daily doses, gives any added protection to patients already taking aspirin; or (2) whether sulfinpyrazone might be used as an alternate agent to aspirin. On first principles, these two agents should be closely similar in their effects. However, for two of the major indications for aspirin, namely unstable angina and threatened stroke in males, sulfinpyrazone (200 mg 4× daily) is not effective.

Indications.   In the USA, the only licensed indication is gouty arthritis, chronic or intermittent. In mitral stenosis, however, a 4 year old prospective blinded study showed that sulfinpyrazone (200 mg 4× daily) decreased thromboembolism and reverted the shortened platelet survival time towards normal.[78] The benefit appeared to include those with mitral valve replacement during the trial. Data from this highly specific trial may not be extrapolated to other situations where there is risk of cardiovascular thromboembolism as in patients with artificial valves, even though sulfinpyrazone does shorten platelet survival times in such patients.

Dose.   "The dose most commonly used, 800 mg/day . . . is at the lower end of the dose-response curve and close to the maximum tolerable level".[67]

Contraindications.   Peptic ulcer, renal impairment, renal stones.[93] Early after AMI, sulfinpyrazone may cause temporary renal failure.[5a]

Drug interactions.   Sulfinpyrazone, being highly bound (98–99 percent) to plasma proteins, may displace warfarin to precipitate bleeding. Sulfinpyrazone may potentiate the effects of sulfa drugs, sulfonylureas, and insulin.

Problems in Postinfarct Prophylaxis

Much confusion has been created by the results of a large postinfarct trial reported in 1980 that appeared to show a dramatic reduction in sudden death.[4] Subsequently, very careful dissection of the data by the FDA led to a rejection of the claim for benefit[83] chiefly because sudden death was imprecisely defined and certain patients were retrospectively excluded from the study. **No amount of subsequent re-analysis and attempted re-instatement of the data has been able to elicit enthusiasm for the use of sulfinpyrazone in postinfarct patients.** It remains to be seen whether interest in postinfarct sulfinpyrazone can be revived by the results of the Italian Anturan trial[3] in which sulfinpyrazone 400 mg 2× daily (started as 200 mg daily to avoid a sudden uricosuric effect) reduced re-infarction in the 19 month postinfarct follow-up period. There was no effect on mortality, possibly the result of selection of patients with no signs of heart failure. Sulfinpyrazone should not be given in high dose (800 mg daily) in the acute phase of myocardial infarction, when it substantially elevates serum urea and creatinine, even though decreasing urate levels.[93]

Sulfinpyrazone—Summary

At present there seems little argument for the use of sulfinpyrazone as a specific antiplatelet agent except in mitral stenosis; even there the benefit of sulfinpyrazone over warfarin is not established. In gouty arthritis, sulfinpyrazone benefits by its uricosuric effect (usual dose 100–200 mg 2× daily with meals). Aspirin may be contraindicated in gout because it impairs urate excretion and interferes with the uricosuric effect of sulfinpyrazone. Except in gout, aspirin is a better platelet-inhibitor than sulfinpyrazone.

PLATELET INHIBITION BY DIPYRIDAMOLE

Dipyridamole (Persantine®) has five effects. First, there are the well-known coronary vasodilator effects mediated by the inhibition of adenosine deaminase, and not yet of clinical value. Second, it inhibits platelet adhesion to the damaged vessel. Third, dipyridamole may potentiate the anti-aggregatory effect of prostacyclin.[57] Fourth, at high and supraclinical doses,[57,67] dipyridamole inhibits phosphodiesterase in platelets, thereby enhancing cyclic AMP formation and lowering platelet calcium (Fig. 9-2). Fifth, dipyridamole by inhibiting the breakdown of adenosine indirectly increases cyclic AMP, thereby inhibiting platelet aggregation.[31,32] **In comparison with aspirin, dipyridamole has far more inhibitory effects on platelet adhesion to the vessel wall and much less on platelet aggregation.** There have been few clinical trials using dipyridamole alone; usually combination with aspirin is undertaken.

Indications.   In the USA, **there are no specific registered indications.** It is classified as "possibly" effective for the long-term therapy of angina pectoris. There is no evidence that dipyridamole alone decreases myocardial re-infarction.

Dose.   Most trials have used 75 mg 3× daily. The manufacturers recommend 50 mg 3× daily, taken at least 1 hour before meals.

Side-effects.   GI irritation; vasodilatory and hypotensive effects such as dizziness, flushing, syncope, occasional angina pectoris ("coronary steal").

Combination Dipyridamole with Aspirin

Because dipyridamole might alter aspirin kinetics to allow increased blood levels of aspirin, it is not clear whether the possible benefits of combination therapy can be ascribed to any specific antiplatelet effect of dipyridamole[66] as suggested by Hanson et al.[32] In *coronary artery saphenous vein grafts*, an important study showed the benefit of dipyridamole, 100 mg 4× daily started 2 days before surgery and continued after operation at 75 mg 3× daily, all in combination with aspirin begun 7 hours postoperatively and then continued as 325 mg 3× daily.[14,15] In another smaller trial,[10] however, combined dipyridamole-aspirin was no better than aspirin itself started within 48 hours of the bypass and continued for 1 year. However, it may be the early administration, pre-operatively, of an antiplatelet agent that confers optimal benefit and aspirin cannot be given pre-operatively because of the effect on bleeding time. The role of aspirin alone, started early in the postoperative phase, is under investigation in a large Veterans Administration Hospitals trial.

In *unstable angina*, dipyridamole is frequently added to aspirin, again only with theoretical substantiation. In the long-term therapy of patients with unstable angina, aspirin is of definite value but the addition of dipyridamole confers no proven added benefit.

> In *postinfarct patients*, the combination dipyridamole 75 mg 3× daily with aspirin 324 mg 3× daily was no different from the results with aspirin alone. Neither agent showed a statistically significant effect by the study criteria, although total mortality and coronary mortality fell by about 20 percent.[68] In another colossal follow-up trial (PARIS II, see reference 39), aspirin-dipyridamole reduced coronary "incidence" (definite nonfatal re-infarction, plus all cardiac deaths) by about 30 percent, without any change in total mortality. It seems doubtful that this result is better than that obtained with aspirin alone (see p 168), although more strict comparisons are required.
>
> In *peripheral vascular disease*, dipyridamole 75 mg—aspirin 330 mg 3× daily limits the progress of the disease, especially in smokers and hypertensives.[34] Aspirin alone is also effective but less so.
>
> In *renal disease* (type 1 membranoproliferative glomerulonephritis[18]), dipyridamole helps to prevent deterioration.

Combination Dipyridamole with Warfarin

In patients with prosthetic valves, this combination may be more effective than warfarin alone in controlling thromboembolism[80] and is less likely than aspirin to provoke bleeding from warfarin.[15]

Dipyridamole—Summary

Dipyridamole theoretically differs in its site of antiplatelet action from aspirin so that combination therapy with aspirin is logical. Nevertheless there are few hard data to substantiate the presumed superiority of combination dipyridamole-aspirin over aspirin especially for the major indications for aspirin, namely unstable angina, postinfarction prophylaxis, and TIAs. In the specific case of patients with coronary artery bypass grafts, dipyridamole may be given pre-operatively and a dipyridamole-aspirin regime is of proven long-term use. In patients with prosthetic valves, dipyridamole-warfarin may be better than warfarin alone, but the data are inconclusive.

OTHER PLATELET INHIBITORS

Indomethacin.   Besides inhibiting cyclo-oxygenase, indomethacin is an anti-inflammatory. Indomethacin is seldom used as a specific antiplatelet agent in patients with cardiovascular diseases, because it seems to inhibit the formation of vasodilatory prostaglandins. The vasoconstrictive action is likely to be worse in the presence of endothelial damage.[45] Thus indomethacin may (1) promote coronary vasoconstriction;[24] (2) attenuate the effects of antihypertensive agents such as β-blockers and diuretics;[90] and (3) cause clinical deterioration in patients with CHF and hyponatremia.[19]

Thromboxane synthetase inhibitors.   Clinical tests are being carried out on new synthetase inhibitors, which have two important theoretical advantages: (1) they might divert precursors from formation of thromboxane to that of prostacyclin by the so-called "endoperoxide steal",[58] although this mechanism does not operate in all models;[73] (2) they specifically inhibit the formation of thromboxane yet not that of prostacyclin. The prototype agent is *dazoxiben*. The major problem with this group of agents is the short half-life of their effect on the synthetase.[23]

Other platelet inhibitors.   These include β-blockers, calcium antagonists, α-receptor antagonists, ketanserin, and nafazatrom (Table 9-1).

ANTICOAGULANTS : HEPARIN

Anticoagulation, when given for an acute indication such as myocardial infarction, or acute venous thrombosis, or acute pulmonary embolism, is usually initiated by IV heparin while awaiting the effect of oral warfarin. Alternatively, in uncomplicated AMI, only heparin may be used till the patient is mobile.[27] Either heparin sodium or heparin calcium may be used. Heparin may be given by infusion, intermittent injection, or subcutaneously but not orally. Fixed-dose regimes are now popular, although strictly speaking the effects of IV heparin should be monitored by the activated partial thromboplastin time and kept at 2–3× the pretherapy value. In patients with bleeding disorders or in whom the effects of bleeding could be serious (subacute bacterial endocarditis, GI or genito-urinary lesions), ultra-low dose heparin (see next section) should be considered.

IV heparin.   The standard IV schedule is usually a 5,000 unit IV injection loading dose, followed by 20,000–40,000 units/day given by an infusion pump. United States Pharmacopeia units may be about 10–15 percent more potent than the international units used in other countries. The heparin may be diluted either in isotonic saline or in dextrose water (which may be better in AMI). *Intermittent injection* may be preferred in AMI to avoid fluid overload; the schedule is 10,000 units given as an initial dose, followed by 5–10,000 units every 4–6 hours. *Ultra-low dose IV heparin* (1 unit/kg/hr for 3–5 days, about 17,000 units/day) seems as effective as other methods in preventing postoperative deep vein thrombosis.[64]

Subcutaneous heparin.   After the initial IV loading dose, heparin may be given as a deep subcutaneous injection 10,000 units 8-hourly or 15,000 12-hourly, using a different site at each rotation. This procedure is as effective as IV heparin in reducing venous thrombosis. The best documented use of subcutaneous heparin is in the prophylaxis of surgical thromboembolism where the schedule is 5,000 units subcutaneously 2–8 hours pre-operation and every 8 hours for 7 days.[38]

Precautions and side-effects.   An increased danger of heparin-induced hemorrhage exists in patients with subacute bacterial endocarditis, hematological disorders including hemophilia, and GI or genito-urinary ulcerative lesions. Platelet plugs are the main hemostatic defence of heparinized patients, and the co-administration of aspirin, sulfinpyrazone, dipyridamole or indomethacin may predispose to bleeding, as may *heparin-induced thrombocytopenia* (in about 10 percent of patients after heparin for 5 days or more,[2a] usually reversible upon heparin withdrawal). Heparin hemorrhage may occur in clinically inapparent sites such as the adrenal glands, which can be life-threatening and demands immediate cortisol replacement therapy. Some patients have a resistance to heparin, and monitoring by coagulation tests every 4 hours during early therapy with full dose heparin is advised. Heparin is derived from animal tissue and occasionally causes allergy; a trial dose of 100–1000 units is required in allergic patients. Patients with severe hepatic disease may be predisposed to bleeding disorders. In renal disease, the dose of heparin is controversial. In AMI, heparin mildly elevates blood free fatty acids that could be potentially harmful; however, the magnitude of this effect may be overestimated.[71]

Heparin overdosage is treated by stopping the drug and, if clinically required, giving protamine sulfate (1 percent solution) at no more than 50 mg very slowly in any 10 minute period as a slow infusion.

Use in Acute Myocardial Infarction

The urgent use of an IV dose of heparin seems logical to initiate protection against venous thrombosis, possibly to help prevent further coronary artery thrombosis, and to prevent mural thrombosis and systemic embolism. Thereafter it is conventional to give high-dose IV infusions, although low-dose subcutaneous heparin may be equally effective.[16a] There are no studies on the possible disadvantage of giving sodium, either in the form of sodium heparin or in the form of isotonic saline used as the diluent. In patients with borderline heart failure, sodium loading can be avoided by the use of calcium heparin (Calciparine®, 5–20,000 USP units/ampoule) and by diluting heparin in dextrose water. Heparin is usually given until the patient is mobile, or until oral anticoagulants take effect. In uncomplicated AMI, the present trend is to give only heparin. When acute thrombolysis is achieved in AMI, heparin is given thereafter in the hope of preventing rethrombosis (see poststreptokinase policy, p 179). Meticulous laboratory control of the heparin dose is required (activated partial thromboplastin time).

ORAL ANTICOAGULANTS: WARFARIN

Warfarin (= Coumarin; Coumadin®; Panwarfarin®) is the most commonly used oral anticoagulant, because a single dose causes a stable anticoagulation as a result of the excellent oral absorption and a circulating half-life of about 36 hours; warfarin also has remarkably few side-effects apart from bleeding.[27] As a group, the oral anticoagulants inactivate vitamin-K in the liver, thereby interfering with the vitamin-K-dependent clotting factors including prothrombin.

Dose.   The usual initial dose of warfarin is 10–15 mg daily, and a maintenance dose of 1–20 mg daily; this wide range means that doses must be individualized. Another standard procedure is to give warfarin 5 mg/day for 5 days and then to check the prothrombin time. Avoiding a large primary dose may also avoid an excess fall of prothrombin and may decrease the risk of skin necrosis (see below). Patients with heart failure or liver disease require lower doses. The effect is monitored by reporting the prothrombin time ratio, which is the treated patient's prothrombin time divided by that of normal plasma. Warfarin has a half-life of 2½ days so that too frequent doses can easily exert an unwanted cumulative effect.

Dose Reduction

Dose reduction of anticoagulants is required in the presence of CHF and liver damage from any source including alcohol, malnutrition, renal impairment, and thyrotoxicosis. The presence of interacting drugs needs to be considered.

Drug Interactions with Warfarin

Warfarin may be subject to something like 80 drug interactions.[79] These include drugs that may reduce vitamin-K absorption or that of warfarin such as cholestyramine, drugs that displace warfarin from its albumin binding sites such as sulfinpyrazone and the previously used agent phenylbutazone, drugs that accelerate warfarin degradation and enhance the anticoagulant effect such as barbiturates or phenytoin, and drugs that decrease warfarin degradation and increase the anticoagulant effect such as a variety of antibiotics including metronidazole (Flagyl®), co-trimoxazole (Bactrim®), and cimetidine. Clofibrate increases the anticoagulant effect by an unknown mean.

Potentiating drugs include the cardiovascular agents allopurinol, quinidine,[40] amiodarone,[55] and phenytoin. Antiplatelet drugs such as aspirin may act by potentiating the risk of bleeding with a big interindividual variation.[65] Very high doses of aspirin (6–8 tablets/day) may act by a different mechanism to potentiate the anticoagulant effect, because synthesis of clotting factors becomes impaired. Sulfinpyrazone powerfully displaces warfarin from blood proteins, to reduce the dose of warfarin required down to 1 mg in some patients.[5] **The safest rule is to tell patients on oral anticoagulation not to take any over-the-counter drugs without consultation, and for the physician to checklist any new drug used.** If in doubt, more frequent measurements of the prothrombin ratio are required. Otherwise, once the warfarin requirement is known, the prothrombin ratio is checked only once every 4–6 weeks.

Contraindications to warfarin.   Stroke, uncontrolled hypertension, hepatic cirrhosis, and potential GI and genito-urinary bleeding points such as hiatus hernia, peptic ulcer, gastritis, colitis, proctitis, and cystitis.[20] If anticoagulation is deemed essential, the benefit-risk ratio must be evaluated carefully. Old age is not of itself a contraindication to anticoagulation that can be successfully carried out.[26] Warfarin in early pregnancy predisposes to abortion.[46a]

Warfarin—associated skin necrosis.   Phenindione has been recommended for this rare but potentially serious hemorrhagic skin condition. The cause of the necrosis is ill-understood, but a vitamin-C deficiency may predispose[37] especially when high-dose warfarin is initiated. Phenindione carries a much higher risk of renal or hepatic toxicity, and may also cause necrosis, so is not frequently the agent of choice. Awareness of vitamin-C deficiency and a low initial dose of warfarin should avoid skin necrosis.

Warfarin overdose.   Excess prothrombinemia without bleeding or with only minor bleeding can be remedied by discontinuation of the warfarin. If bleeding becomes significant, oral or parenteral vitamin-K_1 2–5 mg may be required. In unresponsive patients, plasma 15 ml/kg or fresh, whole blood transfusions are given.

CLINICAL INDICATIONS FOR ORAL ANTICOAGULATION

Although oral anticoagulation, preceded by IV heparin where needed, is established clinical practice, some of the indications for its use remain controversial, as in AMI and postinfarct patients. Logically, anticoagulation therapy should be coupled with a platelet inhibitor to help prevent thrombosis, but added aspirin may lead to bleeding. The evidence that dipyridamole enhances the effect of warfarin is not secure. There are few or no good trials to show the benefit of such combination regimes, so that the use of each agent should be considered on its own merits.

Myocardial Infarction

In the acute stage, the use of full-dose IV heparin followed by standard anticoagulant therapy has been standard during the hospital phase of myocardial infarction,[13] provided that relative or absolute contraindications are absent. A trial aimed at unequivocally documenting the efficiency of this regime in reducing mortality is unlikely to be undertaken. An alternate procedure, usually chosen in uncomplicated AMI, is to use only heparin until the patient is mobile.[27]

Early Postinfarct Anticoagulation

Within the first 3–6 months, there is accumulating evidence that would suggest that mural thrombosis and the subsequent incidence of systemic thromboembolism is more frequent in patients with anterior infarctions, apical dyskinetic areas identifiable echocardiographically (particularly if an intraventricular thrombus is present), large infarctions, and severe left ventricular (LV) dysfunction. Furthermore, the likelihood of systemic thromboembolism is greatest in the first 3 months postdischarge. Although definitive data are unavailable, imperfect evidence supports the use of oral warfarin for a 3–6 month period in these specific postinfarct patients.

Prolonged Oral Anticoagulation

Chronic postinfarct therapy, previously given for years, is unlikely ever to regain its popularity, nor are decisive new large-scale trials likely to be undertaken (for a contrary view, see reference 60). Dogmatic decisions or rules cannot be made. **Successful anticoagulation therapy requires a co-operative patient, meticulous medical supervision, and an excellent laboratory. There must be a constant guard against the use of additional drugs and their interactions. The risks of warfarin therapy are appreciable and must be weighed against the potential benefits for every individual patient.** For most, neither the risk-benefit nor the cost-benefit ratios are in favor of prolonged oral anticoagulation. Even the presence of a LV aneurysm is not an indication for anticoagulation[46] unless there is a history of systemic embolism. Therefore, although selected compliant groups of elderly patients appear to benefit from prolonged anticoagulation,[76] the benefit is only modest and the effort immense.

Postinfarct Anticoagulation versus Aspirin

A French trial[20] compared high-dose aspirin (500 mg 3× daily) with oral anticoagulation; results were similar with an almost identical total mortality with however different side-effects. The incidence of bleeding was 6× higher in the anticoagulant group and the GI problems 5× higher in the aspirin group. The excess bleeding in the anticoagulant group was in non-GI tract bleeding; the incidence of the latter was similar in the two treatment groups. Aspirin may be given with considerably less risk of hemorrhagic complications and without the same degree of supervision. The overall benefit from aspirin postinfarct is still unsettled as is that of anticoagulation. In the case of both agents, however, possible benefits derived from the pooled data are rather similar.[20,27,43] Neither agent has shown clear benefit in good trials. For a prolonged antithrombotic effect postinfarct, aspirin is much simpler and is recommended by the FDA. We do not advise routine postinfarct oral anticoagulation.

Unstable Angina at Rest

In unstable angina (intermediate coronary syndrome), an intracoronary thrombus is found in approximately 40 percent of patients undergoing angiography, thereby focusing on the role of anticoagulation and platelet inhibitor therapy in patients with rest angina.[9] The benefit of heparin is real[82] and the arguments for aspirin are strong (see p 168). Oral anticoagulation is generally not undertaken especially because such patients may come to coronary artery surgery or balloon angioplasty.

In patients with severe repetitive attacks of variant angina, there is a risk of secondary coronary thrombosis following severe coronary artery spasm and oral anticoagulation becomes logical although unproven. In others, low-dose aspirin remains the pragmatic albeit unproven approach to the prevention of spasm-induced platelet stasis and thrombosis.

Venous Thromboembolism

In deep venous thrombosis, warfarin is initiated concurrently with IV heparin as standard therapy for acute episodes. Thereafter, oral anticoagulation alone is continued for a period of 3–6 months. Recurrent venous thrombosis, continuing despite adequate anticoagulant therapy, is uncommon but may be an indication for platelet-inhibitors in addition to warfarin.[77]

For objectively documented *pulmonary embolism*, heparin followed by oral warfarin is used. Warfarin is continued for approximately six months in the absence of recurrences; when the latter occur, indefinite therapy is considered.

Atrial Fibrillation

Atrial fibrillation in the presence of heart disease is strongly associated with thromboembolism.[94] *Cardioversion* in patients with atrial fibrillation probably increases the risk of an embolus. Most cardiologists would anticoagulate patients for 2–3 weeks prior to elective cardioversion (providing this is logistically feasible), followed by a further 2–4 weeks thereafter.[53]

Mitral stenosis or regurgitation. In patients with mitral valve disease, the risk of thromboembolism is greatest in those with atrial fibrillation, marked left atrial enlargement, and previous embolic episodes. Anticoagulation is strongly indicated in this setting. In contrast, in patients with mitral stenosis with sinus rhythm, anticoagulation is usually reserved for secondary prevention after the first episode of systemic embolism.[29] An argument can be made for earlier anticoagulation if the left atrium is dilated.

Hypertensive heart disease. This condition only becomes a candidate for anticoagulation if there is marked left atrial or LV enlargement, or in the presence of atrial fibrillation. These are not, however, firm indications.

Ischemic heart disease. In the presence of good LV function, atrial fibrillation is an unsettled indication for anticoagulation. LV failure strengthens the argument for anticoagulation.[42] However, chronic LV aneurysm is not an indication for oral anticoagulation.[46]

Dilated cardiomyopathy. There is a substantial risk of systemic embolism, particularly if there is atrial fibrillation; anticoagulants substantially reduce thromboembolism.[25] Even in the absence of atrial fibrillation, dilated cardiomyopathy may predispose to mural thrombi and oral anticoagulation with or without platelet inhibitors may be considered, even though statistical evidence for this procedure is lacking.

The tachycardia/bradycardia syndrome. Intermittent atrial fibrillation may have risk of thromboembolism. Anticoagulation may require consideration, especially if there is underlying organic heart disease (ischemic heart disease, hypertension, cardiomyopathy). Once again the evidence is unproven.

Atrial septal defects.   In older patients with atrial septal defects and pulmonary hypertension, anticoagulation is reasonable as prophylaxis against in situ pulmonary arterial thromboses or, rarely, paradoxical emboli.

"Lone" atrial fibrillation.   In the absence of any other cardiac or precipitating condition, including thyrotoxicosis, atrial fibrillation may be a rather rare disease.[8] In the under 60s, it has a risk of thromboembolism no greater than that in an age and sex-matched population, so that the morbidity of anticoagulant therapy outweighs the potential advantages.[41] In a population predominantly over 60 (mostly males), the risk of stroke was about 4× that of controls, so that anticoagulation would need consideration.[8]

Prosthetic Heart Valves

In patients with mechanical prosthetic heart valves, warfarin is standard and preferred to aspirin alone, to dipyridamole-aspirin, or to pentoxifylline-aspirin.[26,62] Adding an antiplatelet agent to warfarin is logical in the hope of further reducing the risk of systemic embolism; however, aspirin increases the risk of bleeding.[15] The benefit of dipyridamole added to warfarin is not clear-cut and is based only on suggestive evidence.[15] When there are relative contraindications to warfarin or platelet inhibitors, then patients with a history of thromboembolism, marked left atrial enlargement, or atrial fibrillation are those most in need of treatment. In children or in others in whom warfarin is difficult to manage, aspirin is a reasonable alternative.[91] In patients with *porcine valves*,[2] the risk of thromboembolism is highest in the first three months and then falls. The ideal agent is not yet sure; aspirin may be a reasonable alternative to warfarin. Arguments for warfarin are strong when mitral porcine valves are combined with atrial fibrillation or a giant left atrium or LV failure.

Marginal or Possible Indications

Cerebral vascular disease.   Anticoagulation in cerebrovascular disease remains a source of fierce debate. Certainly in patients who have had a complete stroke, there is no evidence to support anticoagulation. In patients with TIAs of less than 2 months duration (who do not undergo surgery), warfarin for a period of 3 months has been advised followed by aspirin 1300 mg (approximately) per day. In males with TIAs in whom the last attack was within 2–12 months, treatment with this dose of aspirin until the patient has been free of symptoms for at least a year seems reasonable.[72]

Primary pulmonary hypertension.   This entity includes a variety of histologic appearances and probably, pathogenic mechanisms. Diffuse pulmonary thromboembolism or pulmonary arteriolar thrombosis call for anticoagulation. When the pathogenesis cannot be established, long-term anticoagulation is usually chosen.

Mitral valve prolapse.   In patients with marked mitral valve prolapse and suggestive evidence of thrombotic or thromboembolic events, there might be an indication for warfarin or platelet inhibitors but this remains a moot issue.

Combination of Warfarin with Platelet Inhibitors

Just as there have been few carefully designed studies on the effects of oral anticoagulants by themselves, so are there equally few studies comparing the combination warfarin-antiplatelet agents with either agent separately. Much of the combined use of warfarin with antiplatelet agents such as dipyridamole is based on inferential or indirect evidence; however dipyridamole-warfarin is safer than aspirin-warfarin.[15]

In mitral stenosis with atrial fibrillation, thromboembolism can be reduced by sulfinpyrazone,[78] or by warfarin.[81] However, because the former data were not part of a formal trial and because the latter trial was imperfect, sulfinpyrazone is now frequently combined with warfarin in such patients without satisfactory evidence for the warfarin component (see also sulfinpyrazone-warfarin interaction).

Oral Anticoagulants—Summary

These agents, once the backbone of postinfarct management, are now only used for selected patients thought to be at high risk of thromboembolism. In AMI, their use during the hospital phase is standard, although many other centers give only heparin, limited to the duration of bed rest, for un-complicated AMI. Only a minority of patients qualify for limited anticoagula-tion for 3–6 months, while only a very few require prolonged anticoagulation. Oral anticoagulants are frequently used to prevent systemic embolism espe-cially in selected patients with atrial fibrillation and those with prosthetic heart valves or dilated cardiomyopathy. They are used both in the treatment and prevention of venous thrombosis and pulmonary embolism. Long-term anticoagulation requires meticulous patient compliance and a careful con-sideration of the risk-benefit ratio for the individual patient.

FIBRINOLYTIC THERAPY

Fibrinolytic therapy is used chiefly for hyperacute myocardial infarction and acute pulmonary embolism, but similar principles apply in the case of peripheral vascular emboli. In the case of myocardial infarction, most experi-ence has been gained with streptokinase, an agent that produces both clot-lysis and a systemic lytic state. Many of the early trials can be discounted because the dose of IV streptokinase was too low and the delay from the onset of symptoms too long.[28] Then, in 1979, Rentrop et al[69,70] showed that intra-coronary streptokinase was feasible and interest in this agent was rekindled, especially because the longstanding controversy about the real role of coro-nary thrombosis in causing AMI was settled by an important study by DeWood et al.[17] Thus in the early stages of transmural myocardial infarction, coronary occlusion by a thrombus is the usual mechanism. Logically therefore thrombo-lysis is desirable, its effects being offset only by those of *reperfusion damage*, a poorly evaluated clinical problem apart from reperfusion arrhythmias. Experi-mentally, free radical scavengers and allopurinol limit reperfusion damage.

Recently high-dose streptokinase has been given IV (500,000–1,700,000 units) and within the first few hours after the onset of myocardial infarction to achieve early reperfusion in 50–85 percent of patients.

A recent exciting advance has been the development of a tissue-type plasminogen activator (tPA) that, in clinical doses, produces selective clot lysis usually without a significant systemic lytic state.

Tissue-Type Plasminogen Activator (tPA)

tPA binds to fibrin with a greater affinity than does streptokinase or uro-kinase; once bound it is activated and converts plasminogen to plasmin on the fibrin surface. Experimentally, even in equivalent thrombolytic doses, tPA pro-duces less bleeding than streptokinase[1] and has the further advantage of being non-antigenic. The dose of tPA required to produce nearly complete clot lysis (85 percent) can however produce some delayed bleeding.

Human tPA is now produced by modern recombinant-DNA techniques and is becoming more freely available. In three trials, IV tPA has been very effective, achieving recanalization in about 75 percent of patients with symp-toms of myocardial infarction of less than 6 hours. In the European trial, tPA was infused at 0.75 mg/kg over 90 minutes and was superior to 1,500,000 units of streptokinase given IV over 60 minutes.[88] In the American National Heart, Lung and Blood Institute TIMI trial[84] however, tPA was infused over 3 hours and streptokinase for only 90 minutes, so that strict comparison of effi-cacy may at first sight be difficult. However, 90 minutes after the onset of the tPA infusion, patency was achieved in 66 percent of patients versus 36 percent in the streptokinase group.

Streptokinase and Urokinase

The results of the intracoronary administration of streptokinase are quite variable,[28] partially because of the different doses and variable protocols in-volved, as well as difficulty in obtaining true controls. Furthermore, the benefits of intracoronary streptokinase as opposed to the IV form must be weighed against the inevitable delay caused by catheterization.

In the case of *IV streptokinase* or *urokinase*, an overview of data from 33 randomized controlled trials[95] suggests that the IV treatment produces a highly significant 22 percent reduction in the risk of death, an even larger effect in prevention of re-infarction, and a risk of adverse effects that is much smaller than the benefit obtained. "The apparent mortality reduction in the IV trials was similar whether anticoagulants were compulsory or optional, whether treatment was in a coronary care unit or in an ordinary ward and, surprisingly, whether treatment was begun early (less than 6 hours from the onset of symptoms) or late (generally 12–24 hours)". However, such pooling of data from many different trials with differing protocols is open to question, so that the results of the Italian trial are more definitive and show that **the earlier IV streptokinase is given, the better the result.**[36] Very early thrombolysis (within 1 hour) is much more effective at reducing enzymatic infarct size than thrombolysis 1–2 hours later.[75a] Yusuf et al[95] advocate a simple 1 hour high-dose (dose not stated) IV streptokinase infusion (see also reference 35), without anticoagulation, which will successfully convert virtually all of the available plasminogen into plasmin. IV administration of a thrombolytic agent is going to be increasingly used because (1) the widespread application of intracoronary thrombolysis is logistically not feasible, being applicable to only something like 10 percent of patients; (2) there are appreciable risks including bleeding from the femoral puncture site, requiring substantial transfusion in about 15 percent of patients;[87] and (3) the risk of serious bleeding with IV streptokinase is very low (1–2 percent[95]).

Rate of infusion of streptokinase.   In the Italian trial[36] the rate was 1.5 million units of streptokinase in 100 ml of physiological saline in 1 hour. This dose is less than the rate recommended by Lew et al,[47] although (1) their data are not that clear-cut (see Fig. 1 of their paper) and (2) high rates of infusion may cause hypotension.[48] Therefore the rate of infusion in the Italian trial can be taken as optimal. However, lower doses are also used.

Recognition of reperfusion.   In the absence of early or simultaneous coronary angiography, the criteria are (1) rapid relief of chest pain; (2) accelerated ECG evolution; (3) very high peak blood creatine kinase values as enzyme is washed out from the infarcting myocardium; and (4) *reperfusion arrhythmias* that are common,[52a] and usually respond to lidocaine (theoretically verapamil should work as reperfusion-induced automaticity is calcium-dependent).

Indications for streptokinase other than AMI.   Venous thrombosis, pulmonary embolism, thrombosed arteriovenous shunts. Infusion dose: 250,000 to 600,000 units over 30 minutes, then 100,000 units every hour for up to 1 week.

Contraindications.   Recent hemorrhage or cerebrovascular accident, advancing age with fear of intracranial hemorrhage, coagulation defects, severe uncontrolled hypertension, recent streptococcal infections (bacterial toxins induce resistance to streptokinase), hemorrhagic retinopathy, and high risk of left heart thrombus as in mitral stenosis with fibrillation or subacute bacterial endocarditis. Pregnancy or menstruation.

Precautions.   Ideally check blood count and clotting factors before use. Discontinue heparin (sometimes carefully controlled heparin is used during early PTCA). Give *hydrocortisone* 250 mg IV before streptokinase to prevent allergic reaction.

Side-effects and complications.   Serious reperfusion arrhythmias, allergic reactions, fever, and rashes may all occur. Minor bleeding requires local measures, not cessation of lytic therapy (danger of rebound excess lytic state). Major bleeding requires cessation of fresh frozen plasma or whole blood. Poststreptokinase bleeding diathesis is a risk especially during heparin therapy.

Poststreptokinase policy.   Ideal policy awaits controlled studies (see p 195). After streptokinase, one policy is to start heparin, whilst meticulously and repetitively checking clotting factors. This regime should help to prevent *early rethrombosis,* which may take several days to develop, and is a special risk unless simultaneous intracoronary streptokinase and PTCA are undertaken. When streptokinase is given only IV, early coronary angiography is required within days to select patient for PTCA or coronary bypass grafting. If neither procedure is appropriate, heparin may be stopped. Now aspirin (sometimes with dipyridamole) is logical to prevent rethrombosis. Oral anticoagulants are given if AMI is complicated. Some other workers routinely use warfarin for one month or longer. If despite precautions rethrombosis occurs, urokinase for tPA should be the agent of choice (preferably intracoronary, else IV). Tight coronary stenosis predisposes more to rethrombosis.[52a]

Urokinase. This agent has similar indications, contraindications, and effects to streptokinase. However, being prepared from cultured human renal cells, allergic effects are minimal. Furthermore, a shorter half-life than streptokinase causes less systemic fibrinolysis, and is a safer drug if early coronary bypass is the aim.[83a] Logically rethrombosis after early clot lysis in AMI should respond better to urokinase than streptokinase (blocking antibodies to streptokinase may persist for 3–6 months). A specific indication is for intraocular clot lysis (chosen because of absence of allergic properties). The defect of urokinase is great expense. The *dose* for intracoronary use is 3× that of streptokinase[83a] and for IV use is 2 million units as a bolus.[55a]

Fibrinolytic Therapy: Recommendations

There is a growing consensus that the early (less than 6 hours after the onset of symptoms, ideally within 2 hours[55a]) administration of IV or intracoronary streptokinase improves ventricular function and limits infarct size. The reduction in mortality is best shown when fibrinolysis is really early;[36,75a] even at 6 hours benefits are modest.[35a] It is highly likely that IV fibrinolysis will soon become standard practice in the management of myocardial infarction seen within the first 4–6 hours. At present only IV streptokinase (or urokinase) is widely available, but tPA will soon take its place. Intracoronary and early IV streptokinase will probably continue to be used in specialized centers, especially when early PTCA is considered, as is now increasingly frequent[75] because of the lessened risk of early re-infarction and improved posttherapy ventricular function.[64a]

SUMMARY

Antithrombotic agents include platelet inhibitors, anticoagulants and fibrinolytics. Aspirin irreversibly inhibits the cyclo-oxygenase concerned in the synthesis of prostaglandins with, in practice, a beneficial clinical effect over a wide dose range. Aspirin is now indicated for unstable angina, threatened stroke (TIAs) and postinfarct management. Other indications are less clear. Sulfinpyrazone and dipyridamole have no FDA-approved indications in the USA although both are used in selected patients. In coronary bypass operations, dipyridamole should be started pre-operatively and continued thereafter with the addition of aspirin. When combination of warfarin with an antiplatelet agent is required, dipyridamole is preferred to aspirin (but such combinations are not yet of proven value). Warfarin is now chiefly used in the acute phase of myocardial infarction and in the prevention of venous thromboembolism. In uncomplicated AMI, warfarin may be omitted and only heparin used until the patient is mobile. Prolonged postinfarction anticoagulation is selected only for a limited number of patients at definite risk of thromboembolism. Anticoagulation should be considered for those with prosthetic heart valves and for dilated cardiomyopathy. In atrial fibrillation, anticoagulation should be considered though not necessarily always given. Fibrinolytics such as streptokinase or plasminogen activator are now increasingly seen as logical therapy in the very early stages of AMI and it is likely that IV tPA will soon become part of standard therapy, followed by early coronary angiography. Intracoronary fibrinolytics (combined with early IV use) will be selected whenever early PTCA forms part of the treatment of AMI, as is now increasingly common in specialized centers.

REFERENCES

1. Agnelli G, Buchanan MR, Fernandez F, et al: A comparison of the thrombolytic and hemorrhagic effects of tissue-type plasminogen activator and streptokinase in rabbits. Circulation 72:178–182, 1985
2. Angell WW, Angell JD: Porcine valves. Prog Cardiovasc Dis 23:141–166, 1980
2a. Ansell JE, Price JM, Shah S, et al: Heparin-induced thrombocytopenia. What is its real frequency Chest 88:878–882, 1985
3. Anturan Reinfarction Italian Study: Sulphinpyrazone in post-myocardial infarction. Lancet i:237–242, 1982
4. Anturane Reinfarction Trial Research Group: Sulfinpyrazone in the prevention of sudden death after myocardial infarction. New Engl J Med 302:250–256, 1980

5. Bailey RR, Reddy J: Potentiation of warfarin action by sulphinpyrazone (letter). Lancet i:254, 1980

5a. Boelaert J, Lijnen P, Robbens E, et al: Impairment of renal function due to sulphinpyrazone after coronary artery bypass surgery: A prospective double-blind study. J Cardiovasc Pharmacol 8:386–391, 1986

6. Boerboom LE, Olinger GN, Kissebah AH, et al: Low-dose aspirin is equivalent to aspirin plus dipyridamole in reducing cholesterol in vein grafts. J Am Coll Cardiol 5 (abs):505, 1985

7. Bousser MG, Eschwege E, Haguenau M, et al: Controlled trial of aspirin and dipyridamole in the secondary prevention of atherothrombotic cerebral ischemia. Stroke 14:5–14, 1983

8. Brand FN, Abbott RD, Kannel WB, et al: Characteristics and prognosis of lone atrial fibrillation. JAMA 254:3449–3453, 1985

9. Bresnahan DR, Davis JL, Holmes DR, et al: Angiographic occurrence and clinical correlates of intraluminal coronary artery thrombus: Role of unstable angina. J Am Coll Cardiol 6:285–289, 1985

10. Brown BG, Cukingnan RA, DeRouen T, et al: Improved graft patency in patients treated with platelet-inhibiting therapy after coronary bypass surgery. Circulation 72:138–146, 1985

11. Cairns JA, Gent M, Singer J, et al: Aspirin, sulfinpyrazone or both in unstable angina. New Engl J Med 313:1369–1375, 1985

12. Canadian Cooperative Study Group: A randomized trial of aspirin and sulfinpyrazone in threatened stroke. New Engl J Med 299:53–59, 1978

13. Chalmers TC, Matta RJ, Smith H, et al: Evidence favoring the use of anticoagulants in the hospital phase of acute myocardial infarction. New Engl J Med 297:1091–1096, 1977

14. Chesebro JH, Clements IP, Fuster V, et al: A platelet-inhibitor drug trial in coronary artery bypass operations. New Engl J Med 307:73–78, 1982

15. Chesebro JH, Fuster V, Elveback LR, et al: Trial of combined warfarin plus dipyridamole or aspirin therapy in prosthetic heart valve replacement: Danger of aspirin compared with dipyridamole. Am J Cardiol 51:1537–1541, 1983

16. Dale J, Myhre E, Stortstein O, et al: Prevention of arterial thromboembolism with acetylsalicylic acid: A controlled clinical study in patients with aortic ball valves. Am Heart J 94:101–111, 1977

16a. Davis MJE, Ireland MA: Effect of early anticoagulation on the frequency of left ventricular thrombi after anterior wall acute myocardial infarction. Am J Cardiol 57:1244–1247, 1986

17. DeWood M, Spores J, Berg R Jr, et al: Acute myocardial infarction: A decade of experience with surgical reperfusion in 701 patients. Circulation 68 (suppl II):II-8–II-16, 1983

18. Donadio JV Jr, Anderson CF, Mitchell JC, et al: Membranoproliferative glomerulonephritis. A prospective clinical trial of platelet-inhibitor therapy. New Engl J Med 310:1421–1426, 1984

19. Dzau VJ, Packer M, Lilly LS, et al: Prostaglandins in severe congestive heart failure in relation to activation of the renin-angiotensin system and hyponatremia. New Engl J Med 310:347–352, 1984

20. EPSIM Research Group: A controlled comparison of aspirin and oral anticoagulants in prevention of death after myocardial infarction. New Engl J Med 307:701–708, 1982

21. FDA Drug Bulletin 15:35–36, 1985

22. Fields WS, Lemak NA, Frankowski RF, et al: Controlled trial of aspirin in cerebral ischemia. Stroke 8:301–314, 1977

23. Fitzgerald GA, Reilly IAG, Pedersen AK: The biochemical pharmacology of thromboxane synthase inhibition in man. Circulation 72:1194–1201, 1985

24. Friedman PL, Brown EJ, Gunther S, et al: Coronary vasoconstrictor effect of indomethacin in patients with coronary artery disease. New Engl J Med 305:1171–1175, 1981

25. Fuster V, Gersh BJ, Giuliani ER, et al: The natural history of idiopathic dilated cardiomyopathy. Am J Cardiol 47:525–531, 1981

26. Gadboys HL, Litwak RS, Niemetz J, et al: Role of anticoagulants in preventing embolization from prosthetic heart valves. JAMA 202:134–138, 1967

27. Gallus AS: Indications for oral anticoagulant treatment. Drugs 26:543–549, 1983

28. Gersh BJ: Role of thrombolytic therapy in evolving myocardial infarction. Mod Concepts Cardiovasc Dis 54:13–17, 1985

29. Goodnight SH Jr: Antiplatelet therapy for mitral stenosis (editorial). Circulation 62:466–468, 1980

30. Grayzel AI, Liddle L, Seegmiller JE: Diagnostic significance of hyperuricemia in arthritis. New Engl J Med 265:763–768, 1961

31. Gresele P, Zoja C, Deckmyn H, et al: Dipyridamole inhibits platelet aggregation in whole blood. Thromb Haemost 50:852–856, 1983

32. Hanson SR, Harker LA, Bjornsson TD: Effects of platelet-modifying drugs on arterial thromboembolism in baboons. Aspirin potentiates the antithrombotic actions of di-

pyridamole and sulfinpyrazone by mechanism(s) independent of platelet cyclooxygenase inhibition. J Clin Invest 75:1591–1599, 1985

33. Harter HR, Burch JW, Majerus PW, et al: Prevention of thrombosis in patients on hemodialysis by low-dose aspirin. New Engl J Med 301:577–579, 1979

34. Hess H, Mietaschik A, Deichsel E: Drug-induced inhibition of platelet function delays progression of peripheral occlusive arterial disease. A prospective double-blind arteriographically controlled trial. Lancet i:415–419, 1985

35. Hillis LD, Borer J, Braunwald E, et al: High dose intravenous streptokinase for acute myocardial infarction: Preliminary results of a multicenter trial. J Am Coll Cardiol 6:957–962, 1985

35a. ISAM Study Group: A prospective trial of Intravenous Streptokinase in Acute Myocardial infarction (I.S.A.M). Mortality, morbidity, and infarct size at 21 days. New Engl J Med 314:1465–1471, 1986

36. Italian Group: Effectiveness of intravenous thrombolytic treatment in acute myocardial infarction. Lancet i:397–401, 1986

37. Kazmier FJ: Thromboembolism, coumarin necrosis and protein C. Mayo Clin Proc 60:673–674, 1985

38. Kiil J, Kiil J, Axelsen F, et al: Prophylaxis against post-operative pulmonary embolism and deep-vein thrombosis by low-dose heparin. Lancet i:1115–1116, 1978

39. Klimt CR, Knatterud GL, Stamler J, et al: Persantine-aspirin reinfarction study. Part II. Secondary coronary prevention with persantine and aspirin. J Am Coll Cardiol 7:251–269, 1986

40. Koch-Weser J: Quinidine-induced hypoprothrombinemic hemorrhage in patients on chronic warfarin therapy. Ann Intern Med 68:511–517, 1968

41. Kopecky SL, Gersh BJ, McGoon MD, et al: The natural history of idiopathic "lone" atrial fibrillation: A three decade population-based study. Circulation 72 (suppl III): III-1, 1985

42. Kramer RJ, Zeldis SM, Hamby RI: Atrial fibrillation—a marker for abnormal left ventricular function in coronary heart disease. Br Heart J 47:606–608, 1982

43. Lancet Editorial: Aspirin after myocardial infarction. Lancet i:1172–1173, 1980

44. Lancet Editorial: Aspirin: What dose Lancet i:592–593, 1986

45. Lane GE, Bove AA: The effect of cyclooxygenase inhibition on vasomotion of proximal coronary arteries with endothelial damage. Circulation 72:389–396, 1985

46. Lapeyre AC, Steele PM, Kazmier FJ, et al: Systemic embolism in chronic left ventricular aneurysm: Incidence and the role of anticoagulation. J Am Coll Cardiol 6:534–538, 1985

46a. Lee P-K, Wang RYC, Chow JSF, et al: Combined use of warfarin and adjusted subcutaneous heparin during pregnancy in patients with an artificial heart valve. J Am Coll Cardiol 8:221–224, 1986

47. Lew AS, Laramee P, Cercek B, et al: The effects of the rate of intravenous infusion of streptokinase and the duration of symptoms on the time interval to reperfusion in patients with acute myocardial infarction. Circulation 72:1053–1058, 1985

48. Lew AS, Laramee P, Cercek B, et al: The hypotensive effect of intravenous streptokinase in patients with acute myocardial infarction. Circulation 72:1321–1326, 1985

49. Lewis HD, Davis JW, Archibald DG, et al: Protective effects of aspirin against acute myocardial infarction and death in men with unstable angina. New Engl J Med 309:396–403, 1983

50. Linos A, Worthington JW, O'Fallon W, et al: Effect of aspirin on prevention of coronary and cerebrovascular disease in patients with rheumatoid arthritis. A long-term follow-up study. Mayo Clin Proc 53:581–586, 1978

51. Livio M, Benigni A, Vigano G, et al: Moderate doses of aspirin and risk of bleeding in renal failure. Lancet i:414–416, 1986

52. Lorenz RL, Schacky CV, Weber M, et al: Improved aortocoronary bypass patency by low-dose aspirin (100 mg daily). Lancet i:1261–1264, 1984

52a. MacLennan BA, McMaster A, Webb SW, et al: High dose intravenous streptokinase in acute myocardial infarction—short and long term prognosis. Br Heart J 55:231–239, 1986

53. Mancini GBJ, Goldberger AL: Cardioversion of atrial fibrillation: Consideration of embolization, anticoagulation, prophylactic pacemaker and long-term success. Am Heart J 104:617–621, 1982

54. Marcus AJ: Aspirin as an antithrombotic medication. New Engl J Med 309:1515–1516, 1983

55. Martinowitz U, Rabinovici J, Goldfarb D, et al: Interaction between warfarin sodium and amiodarone. New Engl J Med 304:671–672, 1981

55a. Mathey DG, Sheehan FH, Schofer J, et al: Time from onset of symptoms to thrombolytic therapy: A major determinant of myocardial salvage in patients with acute transmural infarction. J Am Coll Cardiol 6:518–525, 1985

56. May GS, Eberlein KA, Furberg CD, et al: Secondary prevention after myocardial infarction: A review of long-term trials. Prog Cardiovasc Dis 24:331–352, 1982

57. Mehta J, Mehta P, Pepine CJ, et al: Platelet function studies in coronary artery disease. X. Effect of dipyridamole. Am J Cardiol 47:1111–1114, 1981

58. Mehta JL, Mehta P, Lopez L, et al: Platelet function and biosynthesis of prostacyclin and thromboxane A_2 in whole blood after aspirin administration in human subjects. J Am Coll Cardiol 4:806–811, 1984

59. Mielants H, Veys EM, Verbruggen G, et al: Salicylate-induced gastrointestinal bleeding: Comparison between soluble buffered, enteric coated and intravenous administration. J Rheumatol 6:210–218, 1979

60. Mitchell JRA: Anticoagulants in coronary heart disease—retrospect and prospect. Lancet i:257–262, 1981

61. Miwa K, Kambara H, Kawai C: Effect of aspirin in large doses on attacks of variant angina. Am Heart J 105:351–355, 1983

62. Mok CK, Boey J, Wang R, et al: Warfarin versus dipyridamole-aspirin and pentoxifylline-aspirin for the prevention of prosthetic heart valve thromboembolism: A prospective randomized clinical trial. Circulation 72:1059–1063, 1985

63. Moroz L: Increased blood fibrinolytic activity after aspirin ingestion. New Engl J Med 296:525–529, 1977

64. Negus D, Friedgood A, Cox SJ, et al: Ultra-low dose intravenous heparin in the prevention of post-operative deep-vein thrombosis. Lancet i:891–894, 1980

64a. O'Neill W, Timmis GC, Bourdillon PD, et al: A prospective randomized clinical trial of intracoronary streptokinase versus coronary angioplasty for acute myocardial infarction. New Engl J Med 314:812–818, 1986

65. O'Reilly RA, Sahud MA, Aggeler PM: Impact of aspirin and chlorthalidone on the pharmacodynamics of oral anticoagulant drugs in man. Ann NY Acad Sci 179:173–186, 1971

66. Pedersen AK, Fitzgerald GA: Dose-related kinetics of aspirin. New Engl J Med 311:1206–1211, 1984

67. Pedersen AK, Fitzgerald GA: The human pharmacology of platelet inhibition: Pharmacokinetics relevant to drug action. Circulation 72:1164–1176, 1985

68. Persantine-Aspirin Reinfarction Study (PARIS). Persantine and aspirin in coronary heart disease. Circulation 62:449–461, 1980

69. Rentrop KP, Blanke H, Karsch KR, et al: Acute myocardial infarction: Intracoronary application of nitroglycerin and streptokinase. Clin Cardiol 2:354–363, 1979

70. Rentrop KP, Feit F, Blanke H, et al: Effects of intracoronary streptokinase and intracoronary nitroglycerin infusion on coronary angiographic patterns and mortality in patients with acute myocardial infarction. New Engl J Med 311:1457–1463, 1984

71. Riemersma RA, Russel DC, Oliver MF: Heparin-induced lipolysis, an exaggerated risk. Lancet ii:471, 1981

72. Sandok BA, Furlan AJ, Whisnant JP, et al: Guidelines for the management of transient ischemic attacks. Mayo Clin Proc 53:665–674, 1978

73. Schmitz JM, Apprill PG, Buja LM: Vascular prostaglandin and thromboxane production in a canine model of myocardial ischemia. Circ Res 57:223–231, 1985

74. Shea MJ, Driscoll EM, Romson JL, et al: The beneficial effects of nafazatrom (BAYg6575) on experimental coronary thrombosis. Am Heart J 107:629–637, 1984

75. Simoons ML, Serruys PW, van den Brand M: Improved survival after early thrombolysis in acute myocardial infarction. A randomized trial by the Interuniversity Cardiology Institute in the Netherlands. Lancet ii:578–581, 1985

75a. Simoons ML, Serruys PW, van den Brand M, et al: Early thrombolysis in acute myocardial infarction: Limitation of infarct size and improved survival. J Am Coll Cardiol 7:717–728, 1986

76. Sixty-Plus Reinfarction Study Research Group: Risks of long-term oral anticoagulant therapy in elderly patients after myocardial infarction. Lancet i:64–68, 1982

77. Steele P, Ellis J Jr, Genton E: Effects of platelet suppressant, anticoagulant and fibrinolytic therapy in patients with recurrent venous thrombosis. Am J Med 64:441–445, 1978

78. Steele P, Rainwater J: Favorable effect of sulfinpyrazone on thromboembolism in patients with rheumatic heart disease. Circulation 62:462–465, 1980

79. Stratton F, Chalmers DG, Flute PT, et al: Drug interaction with coumarin derivative anticoagulants. Br Med J 285:274–275, 1982

80. Sullivan JM, Harken DE, Gorlin R: Pharmacologic control of thromboembolic complications of cardiac-valve replacement. New Engl J Med 284:1391–1394, 1971

81. Szekely P: Systemic embolism and anticoagulant prophylaxis in rheumatic heart disease. Br Med J 1:1209–1212, 1964

82. Telford AM, Wilson C: Trial of heparin in prevention of myocardial infarction in intermediate coronary syndrome. Lancet i:1225–1228, 1981

83. Temple R, Pledger GW: The FDA's critique of the Anturane reinfarction trial. New Engl J Med 303:1488–1492, 1980

83a. Tennant SN, Dixon J, Venable TC, et al: Intracoronary thrombolysis in patients with acute myocardial infarction: Comparison of the efficacy of urokinase with streptokinase. Circulation 69:756–760, 1984

84. TIMI Study Group: Special Report: The Thrombolysis in Myocardial Infarction (TIMI) Trial. New Engl J Med 312:932–936, 1985

85. Torosian M, Michelson EL, Morganroth J, et al: Aspirin- and coumadin-related bleeding after coronary artery bypass graft surgery. Ann Intern Med 89:325–328, 1978

86. Vanhoutte PM: Peripheral serotonergic receptors and hypertension, in Vanhoutte PM (ed): Serotonin and the Cardiovascular System. New York, Raven Press, 1985, pp 123–133

87. Verheugt FWA, van Eenige MJ, Res JCJ, et al: Bleeding complications of intracoronary fibrinolytic therapy in acute myocardial infarction. Br Heart J 54:455–459, 1985

88. Verstraete M, Bernard R, Bory M, et al: Randomized trial of intravenous recombinant human tissue-type plasminogen activator versus intravenous streptokinase in acute myocardial infarction. Lancet i:842, 1985

89. Wallenburg HCS, Dekker GA, Makowitz JW, et al: Low-dose aspirin prevents pregnancy-induced hypertension and pre-eclampsia in angiotensin-sensitive primigravidae. Lancet i:1–3, 1986

90. Webster J: Interactions of NSAIDs with diuretics and β-blockers. Mechanisms and clinical implications. Drugs 30:32–41, 1985

91. Weinstein GS, Mavroudis C, Ebert PA: Preliminary experience with aspirin for anticoagulation in children with prosthetic cardiac valves. Ann Thorac Surg 33:549–553, 1982

92. Weksler BB, Tack-Goldman K, Subramanian VA, et al: Cumulative inhibitory effect of low-dose aspirin on vascular prostacyclin and platelet thromboxane production in patients with atherosclerosis. Circulation 71:332–340, 1985

93. Wilcox RG, Richardson D, Hampton JR, et al: Sulphinpyrazone in acute myocardial infarction: Studies on cardiac rhythm and renal function. Br Med J 3:531–534, 1980

94. Wolf PA, Dawber TR, Thomas HE Jr, et al: Epidemiological assessment of chronic atrial fibrillation and the risk of stroke: The Framingham study. Neurology 28:973–977, 1978

95. Yusuf S, Collins R, Peto R, et al: Intravenous and intracoronary fibrinolytic therapy in acute myocardial infarction: Overview of results on mortality, reinfarction and side-effects from 33 randomized controlled trials. Eur Heart J 6:556–585, 1985

Reviews

Fuster V, Chesebro JH: Antithrombotic therapy: Role of platelet-inhibitor drugs. I. Current concepts of thrombogenesis: Role of platelets. Mayo Clin Proc 56:102–112, 1981

Fuster V, Chesebro JH: Antithrombotic therapy: Role of platelet-inhibitor drugs. II. Pharmacologic effects of platelet-inhibitor drugs. Mayo Clin Proc 56:185–195, 1981

Fuster V, Chesebro JH: Antithrombotic therapy: Role of platelet-inhibitor drugs. III. Management of arterial thromboembolic and atherosclerotic disease. Mayo Clin Proc 56:265–273, 1981

Goldberg RJ, Gore JM, Dalen JE, et al: Long-term anticoagulant therapy after acute myocardial infarction. Am Heart J 109:616–622, 1985

Harker LA: Clinical trials evaluating platelet-modifying drugs in patients with atherosclerotic cardiovascular disease and thrombosis. Circulation 73:206–223, 1986

L. H. Opie

10

Lipid-Lowering Agents

IDEAL LIPID PROFILE

Blood Cholesterol

The ideal blood cholesterol value may be about 180–200 mg/dL.[1,15,22] Blood cholesterol values above 260–270 mg/dL put a patient over 40 years of age at high risk for coronary artery disease.[1,21] In 1986, the European Atherosclerosis Society[6] set an ideal cholesterol value as below 200 mg/dL (<5.2 mmol/L) and advised that values of 200–250 mg/dL should be treated by dietary advice and correction of other risk factors, with higher cholesterol levels sometimes requiring lipid-lowering drugs (Table 10-1).

Other Lipid Abnormalities

The atherogenic role of lipid abnormalities other than cholesterol is not so clear-cut.[1,6,25] While high blood *triglyceride* levels are common in patients with coronary heart disease (CHD), a specific causative role for hypertriglyceridemia in CHD still remains to be proven, with the exception of some rare abnormalities. An elevated blood triglyceride level may be viewed with special concern when combined with high blood cholesterol values (Table 10-1). *High-density lipoproteins* (HDL) may aid in clearing cholesterol from the diseased arteries. When the HDL-cholesterol falls below 35–30 mg/dL,[1,5] there could be an added reason for lipid-lowering therapy. No specific recommendations are made for *low-density lipoproteins* (LDL).[1,5] The ratio of HDL to LDH, when high, may be one component of a favorable blood lipid profile.

DIETARY THERAPY

Nondrug dietary therapy is basic to the management of all primary hyperlipidemias and frequently suffices as basic therapy when coupled with exercise, cessation of smoking, and treatment of other risk factors such as hypertension or diabetes.

The *dietary recommendations of the American Heart Association*[1] are based on three phases, applied consecutively if needed: *Phase I:* 30 percent of calories as fat; equal amounts of saturated, monosaturated, and polyunsaturated fatty acids; under 300 mg cholesterol. *Phase II:* 25 percent as fat, equal distribution of types of fatty acids, under 200–250 mg cholesterol. *Phase III:* 20 percent of calories as fat, equal distribution of types of fatty acids, 100–150 mg cholesterol. Sodium intake should be limited.

Drugs for the Heart, Second Expanded Edition
Copyright © 1987 by Grune & Stratton, Inc.

ISBN 0-8089-1840-0

TABLE 10-1

BLOOD CHOLESTEROL AND TRIGLYCERIDE VALUES IN MANAGEMENT OF
CARDIAC PATIENTS

	Action
Serum cholesterol level	
<200 mg/dL or 5.2 mmol/L	None
200–250 mg/dL	Dietary; overall risk factor* control
>250 mg/dL[6] or 6.5 mmol/L	As above, then consider use of lipid-lowering
>260 mg/dL[21]	drugs. If triglyceride high, see below.
>268 mg/dL[1]	
Triglyceride level[6]	
<200 mg/dL = 2.3 mmol/L	None
200–250 mg/dL	Loss of weight, dietary therapy, look for cause of
with cholesterol <200 mg/dL	high levels including diuretics and some
	β-blockers
200–500 mg/dL (2.3–5.6 mmol/L)	As above, then consider lipid-lowering drug
with cholesterol 200–300 mg/dL	especially if cholesterol >250 mg/dL
>500 mg/dL	Refer Lipid Clinic for active dietary and drug
with cholesterol >300 mg/dL	therapy
>1000 mg/dL (chylomicronemia)	Urgent therapy needed, risk of pancreatitis

* *Overall risk for coronary heart disease* (CHD): defined by European Atherosclerosis Society as family history of CHD, smoking, hypertension, diabetes mellitus, male sex, and low HDL-cholesterol (<35 mg/dL = <0.9 mmol/L) especially in younger patients.[6] For discussion of cut-off values for blood lipids, see reference 6.

The use of oleic acid as in olive oil and of linoleic acid[27] as in sunflower seed oil may be beneficial. Fish oils as in cod liver oil may also benefit.

There should be an increased intake of fruit, vegetables, and cereal fiber, so that the fiber intake is high. A diet high in oat bran may be part of a high-carbohydrate high-fiber cholesterol-lowering diet.

DRUG-RELATED HYPERLIPIDEMIAS

Drugs Causing Hyperlipidemias

The cardiac patient with hyperlipidemia may be receiving agents such as β-blockers or diuretics which may harmfully influence blood lipid profiles (Table 10-2), especially triglyceride values. β-Blockers with high intrinsic sympathomimetic activity (ISA) or cardioselectivity may have less or no effect. Among the agents with the most consistent changes in triglycerides are chlorthalidone and propranolol as well as the combination propranolol-hydrochlorothiazide. However, total blood cholesterol levels are little changed, by only about 8 percent or less during diuretic therapy and even less with β-blockade. An exception is when diuretics are given to those with low initial cholesterol values as in the young.[8]

Drugs not Causing Hyperlipidemias

Agents appearing to have no harmful effects on blood lipids include the angiotensin-converting enzyme (ACE) inhibitors, the calcium antagonists and the combined α-β-blocker labetalol, besides the ISA-containing β-blocker pindolol. The α-blockers, prazosin and indoramin, appear to favorably influence blood lipid profiles in the case of prazosin, and to cause only modest changes in the case of indoramin. Higher doses of prazosin appear to have similar effects to lower doses.[30] Hydralazine and the centrally acting agents (reserpine, methyldopa, and clonidine) all have little or no effect on blood lipids.[30] Several drug combinations had no effect on lipids (Table 10-2), apart from the unfavorable propranolol-hydrochlorothiazide combination.

Recommendations

β-Blockers given for angina may be replaced by calcium antagonists when there is fear for the consequences of triglyceride elevation. During the therapy of hypertension, β-blockers could likewise be replaced by α-blockers,

α-β-blockers, ACE inhibitors, calcium antagonists, hydralazine, or centrally active agents. If β-blocking therapy is deemed important, then cardioselective agents such as atenolol, metoprolol or acebutolol, or agents with ISA such as pindolol[30] or acebutolol have relatively little effect on blood lipid profiles.

Diuretic doses should be kept low. It may be hoped that with the diuretic dose recommended in this book (25 mg hydrochlorothiazide daily, see pp 117 and 210), few or no adverse effects on blood lipids would be found. However, this expectation requires study. Indapamide 2.5 mg daily, an antihypertensive dose (see p 118), may have relatively little effect although data are conflicting.[10,30]

When *oral contraceptives* are given to patients with ischemic heart disease or those with risk factors such as smoking, possible atherogenic effects of high estrogen contraceptives merit attention. Women receiving oral contraceptives or postmenopausal estrogens must not smoke.[33]

DRUGS FOR TREATMENT OF HYPERLIPIDEMIA

Lipid-lowering drugs may be required when dietary and risk factor management fails, when cardiovascular drugs are not at fault, and when there are no underlying diseases (hypothyroidism, poorly controlled diabetes mellitus, the nephrotic syndrome; excess alcohol intake and obesity for hypertriglyceridemia). In general, lipid-lowering drugs frequently cause side-effects, usually subjective but sometimes serious. Serial blood lipid profiles are required to confirm the benefits of therapy. Failure to improve within 2 months merits drug withdrawal. Sometimes doses less than those usually recommended can be used in conjunction with dietary intervention or in drug combinations.

Bile Acid Sequestrants

Cholestyramine (Questran®) and *colestipol* (Colestid®) bind bile acids so that they interrupt the enterohepatic recirculation. Blood cholesterol and LDL-concentrations fall; there may be a compensatory rise in plasma triglyceride. In the Lipid Research Clinics Primary Prevention Trial,[17] cholestyramine reduced CHD in hypercholesterolemic patients, but had no effect on overall mortality. Low initial doses are increased to cholestyramine 16–24 g daily (maximum 36 g) and colestipol 20–25 g daily, in two divided doses. The major side-effects of these agents are constipation, heartburn, and other gastrointestinal (GI) complaints; with large doses, steatorrhea may occur (rare). Watch for interaction with digoxin (decreased absorption).

Divistyramine, currently available in Holland, Italy, and Switzerland is said to be more palatable than cholestyramine, to avoid the gritty taste of the latter, and to cause fewer abdominal cramps (because divistyramine is less hygroscopic). The dose is of that of cholestyramine.

Inhibition of Liver Lipid Production

Nicotinic acid inhibits secretion of lipoproteins from the liver so that LDL are reduced including the triglyceride-rich component (VLDL). One of the basic effects of nicotinic acid may be decreased mobilization of free fatty acids from adipose tissue. Side-effects include prostaglandin-mediated symptoms such as flushing, dizziness and palpitations, as well as impaired glucose tolerance, increased blood urate, liver dysfunction, and rashes. The dose required for lipid lowering is 1–2 g $3\times$ daily, achieved gradually with a low starting dose (100 mg $3\times$ daily with meals to avoid GI discomfort). Flushing may be lessened by low-dose aspirin.

Nicofuranose (Bradilan®) resembles nicotinic acid with, however, fewer prostaglandin-related side-effects.

Fibric Acid Derivatives: Activators of Plasma Lipoprotein Lipase

As a rule, none of the fibric acid derivatives reduce blood cholesterol as well as does nicotinic acid.[1] However, these agents may be preferable in conditions with high blood triglycerides. Fibrates may also reduce cholesterol and are especially effective in type III lipidemia.

TABLE 10-2   EFFECTS OF ANTIHYPERTENSIVE AGENTS INCLUDING DIURETICS AND β-BLOCKERS ON BLOOD LIPID PROFILES

Agent	Daily Dose	Duration	Total Cholesterol (percent)	HDL-Cholesterol (percent)	LDL-Cholesterol (percent)	Triglycerides	References
Diuretics							
HCTZ	50 mg	2 wks	0	0	0	up to 10	24
HCTZ	50 mg	10–12 wks	up to 10	0	0	0	10,14
HCTZ	100 mg	6 wks	+6	0	(+9)	+17	9
Chlorthal	Variable	8–12 wks	+5	ND	ND	+25	2
Chlorthal	100 mg	6 wks	+8	0	+3	+15	9
Chlorthal	50–100 mg	1 yr	+5	0	+10	+10	8
Various	(. + prop)	Long-term	+10	0	0	+27	3
Loop	ND	4–12 mths	(+4)	(−15)	ND	(+15)	30
Indapamide	2.5 mg	Various	0	0	ND	0	30
Indapamide	2.5 mg	12 wks	+8	ND	ND	ND	10
β-Blockers							
Propranolol	160 mg	8–12 wks	0	−14	0	+37 (+25)*	5,14
Oxprenolol	160 mg	5–15 wks	0	(−5)	0	+18	5,14
Pindolol	7.5–15 mg	10–12 wks	0	+10	0	0 (+11)†	14,25
Nadolol	ND	12 wks	0	ND	ND	+22	31
Sotalol	160–640 mg	1 yr	+16	−28	+32	+66	12,13
Acebutolol	400 mg	24 wks	0	ND	ND	0	12
Atenolol	100 mg	5–12 wks	(−3)	(−4)	0	+8	5,14,28
Metoprolol	200 mg	8–12 wks	(−1)	0	0	+10	5,19,25,28
α-Blockers							
Prazosin	4 mg	8 wks	−9	0	−10	−16	14
Indoramin	50–100 mg	8 wks	0	0	−10	(+9)	19

	Dose	Time					
α-β-Blockers							
Labetalol	300–1200 mg	12 wks; 1 yr	0	0	0	0	7,20
ACE inhibitors							
Captopril	50–100 mg	6–12 wks	0	0	0	0	(Manuf)
Enalapril	10–40 mg	1 yr	0	ND	ND	0	18
Ca^{2+} antagonists							
Nifedipine	40 mg SR‡	48 wks	0	ND	ND	0	11
Verapamil	240–720 mg	12 wks	0	0	0	0	16
Diltiazem	90–180 mg	<12 wks	0	0	0	0	4
Combination therapy							
Methyldopa	250–300 mg						
+ HCTZ	50 mg	3 yrs	0	0	0	0	14
Propranolol	80–320 mg						
+ HCTZ	50 mg	3 yrs	0	–18	0	+44	14
Pindolol	10–20 mg						
+ HCTZ	50 mg	6–18 mths	0	+17	–4	0	29
Prazosin	1–8						
+ HCTZ	50 mg	14 wks	0	0	0	0	24
Prazosin	4 mg						
+ propranol	160 mg	8 wks	0	–8	0	0	14
Enalapril	10–40 mg						
+ HCTZ	50 mg	1 yr	0	ND	ND	0	18
Captopril	50–100 mg						
+ HCTZ	50 mg	6 wks	0	ND	ND	ND	32

* = after 6 years of propranolol[30]
† = after 5 years of pindolol[30]
‡ = nifedipine capsules have no effect on blood lipids over 8 weeks[30]
Changes in brackets = not significant; HCTZ = hydrochlorothiazide; Chlorthal = chlorthalidone; Prop = propranolol; ND = no data; Manuf = Manufacturers information; SR = slow release form of nifedipine

Clofibrate (Atromid-S®) promotes lipolysis of VLDL triglycerides by activating lipoprotein lipase, with variable secondary effects on blood cholesterol. In addition, excretion of sterol in the bile is enhanced. Dose: 500 mg 2–3× daily after meals. Side-effects include abdominal discomfort, muscle pains, and cholesterol gallstones. Watch for warfarin potentiation. Initial enthusiasm for prophylaxis of CHD in the general population by clofibrate rapidly cooled when it became evident that a massive European Trial showed no improvement in mortality:[23] in fact, the improved cardiovascular mortality was more than offset by the increased mortality from operations required for cholesterol gallstones, and because of pancreatitis. Contraindications to clofibrate include biliary tract or hepatic disease, or severe renal disease. Presently, clofibrate is used chiefly for specific indications as when hypertryglyceridemia has risk of pancreatitis.

Bezafibrate (Bezalip®) may be more effective than clofibrate in raising HDL cholesterol. Indications, contraindications, and side-effects are similar to clofibrate. In addition, myositis, renal failure, and alopecia may rarely occur. The dose is 200 mg 2–3× daily: reduce if serum creatinine rises.

Gemfibrozil (Lopid®) also acts similarly to clofibrate, with in addition inhibition of the synthesis of VLDL. Indications, contraindications, and side-effects are similar to clofibrate. Also watch for warfarin potentiation. The usual dose is 600 mg 2× daily, 30 minutes before meals (up to 1500 mg total daily dose).

Clearance of Cholesterol from Circulation

Probucol (Lurselle®, Lorelco®). This agent, reserved for hypercholesterolemia, promotes clearance of HDL and LDL-cholesterol from the circulation without any effect on triglycerides, possibly acting by increased excretion of cholesterol in the bile. The dose is 500 mg 2× daily with food. The side-effects although potentially many are not usually serious are as follows. GI: nausea, vomiting, flatulence, diarrhea and abdominal pain. Cardiovascular: QT-prolongation has been reported; therefore check for possible interaction with other agents prolonging QT (thiazide diuretics, group IA and III antiarrhythmics, see Fig. 4-5). Because probucol persists in adipose tissue for up to 6 months, pregnancy should not be embarked on until the drug has been withdrawn for that period.

HMG CoA Reductase Inhibitors

Several agents in this group are under development, including mevinolin, synvinolin, compactin, and eptastatin. Such agents enhance removal of LDL from the circulation, and in the long run may emerge as a very promising group.

Pregnancy and Lipid-lowering Drugs

As a group, lipid-lowering drugs are contraindicated during pregnancy; the bile acid sequestrants may be safest. Women desiring to become pregnant should stop other lipid-lowering drugs for about 6 months before conception.

SUMMARY

The basis for the usual therapy of hyperlipidemias, apart from the severe and hereditary types, is dietary. Lipidemias secondary to drugs and diseases must be excluded. Among the cardiac drugs tending to cause hyperlipidemias are β-blockers (especially nonselective agents such as propranolol) and thiazide diuretics. Careful attention to all other coronary risk factors is essential. No ideal lipid-lowering drug has yet been evolved, but several are in the pipeline. Of the existing agents, each can be used with success for specific indications when dietary management fails or is inappropriate. The ideal blood cholesterol level appears to be falling lower and lower, emphasizing the virtues of dietary advice for all cardiac patients.

ACKNOWLEDGMENT

This chapter was reviewed with the kind assistance of G.M. Berger.

REFERENCES

1. AHA Special Report: Recommendations for treatment of hyperlipidemia in adults. Circulation 69:1067A-1090A, 1969

2. Ames RP, Hill P: Increase in serum lipids during treatment of hypertension with chlorthalidone. Lancet i:721–723, 1976

3. Ames RP, Hill P: Improvement of glucose tolerance and lowering of glycohemoglobin and serum lipid concentrations after discontinuation of antihypertensive drug therapy. Circulation 65:899–904, 1982

4. Chaffman M, Brogden RN: Diltiazem. A review of its pharmacological properties and therapeutic efficacy. Drugs 29:387–454, 1985

5. Day L, Metcalfe J, Simpson CN: Adrenergic mechanisms in control of plasma lipid concentrations. Br Med J 284:1145–1148, 1982

6. European Atherosclerosis Society: Report of the 47th Annual Meeting, Naples, Italy, 1986. Eur Heart J, in press, 1986

7. Frishman W, Michelson E, Johnson B, et al: Effects of beta-adrenergic blockade on plasma lipids: A double-blind randomized placebo-controlled multi-center comparison of labetalol and metoprolol in patients with hypertension. Am J Cardiol 49 (abs):984, 1982

8. Goldman AI, Steele BW, Schnaper HW, et al: Serum lipoprotein levels during chlorthalidone therapy. JAMA 244:1691–1695, 1980

9. Grimm RH Jr, Leon AS, Hunninghake DB, et al: Effects of thiazide diuretics on plasma lipids and lipoproteins in mildly hypertensive patients. Ann Intern Med 94:7–11, 1981.

10. Kreeft JH, Langlois S, Ogilvie RI: Comparative trial of indapamide and hydrochlorothiazide in essential hypertension, with forearm plethysmography. J Cardiovasc Pharmacol 6:622–626, 1984

11. Landmark K: Antihypertensive and metabolic effects of long-term therapy with nifedipine slow-release tablets. J Cardiovasc Pharmacol 7:12–17, 1985

12. Lehtonen A: Effects of beta blockers on blood lipid profile. Am Heart J 109:1192–1196, 1985

13. Lehtonen A, Viikari J: Long-term effect of sotalol on plasma lipids. Clin Sci 57:405s–407s, 1979

14. Leren P, Eide I, Foss A, et al: Antihypertensive drugs and blood lipids: The Oslo Study. Br J Clin Pharmacol 13:441S–444S, 1982

15. Lewis B, Mann JI: Reducing the risks of coronary heart disease in individuals and in the population. Lancet i:956–959, 1986

16. Lewis GRJ: Long-term results with verapamil in essential hypertension and its influence on serum lipids. Am J Cardiol 57:35D–38D, 1986

17. Lipid Research Clinics Coronary Primary Prevention Trial Results: I. Reduction in incidence of coronary heart disease. II. The relationship of reduction in incidence of coronary heart disease to cholesterol lowering. JAMA 251:351, 1984

18. Malini PL, Strocchi E, Ambrosioni E, et al: Long-term antihypertensive, metabolic and cellular effects of enalapril. J Hypertens 2 (suppl 2):101–105, 1984

19. Martinez TLR, Auriemo CRC, Machado AMO, et al: Effects of indoramin and metoprolol on plasma lipids and lipoproteins. J Cardiovasc Pharmacol 8 (suppl 2):S76–S79, 1986

20. McGonigle RJS, Williams L, Murphy MJ, et al: Labetalol and lipids. Lancet i (letter):163, 1981

21. NIH Consensus Conference: Lowering blood cholesterol to prevent heart disease. JAMA 253:2080–2086, 1985

22. Oliver MF: The optimum serum cholesterol. Lancet ii:655, 1982.

23. Oliver MF, Heady JA: WHO Cooperative Trial on Primary Prevention of Ischaemic Heart Disease with Clofibrate to Lower Serum Cholesterol: Final mortality follow-up. Lancet ii:800–804, 1984

24. Overlack A, Stumpe KO: Comparison of the effect of indoramin and prazosin on blood pressure and lipid profiles in essential hypertension. J Cardiovasc Pharmacol 8 (suppl 2):S53–S55, 1986

25. Pasotti C, Capra A, Fiorella G, et al: Effects of pindolol and metoprolol on plasma lipids and lipoproteins. Br J Clin Pharmacol 13:435S–439S, 1982

26. Pocock SJ, Shaper AG, Phillips AN, et al: High density lipoprotein cholesterol is not a major risk factor for ischaemic heart disease in British men. Br Med J 292:515–519, 1986

27. Riemersma RA, Wood DA, Butler S, et al: Linoleic acid content in adipose tissue and coronary heart disease. Br Med J 292:1423–1427, 1986

28. Rossner S, Weiner L: A comparison of the effects of atenolol and metoprolol on serum lipoproteins. Drugs 25 (suppl 2):322–325, 1983

29. Samuel P, Chin B, Fenderson RW, et al: Improvement of the lipid profile during long-term administration of pindolol and hydrochlorothiazide in patients with hypertension. Am J Cardiol 57:24C–28C, 1986

30. Weidmann P, Uehlinger DE, Gerber A: Editorial Review. Antihypertensive treatment and serum lipoproteins. J Hypertens 3:297–306, 1985

31. Weinberger MH: Antihypertensive therapy and lipids: Evidence, mechanisms, and implications. Arch Intern Med 145:1102–1105, 1985

32. Weinberger MH: Influence of an angiotensin converting enzyme inhibitor on diuretic-induced metabolic effects in hypertension. Hypertension (suppl III):132–138, 1983

33. Wilson TWF, Garrison RJ, Castelli WP: Postmenopausal estrogen use, cigarette smoking and cardiovascular morbidity in women over 50. New Engl J Med 313:1038–1043, 1985

B. J. Gersh
L. H. Opie
N. M. Kaplan

11

Cardiovascular Diseases and Hypertension: Which Drug for Which Condition?

ANGINA PECTORIS

For *exertional angina pectoris*, initial treatment requires attention to precipitating factors (hypertension, anemia, congestive heart failure (CHF), tachyarrhythmias, and valve disease). Sublingual nitroglycerin (Chapter 2) in combination with either a β-blocker (Chapter 1) or calcium antagonist (Chapter 3) remains standard therapy. Thereafter, the addition of long-acting nitrates or the combination of β-blockers with calcium antagonists is indicated. Nifedipine plus β-blocker may be better than isosorbide dinitrate plus β-blocker. The latter combination appears safest in the case of nifedipine, provided that hypotension is excluded. In the case of verapamil or diltiazem, special caution is needed (although these combinations are freely used) particularly in patients with a history of heart failure or conduction disturbances or bradycardia, in whom there is the potential for serious side-effects. "Triple therapy" with nitrates, calcium antagonists, and β-blockade should not be an automatic next step; individual reactions vary (see p 29).

In *variant angina*, due to transient spasm of one or more of the coronary arteries as originally proposed by Prinzmetal, the calcium antagonists are undoubtedly effective, as are nitrates, but patients may require the combination for optimal results.[95] β-Blockers are inferior to calcium antagonists in the treatment of true Prinzmetal's angina and may aggravate the condition.[22] Prazosin occasionally works. In refractory cases of Prinzmetal's angina associated with coronary artery disease, bypass grafting combined with cardiac sympathetic denervation (plexectomy) appears superior to bypass alone.[41]

In *unstable angina and angina at rest,* the nearer the patient is to threatened myocardial infarction, the stronger is the case for β-blockers, whereas the nearer the patient is to true Prinzmetal's angina, the stronger is the case for calcium antagonists. In the absence of coronary spasm, the case for routine nifedipine is weak and a randomized trial showed that it might even harm, presumably because of excess hypotensive or tachycardiac effects, unless combined with propranolol.[79] Calcium antagonists, especially nifedipine are frequently used together with β-blockers and high-dose nitrates (see p 43); careful attention to the development of side-effects is mandatory.

The common clinical practice of giving nasal oxygen may prevent nitrate-induced arterial hypoxemia. Anticoagulants (heparin) and antiplatelet agents especially aspirin (see pp 168 and 173) are logical, because of the high incidence of intracoronary thrombus in some of these patients.[45] Hospital admission and complete bed rest may be helpful.

Coronary Artery Bypass Surgery and PTCA for Angina Pectoris

The indications for coronary bypass surgery have expanded widely, reflecting refinements in techniques and improved results. The Coronary Artery Surgery Study (CASS) randomized trial, confined to patients with mild stable angina under the age of 65 years, showed no benefit of bypass on survival except in patients with triple vessel disease and mild to moderate impairment of left ventricular (LV) function.[80] Bypass is more likely to benefit patients at higher risk, having moderate or severe or unstable angina, left main coronary disease, LV dysfunction, and an age of 65 years or more.[50] The European trial also gave benefit to double vessel disease that included the proximal left main coronary.[63] **The decision about surgery must be tailored to the individual and needs to take into account complex factors** including the effect of angina on the patient's lifestyle and occupation, the severity of symptoms, the type of coronary artery disease, LV function, the presence of other medical conditions, and the tolerance of medical therapy. Even in some higher risk patients, careful medical therapy may lead to improved symptoms.[50]

Percutaneous transluminal coronary angioplasty (PTCA) is a promising alternative to coronary bypass in patients with a dilatable lesion in whom operation can be avoided. Further evaluation of this technique is urgently needed; restenosis remains a significant problem. There have been no randomized trials comparing angioplasty with coronary bypass surgery or medical therapy.

ACUTE MYOCARDIAL INFARCTION (AMI)

Morphine (5–10 mg slow IV at 1 mg/min) combines a potent analgesic effect with hemodynamic actions that are particularly beneficial in reducing myocardial oxygen demand (MVO_2), namely: a marked venodilator action reducing ventricular preload, an ability to decrease heart rate, and a mild arterial vasodilator action that may reduce afterload.[32] In the presence of hypovolemia, morphine may cause profound hypotension. Unlike morphine, *nalbuphine hydrochloride* (Nubain®, 10 mg slow IV) has few hemodynamic effects and appears to be an effective analgesic with a ceiling for respiratory depression even at higher doses.[17] *Atropine* (IV 0.3 mg aliquots to maximum of 2.0 mg) has a vagolytic effect that is useful for the management of bradyarrhythmias with atrioventricular (AV) block (particularly with inferior infarction), sinus or nodal bradycardia with hypotension, or bradycardia-related ventricular ectopy.[21] Small doses and careful monitoring is essential since the elimination of vagal overactivity may unmask latent sympathetic overactivity, producing sinus tachycardia and rarely ventricular tachycardia (VT) or fibrillation (VF).[27] The role of prophylactic atropine for uncomplicated bradycardia is questionable.

Sinus tachycardia is a common manifestation of the autonomic instability characteristic of the early phase of acute infarction. Sympathetic overactivity may reflect underlying pump failure, but as a cause of increased myocardial oxygen demand (MVO_2) and tachyarrhythmias, warrants treatment. **The first step is to treat the underlying cause,** for example, pain, anxiety, hypovolemia or pump failure, but in the absence of these IV propranolol (Inderal®) in 0.5 mg increments into a total dose of 0.1 mg/kg or IV metoprolol (Lopressor®) 5 mg increments every 2 minutes up to 15 mg is safe and effective provided the patient is carefully observed. In Europe, other β-blockers such as atenolol[60] or sotalol have been extensively used. In the absence of LV failure, sinus tachycardia and hypertension with its attendant demand on MVO_2 is an urgent indication for β-blockade.

Acute hypertension also increases afterload and MVO_2 while improving perfusion of the ischemic zone. Thus the benefits of blood pressure (BP) reduction in AMI are not clear unless there is LV failure (frequent in severe infarcts). Nor is the ideal rate of BP reduction known; a smooth and careful reduction by IV nitroglycerin or nitroprusside seems best; other tested drugs include IV labetalol, IV β-blockers, and sublingual nifedipine. In experimental coronary stenosis without infarction, the lower the heart rate the higher the BP that can be tolerated, and the ratio of mean BP to heart rate should exceed one.[45a]

Acute Reperfusion Therapy

An increase in blood supply remains the most effective mode of preservation of ischemic myocardium. The concept of acute clot lysis in evolving myocardial infarction has the potential radically to alter the management of this condition. This is a rapidly changing area of investigation and poses some pivotal issues relevant to current clinical practice. Fibrinolytic therapy, once limited to centers with facilities for emergency intracoronary administration, can now be given intravenously which has the major advantage of earlier administration. Thereafter angiography must follow to select patients for PTCA or bypass grafting (see p 179). Clot selective agents such as tPA offer most promise (see p 178).

There is, however, an increasing awareness that **successful thrombolysis is not an end in itself.** Residual pre-existing stenosis of the vessel may impair the recovery of LV function and predispose to re-occlusion. Thus whenever possible early PTCA warrants consideration, although still not unequivocally of proven value. The ideal approach to *postthrombolytic therapy* in unknown, including the role of PTCA (early or late), coronary artery bypass, and anticoagulant or antiplatelet therapy. These crucially important issues should be subjected to the rigorous scrutiny of large clinical trials. The results of these will have a major impact upon cardiology in the future.

Therapy of Ventricular Arrhythmias in Acute Infarction

Lidocaine (lignocaine)(Chapter 4) is widely used in the prophylaxis and therapy of early postinfarction arrhythmias. The role of prophylactic lidocaine therapy in abolishing "warning arrhythmias" and consequently VF is controversial. Because lidocaine is reasonably safe and may benefit, it may be given to all patients suspected of acute infarction (for contrary arguments, see p 67), providing they are not allergic to lidocaine or its analogs. In patients in the prehospitalization phase of AMI, 400 mg of intramuscular (deltoid) lidocaine protected them against primary VF from 15 minutes after the injection.[71] However, about 250 patients with suspected AMI had to be treated to prevent VF in only one.

It is rational to use *β-blocking agents*, in the absence of contraindications, for the treatment of ventricular arrhythmias related to persistent or recurrent ischemia, or when there is overt evidence of sympathetic overactivity; several studies have shown that β-blockers can have wider antiarrhythmic use in AMI.[24]

Treatment of LV failure is an essential adjunct to antiarrhythmic therapy, and the possibility of drug-induced VT or hypokalemia should always be borne in mind. Pacing techniques (atrial or ventricular), stellate ganglion blockade or programmed ventricular stimulation may occasionally be lifesaving.

Supraventricular Arrhythmias in AMI

Atrial fibrillation, flutter or paroxysmal supraventricular tachycardia are usually transient but are recurrent and troublesome. Precipitating factors requiring treatment include hypoxia, acidosis, heart failure with atrial distention, pericarditis, and sinus node ischemia. Initial therapy should be carotid sinus massage or other vagal maneuvers in the case of supraventricular tachycardia. In the absence of LV failure, verapamil or IV β-blockade is acceptable and effective, particularly in controlling the ventricular rate and may be combined with digoxin. The new ultrashort-acting β-blocker, esmolol, is likely to be used when β-blockade may be a potential hemodynamic danger. Cardioversion is limited to resistant cases with hemodynamic compromise. Recurrent atrial flutter may respond to atrial overdrive pacing.

LV Failure with Pulmonary Congestion

Swan-Ganz catheterization to measure LV filling pressure and cardiac output allows a rational choice between various IV agents that reduce both preload and afterload (nitroprusside, see p 136) or chiefly the preload (nitrates, see p 137). Of the specific afterload reducers (hydralazine and nifedipine) only hydralazine (see p 138) can be given intravenously; however, both may cause tachycardia so are usually contraindicated. Amrinone (see p 106), an inotropic-vasodilator, is contraindicated because it may promote arrhythmias. Heart failure with recurrent angina pectoris in AMI is particularly amenable to therapy with IV nitroglycerin (see p 27) or nitroprusside. Captopril or enalapril (Chapter 8) are now increasingly used for CHF in AMI, although limited by oral administration. The diuretic furosemide (see p 112) is standard therapy and acts by rapid vasodilation as well as by diuresis. In the patient with AMI and pulmonary edema, excessive diuresis, preload reduction, and relative volume depletion must be avoided. These patients have reduced ventricular compliance and require higher filling pressures to maintain cardiac output.

The role of *digitalis in AMI is controversial* (see p 96). An increase in contractility and coronary vasoconstriction mediated by digitalis may increase myocardial oxygen demand, which may again fall as failure is treated and the heart volume decreases. The benefits of digoxin in AMI are probably small so that its use is restricted to patients with frank LV failure not responding to furosemide or nitrates, or angiotensin-converting enzyme (ACE) inhibitors, or with atrial tachyarrhythmias in whom verapamil fails or is contraindicated.

Where there are no intensive care facilities, IV unloading agents such as nitroprusside and nitrates are best avoided. In theory, sublingual agents that reduce preload (short-acting nitrates) or afterload (nifedipine) should be useful here.

"Forward Failure" in AMI

When cardiac output is low in the absence of an elevated wedge pressure or clinical and radiographic evidence of LV failure, it is crucial to exclude hypovolemia (possibly drug-induced), or right ventricular infarction. In the absence of these, the best strategy is to employ afterload reducing agents alone or in combination with a positively inotropic agent such as dopamine or dobutamine. Inodilator therapy (see pp 104–107) is logical. Monitoring the hemodynamic response invasively is indispensible in this situation. Nitrates are usually contraindicated because their main effect is reduction of preload.

Limitation of Infarct Size

Since myocardial infarction is ultimately the consequence of an imbalance between myocardial oxygen supply and demand, it is logical and prudent to employ measures aimed at redressing this. These include the treatment of arrhythmias, hypoxia, heart failure, hypertension and tachycardia. Hypokalemia should be sought and treated. Despite much experimental evidence that numerous pharmacologic agents such as β-blockers, hyaluronidase or nitrates, or metabolic agents such as glucose-insulin-potassium or free radical scavengers will reduce infarct size, clinical proof of benefit has been difficult to obtain.

Pooled data from several randomized trials would suggest that the early administration of *IV nitroglycerin or nitroprusside* (see pp 29 and 136) may favorably influence infarct size in various specific subgroups of patients.[97] The beneficial effect of early IV metoprolol in AMI suggested by two studies[10,77] is probably multifactorial in nature and confined to high risk patients.[77] The massive ISIS study on over 16,000 patients showed that IV atenolol (5–10 mg) followed by 7 days of oral atenolol (100 mg/day) reduces mortality by about 15 percent, which is only one life saved for 150 patients treated.[60] In another study, early metoprolol did not reduce early VF.[84] **Whether these somewhat modest benefits of early IV β-blockade are really worthwhile in the absence of another added indication such as sinus tachycardia or hypertension, remains a moot point, especially because of the negative inotropic and chronotropic potential.** Heart rate reduction is required for infarct size limitation.[69a] In a borderline hemodynamic situation, an "on-off" test of transient β-blockade can be achieved by *esmolol.* When β-blockade needs abrupt cessation, there is no major withdrawal rebound.[47a]

IV hyaluronidase, previously thought to be effective, is discounted by a recent study on nearly 1,500 patients showing that the mortality at 6 months was not decreased.[64] In a randomized trial of glucose-insulin-potassium (GIK) or saline infusions in AMI, GIK appeared to reduce the frequency of premature ventricular systoles and in-hospital mortality in patients in Killip functional classes I-III.[23] Lack of a commercial backer seems to limit interest in GIK. However, it should be considered that insulin by itself has a positive inotropic effect.

LONG-TERM THERAPY AFTER AMI

β-Blockade

Three important randomized double-blind studies in 1981 showed a clear-cut benefit in the secondary prevention of death following myocardial infarction in subjects treated with timolol,[20] metoprolol,[10] and propranolol.[2] Obvious contraindications are overt heart failure, severe bradycardia, hypotension, asthma, and heart block greater than first degree. Approximately half the patients entering these trials were excluded.

Several questions remain unanswered (see p 7): Does the effect apply to all other β-blockers except those with intrinsic sympathomimetic activity (ISA) as suggested by Yusuf et al [96]? What is the mechanism of the reduction in mortality? When should therapy be initiated and for how long? Further information about subsets of patients more likely to benefit from β-blockade is needed. **There seems little point in giving β-blockade to patients with good LV function and at low risk of mortality.** In others, it would appear reasonable to give β-blockers to patients in the 30–70 year age group who have no contraindications. Mild to moderate compensated congestive heart failure is not a contraindication to postinfarct β-blockade, and a history of prior CHF renders β-blockade more rather than less effective.[45b] For β-blockade to be of benefit, it should be initiated within the first four months postinfarction (probably within the first few weeks); it can be continued for up to six years.[30] The timolol and sotalol studies show that in these circumstances β-blockade can be discontinued abruptly.

Digitalis

The controversy whether digitalis contributes independently to cardiac death in the first year postinfarction has not been settled (see p 96). While it should not be withheld from patients with LV failure in the postinfarct phase, digitalis should not be given without careful evaluation of the risk-benefit ratio. Special consideration should be given to the earlier use of ACE inhibitors rather than digitalis, and to monitoring plasma potassium during combined digitalis-diuretic therapy.

Platelet Inhibitor Agents

In survivors of AMI, these drugs (aspirin, sulfinpyrazone, and dipyridamole) have been the focus of several large clinical trials (see pp 168, 170, 172). Sulfinpyrazone and dipyridamole have shown marginal benefit at best and on the basis of currently available data, their routine use in postinfarction patients cannot be recommended.[6] **Aspirin, the simplest and safest agent, is now approved by the FDA to reduce the risk of sudden death or re-infarction** (dose: 1 tablet daily, 300–325 mg). Aspirin may also be selected for those patients thought to be at risk of thromboembolism in whom oral anticoagulation is either not advisable or the patient is not likely to comply with the stringent requirements for prolonged oral anticoagulation therapy.

Ventricular Arrhythmias in Myocardial Infarction Survivors

Complex ventricular ectopy and VT in the late-hospital phase of myocardial infarction are well described as predictors of subsequent sudden death after discharge,[25] independently of their frequent association with LV dysfunction.[28] Treatment of these is logical, providing that drug efficacy is established under monitoring conditions (Fig. 4-6). **Yet any effect of antiarrhythmic therapy on postinfarct mortality is as yet unproven;** preliminary data are discouraging.[58,86] The role of programmed ventricular stimulation in the identification of infarct survivors at high risk of sudden cardiac death is currently unresolved but is a promising avenue for further investigation.

MANAGEMENT OF ARRHYTHMIAS

Paroxysmal Atrial Fibrillation

Severely symptomatic patients in shock or cardiac failure need immediate cardioversion. If a rapid reduction in rate is needed, for instance, when the tachycardia has precipitated ischemia, IV verapamil will slow the rate pending a response to digoxin. If the objective is to restore sinus rhythm, IV procainamide (or disopyramide in Europe) may circumvent the need for electrical cardioversion. In the prevention of paroxysmal atrial fibrillation, quinidine is most commonly used, but with mixed success. Of the investigational agents, propafenone appears very promising and has fewer side-effects than amiodarone. Anticoagulation is discussed in Chapter 9 (see p 176).

Recent Onset Atrial Fibrillation

Patients are first given oral quinidine (or disopyramide) in a standard dose, which will convert about one-third of patients to sinus rhythm; electrocardioversion is used for the others. Digitalization is standard in combination with quinidine but usually stopped before cardioversion. When there is possible risk of embolization at the time of rhythm conversion, prophylactic anticoagulation is usual.

Chronic Atrial Fibrillation

When the ventricular rate seems not to respond to digitalis compounds, the first move is to check the patient's compliance, the digoxin blood level, and to reassess for thyrotoxicosis or other systemic or cardiac diseases. Thereafter the digitalis dose may be cautiously increased; however, optimal control of exercise heart rate usually needs added oral verapamil[39] or diltiazem.[83a] In patients without LV failure, verapamil or diltiazem is logical first-line therapy. If it is necessary acutely to reduce the ventricular response, IV verapamil or β-blockade is effective, but may be dangerous in patients who are already digitalized and neither should be given to patients receiving the other.

In the case of atrial fibrillation or flutter with antegrade *pre-excitation* via an accessory pathway (Wolff-Parkinson-White syndrome), digitalis, which shortens the refractory period of the bypass tract, is *absolutely* contraindicated. Verapamil, diltiazem, and β-blockade may sometimes be hazardous and should be avoided. The treatment of choice is cardioversion if the patient is shocked, or IV procainamide. IV disopyramide may be effective (exclude heart failure first) but is not yet available in the USA. The new Class IC antiarrhythmics such as flecainide, encainide, or propafenone may therefore be used. In the prevention of paroxysmal atrial fibrillation with a rapid ventricular response due to pre-excitation, low-dose amiodarone may first be tried before surgical ablation of the accessory pathway which has been highly successful in a few specialized centers.

Atrial Flutter

In the patient with stable atrial flutter, the ventricular rate may be controlled by digitalis, verapamil, or β-blockade, or a double or triple combination of these drugs. Satisfactory control of the ventricular rate may be extremely difficult to achieve but the rhythm is easily converted by a low-energy countershock and is highly responsive to atrial pacing techniques. The use of temporary atrial pacing electrodes for rapid atrial pacing is particularly helpful in the management of paroxysmal atrial flutter, postoperatively after cardiac surgery. In the prevention of recurrent atrial flutter, one or more of these drugs are used, frequently with quinidine. When atrial flutter complicates congenital heart disease,[49] digoxin plus quinidine or procainamide is frequently effective; in selected cases amiodarone gives excellent results.

Supraventricular Tachycardia

Newer drugs, antitachycardia pacing techniques, and innovative surgical approaches have radically improved treatment. Patients with supraventricular arrhythmias that are very rapid or refractory to standard drugs, or associated with a wide QRS complex on the standard electrocardiogram (implying either aberration, antegrade pre-excitation, or VT) warrant an invasive electrophysiologic study. Yet in the majority of patients, management can be guided by clinical principles.

Vagotonic procedures (Valsalva maneuver, facial immersion in cold water, or carotid sinus massage) may terminate the tachycardia. Always auscultate the carotid arteries before performing carotid sinus massage. If these measures fail, *IV verapamil* (see p 38) is the simplest and most effective treatment (providing the patient is not already receiving digitalis or β-blockers). *IV adenosine* may soon become the drug of choice. Alternatively, cholinergic stimulation by tensilon (Edrophonium®) is given as 2 mg IV; wait for 45 seconds to exclude hypersensitivity, then 8 mg IV; atropine should be at hand for occasional excess cholinergic reaction. Another way of augmenting vagal tone, occasionally used, is by gradual elevation of the systolic pressure with α-adrenergic drugs such as phenylephrine or methoxamine. IV β-blockade is another alternative but less effective than verapamil and is contraindicated if the patient has already received verapamil.

If these steps fail, vagotonic maneuvers are worth repeating. Thereafter the choice lies between IV digitalization, IV procainamide (or disopyramide in Europe), or cardioversion and should be tempered by the clinical condition of the patient.

For the *prevention of paroxysmal supraventricular tachycardia*, the simplest drug is digoxin, but verapamil (or diltiazem) and β-blockers are suitable alternatives and preferable to quinidine, procainamide, or disopyramide; the latter drugs all have a higher incidence of side-effects. Prevention may result from abolition of the initiating ectopic beats or by altering the characteristics of the re-entrant pathway in such a way that tachycardia cannot be sustained. Amiodarone is highly effective for supraventricular arrhythmias including paroxysmal atrial fibrillation and arrhythmias involving accessory pathways; severe side-effects may be limited by a low dose (see p 75).

Bradyarrhythmias

Asymptomatic sinus bradycardia does not require therapy and may be normal in many patients. For symptomatic sinus bradycardia, probanthine and chronic atropine are unsatisfactory in the long run so that pacing may be needed; first exclude the effects of drugs such as β-blockers, digitalis, verapamil, diltiazem, quinidine, procainamide, amiodarone, lithium carbonate, lidocaine, guanethidine, and clonidine.

Intrinsic sinus node dysfunction, often characterized by the *tachycardia/bradycardia syndrome* is difficult to treat, but in most cases digitalis is not contraindicated. β-blockers aggravate the bradycardic component of the syndrome. An exception is pindolol with its ISA, which may help to dampen down the tachycardia episodes while limiting the bradycardia; however, Holter monitoring is required to show its efficacy before long-term use. Nonetheless, patients usually end up with a combination of permanent cardiac pacing and antiarrhythmic drugs. For AV block with syncope or excessively slow rates, drug therapy (isoproterenol) is used as an emergency but temporary measure, pending pacemaker implantation.

Digitalis Toxicity

This should always be considered when arrhythmias develop in a patient on digitalis, particularly in the presence of an accelerated nodal or idioventricular tachycardia (see p 99).

Ventricular Arrhythmias

The therapy of ventricular arrhythmias is a complex, rapidly changing area that cannot readily be simplified (Fig. 4-6). The criteria for instituting therapy are not clear-cut, although patients with sustained VT, survivors of previous arrhythmia-related cardiac arrest, and those with symptomatic arrhythmias, all require treatment. Antiarrhythmic drugs are costly and potentially highly toxic by their pro-arrhythmic effect,[33] especially Class III or IA agents causing torsades de pointes. Therefore the serum potassium and magnesium and QT-interval must be monitored during co-therapy with diuretics, and the serum digoxin level during co-therapy with digitalis. Documentation of the efficacy of antiarrhythmics is essential prior to their long-term use. This requirement means the selection of a model, whether based on the combination of Holter monitoring and exercise testing or the inducibility of ventricular arrhythmias during an invasive electrophysiologic study. The intensive investigation and treatment of symptomatic ventricular arrhythmias is time-consuming and a task for specialized units, but the stakes are high.

Does therapy alter the *prognosis* of malignant symptomatic ventricular arrhythmias Accumulating evidence says yes, provided that extensive investigation is followed by meticulous assessment of drug efficacy. Using programmed ventricular stimulation in patients with malignant ventricular arrhythmias or in survivors of out-of-hospital cardiac arrest, drug suppression of inducible arrhythmias is strongly associated with a favorable long-term outcome. In patients in whom a successful drug was not identified by electrophysiologic testing, the recurrence rate appears high.[51,83,89] **There is no evidence that therapy of asymptomatic ventricular arrhythmias, even in the presence of heart disease, prolongs life or prevents sudden death.**

The *choice of drug* for chronic use is ideally based on prior demonstration during acute and chronic testing that the drug actually works and on its potential for toxicity in the individual under study. Quinidine, procainamide, tocainide, and disopyramide are first-line drugs in the USA, but the use of the latter agent is limited by its negative inotropic potential. In Europe, mexiletine, propafenone, encainide, and flecainide are widely used; all of these except propafenone are or will soon be available in the USA. Class IC agents may be particularly prone to pro-arrhythmic effects. Amiodarone remains the last-ditch stand. Deciding between the agents currently available is somewhat of a personal choice and not entirely logical (Fig. 4-6).

Treatment of heart failure, hypoxia, electrolyte imbalance, and ischemia are essential adjuncts to antiarrhythmic therapy. Coronary bypass surgery helps selected patients.[91] β-Blockade alone is relatively ineffective but may be useful in arrhythmias accompanying myocardial ischemia or mitral valve prolapse. Phenytoin has little role to play except for digitalis toxicity and in children. The side-effects of bretylium limit its long-term use.

Nonpharmacological approaches to the management of ventricular arrhythmias include sophisticated pacing modalities and surgery in conjunction with electrophysiologic mapping. Excellent results can be achieved in selected patients. The automatic implantable cardioverter defibrillator could be the harbinger of an entirely new approach to the management of patients with malignant ventricular arrhythmias. Results with this device, while confined to specialized centers, are most encouraging and exciting.[78]

CONGESTIVE HEART FAILURE

Despite newer agents (particularly the vasodilators), the long-term prognosis of CHF remains poor, unless a reversible cause, for instance valvular heart disease, is present. The initial steps in a patient with heart failure are to investigate the cause and treat associated conditions such as hypertension and anemia. The usual policy is to initiate treatment with diuretics, salt restriction, and then digitalis before proceeding to conventional vasodilators—this is changing with the earlier use of ACE inhibitors. **The role of digitalis remains contentious; nonetheless, its use should not be withheld in patients with objective signs of CHF, especially after introduction of diuretic therapy** (see pp 94 and 126).

In *severe intractable CHF*, hemodynamic monitoring is required both to evaluate the hemodynamic status and, usually, to initiate IV therapy before going on to oral agents. Theoretically, inotropic vasodilators ("inodilators," Table 5-8) such as *amrinone* and *milrinone* should have different indications from predominant inotropes such as dobutamine; yet a recent multicentered randomized study showed that *milrinone* (50 μg/kg bolus, followed by 0.5–0.625 μg/kg/min) gave very similar clinical effects to *dobutamine* with somewhat less initial chronotropic effect.[70] Once benefit has been achieved by IV inotropes, therapy should not be continued without re-evaluation because in the case of dobutamine there is loss of a sustained effect during one week of IV infusion[72] and in the case of milrinone a preliminary study suggests that long-term oral use appears to be associated with an adverse outcome.[52]

Oral Vasodilator Therapy

Ideally vasodilator therapy should be governed by the hemodynamic status, measured invasively (not in mild heart failure). The problems of drug tolerance are common to many vasodilators, especially prazosin, although less frequent during ACE inhibitor therapy. Another common problem is the precipitation of hypotension. Conventionally patients with predominantly elevated LV filling pressures require long-acting nitrates, with the addition of hydralazine or nifedipine (precautions, see pp 138 and 142) for an elevated systemic vascular resistance. When both are elevated, then short-term prazosin, captopril, or enalapril may be used. Such "rules" may not work so that a flexible pragmatic approach is needed. Prolonged nitrate-hydralazine therapy may benefit mortality (see pp 27 and 138). **In patients without pulmonary congestion, it is essential to avoid excessive preload reduction that may precipitously reduce filling pressures.** In such patients, agents working only on the arteriolar bed such as hydralazine might be best; again, hypotension remains a risk. Hydralazine should be avoided in patients with ischemic cardiomyopathy (risk of tachycardia-induced angina).

Diastolic Heart Disease

Traditional concepts of heart failure emphasize the primary role of systolic ventricular dysfunction. Two recent studies of patients with a clinical diagnosis of heart failure found well preserved LV systolic function in 36 percent and 42 percent respectively and draw attention to the entity of "diastolic dysfunction".[54,85] The role of calcium antagonists and β-blockers in this syndrome needs evaluation; experience with hypertrophic cardiomyopathy suggests that diastolic function can be improved by calcium antagonists.

ACUTE PULMONARY EDEMA

In acute pulmonary edema of cardiac origin, the initial management requires positioning the patient in an upright posture and oxygen administration. If the underlying cause is an arrhythmia, restoration of sinus rhythm takes priority. *Morphine sulfate* is highly effective in relieving symptoms. Its mechanism of action is not precisely understood, but a venodilator action and a central sedative effect are likely.[31] *IV furosemide*, which acts both as a diuretic and a vasodilator, is the other basic therapy (see p 112).

Because of the potential hazards of giving digitalis to the acutely ill hypoxic patient (Chapter 4), **there is much to be said for load reduction with sublingual or IV nitrates, IV sodium nitroprusside, or nifedipine.** Particular caution is necessary in the patient with a systolic blood pressure of less than 90 mmHg, if *vasodilators* are contemplated. In patients with pulmonary edema secondary to severe acute or chronic mitral or aortic regurgitation, IV nitroprusside (see p 136) is probably the agent of choice. Once acute pulmonary edema has been relieved and in the absence of AMI, *cautious digitalization* is started (1 mg digoxin intravenously over 30 minutes, providing the patient is not already receiving digitalis). When there is risk of arrhythmia as in AMI,[18] *aminophylline* or theophylline or the related xanthine compounds are also best avoided (bronchospasm will usually respond to diuresis or load reduction). If IV xanthine compounds must be used, they should be given slowly (side-effects on respiration and the central nervous system) with monitoring for arrhythmias. Aminophylline may be given at 6 mg/kg intravenously over 30 minutes followed by 0.5 mg/kg/hr.

In refractory cases, resort to rotating tourniquets or intubation with mechanical ventilation. Pulmonary edema of cardiac origin must be differentiated from the adult respiratory distress syndrome, which requires specific therapy.

CARDIOMYOPATHY

Hypertrophic Cardiomyopathy (IHSS)

Although many patients are asymptomatic, there is risk of sudden cardiac death, which mandates avoidance of competitive sports even in the absence of symptoms. **The cornerstone of drug therapy in symptomatic patients is to avoid agents that increase cardiac contractility,** such as digitalis, or reduce ventricular preload, such as nitrates (which should be given with care to patients with added angina).

Three basic therapies have been used: β-blockade, calcium antagonists (especially verapamil), and disopyramide. Each has its advocates. *High-dose propranolol* is most widely used and frequently reduces symptoms. Verapamil may be more useful than β-blockade in patients with pulmonary symptoms or other contraindications to β-blockade and is usually well tolerated. *Verapamil or diltiazem* is increasingly seen as a logical therapy to relieve the diastolic relaxation problems found in hypertrophic cardiomyopathy.[43,88] Occasional dangerous or even lethal side-effects with verapamil have been reported, presumably because the afterload reducing effect is more vigorous than the negative inotropic effect so that outflow tract obstruction is precipitated. For that reason nifedipine, a stronger peripheral dilator, is contraindicated in patients with resting obstruction.[42]

Antiarrhythmics

Disopyramide (see p 64) is used chiefly for its negative inotropic effect, but should also have antiarrhythmic potential. Strict comparisons with verapamil are lacking. When severe arrhythmias intervene or are feared, *amiodarone* is the antiarrhythmic of choice.[75] In patients with a family history of sudden death, a history of syncope or severe dyspnea, or in patients in whom malignant arrhythmias are suspected for other reasons, Holter monitoring is required to evaluate antiarrhythmic therapy.

Surgery

For refractory symptoms, septal myectomy is effective therapy,[38] although the exact indications are not widely agreed upon nor is the mechanism of benefit settled.

In older patients the entity of *hypertensive hypertrophic cardiomyopathy* has now been recognized and β-blockers or calcium antagonists are used in therapy. Digitalis is contraindicated.[90]

Dilated Cardiomyopathy

Standard therapy for idiopathic dilated cardiomyopathy consists of inotropic support, diuretics, and vasodilators, as in the case in most other forms of CHF. Arrhythmias are frequent in patients with cardiomyopathy and sudden cardiac death is a common mode of death in this condition. Antiarrhythmic therapy is, therefore, logical but data confirming therapeutic efficacy in this area are needed. For atrial fibrillation, anticoagulants are usual (see p 176).[7]

β-**Blockers remain controversial.** Several studies have provided inconsistent but provocative results on the value of treating heart failure in dilated cardiomyopathy with β-blocking agents.[36] Some patients may respond dramatically to the cautious addition of low-dose metoprolol to pre-existing therapy, especially when tachycardia is excessive; in others, there is unexpected deterioration.

An autoimmune etiology in dilated cardiomyopathy with the potential for immunosuppressive therapy is another area of controversy and intense investigation.[74]

Cardiac Transplantation

In patients with cardiomyopathy failing to respond to conservative therapy (diuretics, vasodilators) including cautious β-blockade, a severely impaired left ventricle may require cardiac transplantation. The important points are to go to a surgical center well experienced in all phases of care, and not to wait until there is deterioration in the patient's general health.

VALVULAR HEART DISEASE

General Approach

In most patients with symptomatic valvular regurgitation (= incompetence) or stenosis, valve replacement or repair is indicated. As surgical techniques and the performance of prosthetic valves have improved, so have the surgical indications become less stringent. **Now most patients with LV dysfunction are operated on even if asymptomatic.** The indications for surgery for other patients with severe but asymptomatic valvular regurgitation are less clearly established. Concomitant therapy in patients with valvular heart disease may include diuretics, digitalis and for certain nonstenotic lesions, vasodilators. Attention to arrhythmias, particularly atrial fibrillation, is essential. (For anticoagulants in valvular heart disease, see pp 176 and 177).

Aortic or Mitral Stenosis

In valvular stenosis, the basic problem is obstructive and requires surgical relief. When heart failure or hypertension are complications, vasodilator therapy is contraindicated.

In mitral stenosis, *paroxysmal atrial fibrillation* precipitating left-sided failure may require carefully titrated IV verapamil, provided that the left ventricle itself is not depressed in function (associated mitral regurgitation).

In established *atrial fibrillation*, digitalization is usually not enough to prevent an excessive ventricular rate during exercise, so that digoxin should be augmented by verapamil[39] or by β-blockade to slow the ventricular rate adequately during exercise. In patients at high risk for emboli (previous thromboembolism or atrial paroxysmal arrhythmias or advanced disease) anticoagulation is required; sulfinpyrazone may be added.[53]

In *mitral stenosis with sinus rhythm*, β-blockade by atenolol improves exercise capacity and is preferable to propranolol to lessen possible pulmonary symptoms. Digitalization in patients with mitral stenosis in sinus rhythm is used chiefly "prophylactically" to avoid a high ventricular rate during intermittent atrial fibrillation; good evidence for this indication is not yet available.

In *aortic stenosis with angina*, therapy without surgery is difficult because the angina is at least partially based on the increased demand of the hypertrophic left ventricle (there may also be accompanying coronary artery disease).

Mitral or Aortic Valve Regurgitation

Afterload reduction is much more effective in regurgitation than in stenosis (although sometimes used cautiously in mitral stenosis). In severe or symptomatic regurgitation, valve replacement is required.

Mitral Valve Prolapse

Prophylactic antibiotic (Tables 11-1 and 11-2) cover is advised for patients undergoing dental or urogenital procedures, provided that the degree of prolapse is significant (combined click and murmur).

INFECTIVE ENDOCARDITIS

The management of acute or subacute endocarditis varies with the etiology and virulence of the infecting organism and the clinical manifestations of the episode. Consideration should be given to differences in the prognosis, bacteriologic spectrum and the response to therapy between "early" and "late" prosthetic valve endocarditis and native valve endocarditis.

TABLE 11-1
AMERICAN RECOMMENDED ANTIBIOTIC REGIMENS FOR DENTAL/RESPIRATORY TRACT PROCEDURES

Standard regimen For dental procedures that cause gingival bleeding, and oral/respiratory tract surgery	Penicillin V 2.0 g orally 1 hr before, then 1.0 g 6 hr later. For patients unable to take oral medications, 2 million units of aqueous penicillin G IV or IM 30–60 min before a procedure and 1 million units 6 hr later may be substituted
Special regimens Parenteral regimen for use when maximal protection desired; eg. for patients with prosthetic valves	Ampicillin 1.0–2.0 g IM or IV *plus* gentamincin 1.5 mg/kg IM or IV ½hr before procedures, followed by 1.0 g oral penicillin V 6 hr later
Oral regimen for penicillin-allergic patients	Erythromycin 1.0 g orally 1 hr before, then 500 mg 6 hr later
Parenteral regimen for penicillin-allergic patients	Vanomycin 1.0 g IV *slowly* ovr 1 hr starting 1 hr before. No repeat dose is necessary.

From Shulman ST, Amren DP, Bisno AL, et al: Prevention of bacterial endocarditis. Circulation 70:1123A–1127A, 1984. Reproduced with permission of the American Heart Association.

Optimal therapy requires identification of the *causative organism*, and in subacute endocarditis therapy may be delayed for a short period prior to the microbiologic diagnosis. **Definitive antibiotic therapy is based upon susceptibility testing, although in culture-negative endocarditis therapy is empiric.** The duration of antibiotic therapy is still under debate but a 4–6 week period is generally accepted. Attention should be paid to conditions predisposing the patient to infective endocarditis, e.g. poor dental hygiene or genito-urinary tract pathology.

An increasing aggressive approach to *early cardiac surgery* has favorably influenced the outcome of infective endocarditis.[68] In patients with *native valve endocarditis*, the indications for surgery are: heart failure resulting from valve dysfunction, uncontrolled infection, new conduction disturbances suggestive of ring abscess formation, fungal infection, relapse after initially successful therapy, and possibly recurrent emboli.[68,94] The approach to *prosthetic valve endocarditis*, particularly within three months of the initial operation, is also aggressive with surgery indicated for any signs of prosthetic valve dysfunction or any of the indications for surgery in native valves.[67] In the face of hemodynamic decompensation, surgery should not be delayed pending completion of antibiotic therapy.

Anticoagulant Therapy

The decision to initiate or continue anticoagulant therapy in patients with infective endocarditis is often difficult. In those patients already on anticoagulants, e.g. patients with mechanical prostheses or those in whom there are other indications for anticoagulation, e.g. thrombophlebitis, anticoagulant therapy should be continued or initiated. In the event of a cerebral thromboembolic complication, the risk of anticoagulant-induced hemorrhage must be balanced against the alternate risk of recurrent embolism.

TABLE 11-2
EUROPEAN RECOMMENDATIONS: ANTIBIOTIC PROHYLAXIS OF INFECTIVE ENDOCARDITIS FOR ADULTS DURING DENTAL PROCEDURES

Not Allergic to Penicillin		Allergic to Penicillin	
Oral Amoxycillin	IV or IM Amoxycillin	Oral Erythromycin	IV Erythromycin
3 g 1 hr before	1 g just before 0.5 g 6 hr later	1.5 g 1 hr before 0.5 g 6 hr later	1 g just before

From Delaye J, Etienne J, Feruglio GA, et al: Prophylaxis of infective endocarditis for dental procedures. Eur Heart J 6:826–828, 1985. Reproduced with permission of the European Heart Journal and the Academic Press.

Antibiotic Prophylaxis

Chemoprophylaxis is indicated for patients with increased susceptibility to infective endocarditis, who must undergo surgical or other procedures that may produce a bacteremia. Cardiac conditions for which antibiotic prophylaxis is recommended are rheumatic or other acquired valvular heart disease, prosthetic heart valves or a prosthetic patch, hypertrophic obstructive cardiomyopathy, prior infective endocarditis, and congenital heart disease with the exception of uncomplicated secundum atrial septal defects and a previously repaired patent ductus arteriosus. **In uncomplicated mitral valve prolapse with only a click, antibiotic prophylaxis is debatable; when there is a murmur and mitral regurgitation, prophylaxis is definitely desirable.** Table 11-1 lists the recommendations of the American Heart Association for antibiotic prophylaxis, and Table 11-2 lists current European practice.

COR PULMONALE

Therapy of right heart failure is similar to that of left heart failure, except that digitalis appears to be less effective because of a combination of hypoxemia, electrolyte disturbances, and enhanced adrenergic discharge. Thus when atrial fibrillation develops, cautious use of verapamil may both benefit the ventricular rate in atrial fibrillation, may cause bronchodilation, and may help relieve pulmonary artery pressure. However, there appear to be no formal trials about the use of verapamil in such conditions.

In general, β-blockers should be avoided because of the risk of bronchospasm. Bronchodilators should be β_2-selective such as salbutamol (albuterol in the USA), which have relatively little effect on the heart rate, while causing peripheral vasodilation and thereby unloading the left side which may also be compromised (see p 143).

When right ventricular failure is accompanied by LV failure, and the latter is not caused by hypoxemia, then digitalis is again added to diuretic therapy.

PULMONARY HYPERTENSION

Primary pulmonary hypertension includes a variety of histological appearances and probably pathogenic mechanisms, while excluding pulmonary hypertension secondary to chronic pulmonary disease. Diffuse pulmonary thromboembolism or pulmonary arteriolar thrombosis in situ occur in some patients. Unless lung biopsy is performed, the pathogenesis cannot be established and **long-term anticoagulants are frequently used** on the assumption that there is thromboembolism.

Calcium antagonists are increasingly being tried, with nifedipine one of the best documented, but the results are unpredictable and generally disappointing. Pulmonary vasodilators should only be given under stringent monitoring.

PERIPHERAL VASCULAR DISEASE

Here the basic problem is vascular atheroma, added to which are (1) variable degrees of arterial spasm and (2) variable severities of arterial thrombosis and platelet aggregation and embolization. Thus far the only effective attack on atheroma has been by surgery, when appropriate. Correction of "coronary risk factors" appears to play little or no role, except for the role of smoking in some types of active peripheral vascular disease (previously called Burger's disease). **In general, β-blockers are said to be contraindicated in the presence of active peripheral vascular disease although the evidence is not firm.**[56]

Calcium antagonists are preferred therapy for patients with peripheral vascular disease plus angina and hypertension; these agents are now being evaluated for their possible role in improvement of arterial blood flow. *Flunarizine* (not in the USA or UK) (see p 47), with little or no central cardiac effects, may be tried. Experimentally, all calcium antagonists including verapamil, nifedipine, and diltiazem can stop the progression of atheroma in rats, presumably by inhibition of calcium deposits in the atheroma; however, huge doses are required and the relevance to man is as yet unknown.

Pentoxifylline (Trental®) is an agent said to protect against red cell deformability, which may occur as the erythrocytes are "squeezed" through the narrowed arterioles. It improves claudication distance and is **licensed for use in intermittent claudication**[82] in the USA (600–1200 mg daily in three divided doses with meals; side-effect nausea).

Platelet active agents and prostaglandin inhibitors have all been tried; only recently has objective **angiographic data favoring aspirin** (330 mg daily) **plus dipyridamole** (75 mg 3× daily) become available.[55] The serotonin antagonist, *ketanserin*, has proved to be of marginal benefit.[44]

In such chronic diseases where conventional therapy has relatively little to offer, various "borderline" therapies are frequently used, including *vitamin E*. Again, proof of efficacy is lacking.

In summary, medical therapy is generally not regarded as giving substantial benefit in most patients with peripheral vascular disease, unless there is associated vascular spasm when calcium antagonists and avoidance of β-blockers are logical therapy. Smoking and hypertension must be controlled.[55] New approaches center on agents regulating red cell shape and the use of aspirin-dipyridamole.

RAYNAUD'S PHENOMENON

Once a secondary cause has been excluded (for example vasculitis, scleroderma, or lupus erythematosus), then **calcium channel antagonists** (nifedipine, verapamil, or diltiazem) are logical. Nifedipine is considerably more effective than prazosin.[65] β-Blockers are traditionally contraindicated in Raynaud's phenomenon, but one recent trial showed that low-dose propranolol or metoprolol did not exaggerate primary Raynaud's phenomenon.[46]

HYPERTENSION

The therapy of hypertension is usually simple, since many patients have minimally or moderately elevated pressures that usually respond adequately to one or two drugs (Table 11-3). More effective, less bothersome, and longer-acting agents have become available so that for most hypertensives one or two pills every morning work quite well. Asymptomatic patients, however, often will not stay on therapy, particularly if it makes them feel weak, sleepy, or impotent. A small proportion have resistant hypertension, which may only respond to multiple therapies.

The Decision to Treat

Before any drug is begun, persistence of the patient's hypertension should be ascertained by multiple measurements over at least a few weeks, preferably at home and at work, unless the pressure is so high (e.g. >180/110 mmHg) as to mandate immediate therapy. **Nondrug therapies, particularly weight reduction for the obese and moderate dietary sodium restriction such as 75 to 100 mmole/day or a 2 g sodium diet, should be used before drugs in those with minimal elevations, and with drugs in those with higher levels. Weight reduction also helps to prevent LV hypertrophy.**[73a]

A careful general work-up is required before therapy is started. The presence of prominent risk factors for ischemic heart disease or renal impairment argues for tighter control of the blood pressure.

In the USA, a more aggressive approach to the active drug therapy of even minimally elevated pressures, such as diastolics in the 90–100 mmHg range, has become "accepted medical practice". In most of the rest of the world, drug therapy is usually reserved for those with diastolics over 100 mmHg. Voices for a less aggressive approach are being heard in the USA[1,8,12] and the current therapeutic enthusiasm may cool. The giant British trial, recently published in detail,[76] gave only **very modest benefit for therapy in mild to moderate hypertension;** one stroke was prevented by treating 850 patients for one year. **Likewise the aim of therapy should not be over-idealistic.** Even diastolics of 105 mmHg during treatment were associated with only a margin-

TABLE 11-3
SPECIFICS ABOUT ORALLY EFFECTIVE ANTIHYPERTENSIVE DRUGS

Drug	Trade name® (in USA)	Total Dosage (mg/day)	Doses/Day
Diuretics (see Table 6-3)			
Adrenergic inhibitors			
Rauwolfia derivatives			
Reserpine	Serpasil	0.05–0.25	1
Whole root	Raudixin	50 100	1
Guanethidine	Ismelin	10–150 or more	1
Guanadrel	Hylorel	10–75	2
Methyldopa	Aldomet	500–3000	2
Clonidine	Catapres	0.5–1.5	1–2
Guanabenz	Wytensin	8–64	2
Prazosin	Minipress	2.0–20.0	2
β-Blockers			
Acebutolol	Sectral	400–800	1
Atenolol	Tenormin	50–100	1
Labetalol	Normodyne, Trandate	200–800	2
Metoprolol	Lopressor	100–450	2
Nadolol	Corgard	40–320	1
Pindolol	Visken	10–60	2
Propranolol	Inderal	80–480	2
Timolol	Blocadren	20–60	2
Vasodilators			
Hydralazine	Apresoline	50–400	2
Minoxidil	Loniten	5–60	1
ACE inhibitors			
Captopril	Capoten	25–150	3
Calcium antagonists			
Nifedipine	Procardia, Adalat	20–120	2
Verapamil	Isoptin, Calan	360–480	2–3

ally higher incidence of stroke or of cardiac events than lower values[59] and the effort involved and discomfort to the patient in achieving a lower diastolic might not be worth it. The cost, both in financial terms and in symptoms, needs to be balanced against the expected benefits. Even with agents such as the ACE inhibitors (Chapter 8) which preserve the quality of life, evaluation of the cost-benefit ratio is not easy and requires specific evaluation for each patient.

Choice for Initial Drug

Until recently a *diuretic* has been the first drug advocated by authorities and chosen by most practitioners,[3,11,14,29,35] but β-blockers have been increasingly used and other suitable choices are now available for initial therapy. If the first drug is not enough, one of another class, particularly a diuretic if that was not the initial choice, is then added and, for about 10 percent of patients, a third is needed. The diuretic first "step-care" approach has been used in most large therapeutic trials in the USA. With it, the vascular complications more directly related to the height of the blood pressure per se (strokes, CHF, renal damage) have been reduced, but the frequency of the most common cause of disease and death among hypertensives, coronary artery disease, has not been significantly altered, except in the diuretic-based trial in elderly hypertensives wherein a potassium-sparing agent was also used.[37] The recently completed British MRC trial[76] compared a diuretic (bendrofluazide) to a β-blocker (propranolol). Neither had a significant impact on coronary disease except for propranolol among men who did not smoke.

Awareness of the biochemical derangements often induced by chronic diuretic therapy, including an average 0.6 mmol/L fall of serum potassium, a rise in triglycerides and cholesterol (Table 10-2), and a worsening of glucose tolerance, all of which could add risks for coronary disease, has raised **concern over the appropriateness of a diuretic as the routine choice as initial therapy.**[66] Therefore, the alternative initial approach of an adrenergic inhibitor, particularly a β-blocker, has been advocated.[5,15] Laragh[16] has long argued for the wisdom of starting with a β-blocker, but his emphasis on renin-profiling has probably held back acceptance of his argument.

Younger hypertensives especially have often been started on a *β-blocker*. Many clinicians assume, without evidence, that the partial protection β-blockers provide against recurrent heart attacks may serve to prevent initial coronary events, but this was shown neither in the British Medical Research Council (MRC) trial with propranolol[76] nor in the International Prospective Primary Prevention Study in Hypertension (IPPPSH)[59] with oxprenolol. In both trials, the β-blocker protected only nonsmoking men from coronary disease. **In addition to concern about the overt side-effects of β-blockers (in particular their reduction of exercise ability), their covert action to raise an already high peripheral resistance** (which is responsible for their most common side-effect, cold extremities; exceptions: acebutolol, pindolol) **and their tendency to raise serum triglycerides and lower HDL-cholesterol levels** (Table 10-2) **have prompted advocacy of other agents as initial therapy** (Table 11-4). **As a result, other agents such as α-blockers including prazosin, ACE inhibitors, and calcium antagonists are being used earlier and earlier.**

Factors in the Choice of Drug

A moderate dose of any of these drugs will lower the blood pressure to about the same degree in most patients.[3] Blacks may be more responsive to

TABLE 11-4
PERSPECTIVES ON ORALLY EFFECTIVE ANTIHYPERTENSIVE AGENTS

Advantages	Disadvantages

Thiazides and Other Diuretics
Once a day (usually)
  Potentiate effects of other agents
  Prevent reactive fluid retention
	Effectiveness reduced by heavy sodium intake or renal insufficiency (furosemide and metolazone effective)
	Hypokalemia-arrhythmias
	Hypercholesterolemia—accelerate atherosclerosis
	Abnormal glucose tolerance
	Hyperuricemia—gout

Potassium-sparing agents Given in combination with diuretic Few overt side-effects	Potential for hyperkalemia (avoid use with potassium supplements, particularly in presence of renal insufficiency; avoid co-therapy with captopril or enalapril)

Adrenergic inhibitors
Reserpine
  Ultralong NE depletion
  Inexpensive
  Minimal titration needed
	Slow onset of action
	Common side-effects: sedation, nasal stuiffiness
	Rare: depression, increased gastric acidity

Guanethidine
  Steep dose-response curve
  Once a day
  No central effects
	Frequent orthostatic hypotension
	Occasional diarrhea, retrograde ejaculation
	Not with MAO inhibitors

Guanadrel No central nervous effects	Side-effects: Similar but less severe than guanethidine. Not with MAO inhibitors

Methyldopa
  Twice a day
  Maintains renal blood flow
  Proven long-term safety
	Common side effects: sedation, dry mouth
	Rare: autoimmune reactions

Clonidine Available in patch for once-a-week use	Common side-effects: sedation, dry mouth Rare: rebound of blood pressure

Guanabenz
  Twice a day
  May cause less reactive fluid retention
	Side effects: sedation, dry mouth

α-Blockers: Prazosin
  Lack of sedation, dry mouth
  Decrease in peripheral resistance
  No fall in cardiac output
  No alterations of plasma lipids
	First-dose hypotension (minimized by small doses and deletion of diuretics)
	Lassitude

TABLE 11-4 *(Continued)*
PERSPECTIVES ON ORALLY EFFECTIVE ANTIHYPERTENSIVE AGENTS

Advantages	Disadvantages
β-Blockers	
Once a day: acebutolol, atenolol, nadolol, others in high doses	Side efffects (less with more cardioselective or high intrinsic sympathomimetic activity)
Lack of sedation, dry mouth	
Relief from anxiety-related symptoms	
Less reactive volume retention	Serious: bronchospasm, prollongation of insulin-induced hypoglycemia, heart failure
Possible protection from coronary disease (shown only for nonsmoking men)	
Antianginal and antiarrhythmic	Others: cold extremities, reduced exercise tolerance, fatigue
	Unknown consequences:
	Increased triglycerides
	Decreased HDL-cholesterol
	Increased peripheral resistance
	Less effect in elderly and blacks (when used alone)
Direct vasodilators	
Hydralzine	
Increased in cardiac output and renal blood flow	Reflex sympathetic tachycardia and increased cardiac output—prevent by adrenergic inhibitor
	Lupus-like reaction (rare below 200 mg/day)
Minoxidil	
Once a day	Reactive fluid retention
Greater potency	Reflex sympathetic stimulation (as with hydralazine)
Effective in patients with renal insufficiency	Hirsutism in 80 percent
ACE inhibitors	
Captopril	
No sedation; good quality of life	Side-effects: Hypotension, rash, loss of taste; renal
May be particularly effective in high-renin patients	Rare: proteinuria, leukopenia
Enalapril	
Similar effects, longer acting	Side-effect: Hypotension; renal
Calcium antagonists	
Nifedipine	
Powerful, rapid effect	Occasional flushing, pedal edema, headaches
Easy combination with β-blockers	
No lupus or hirsitusm	
Verapamil	
Few serious side-effects	Occasional negative inotropic interaction with β-blockade; AV block; constipation
Diltiazem	
Few side-effects	Bradycardia in elderly patients; AV block

MAO inhibitors = monoamine oxidase inhibitors such as isocarboxazid (Marplan®), phenelzine (Nardil®) and tranylcypromine (Parnate®); NE = norepinephrine

diuretics or to combined α-β-blockers (see p 14), and older patients less responsive to β-blockers and more responsive to calcium antagonists. Patients with very high renin levels may do better with renin inhibition by either a β-blocker or an ACE inhibitor.

Too often the choice of drug is based upon habit (e.g. the continued widespread use of methyldopa) or the intensity of promotional advertisement (e.g. the minimal use of low-dose reserpine, which has no commercial advocate). New drugs promise therapeutic breakthroughs, such as captopril or enalapril with few symptomatic side-effects and a new mechanism of action.[93] At present such agents and calcium antagonists seem to be gaining the spotlight.

Diuretics

A single morning dose of 25 mg of hydrochlorothiazide or its equivalent will provide a 10 mmHg fall in the blood pressure of most uncomplicated hypertensives, requiring several weeks to act. Diuretics, preferred initial treatment in the elderly, obese, or in blacks, have been shown to reduce stroke than coronary events.[76] Lower doses (12.5 mg hydrochlorothiazide) are probably equally effective especially when combined with β-blockade.[19] Higher doses lead to no greater fall in blood pressure and may enhance side-effects. High doses of thiazide are contained in many combination agents (Table 6-5). Longer acting diuretics (e.g. chlorthalidone) may provide slightly more antihypertensive effect but are more likely to cause more hypokalemia and nocturia. The shorter acting loop diuretics, furosemide or bumetanide, usually reserved for those with edema or renal insufficiency are also effective antihypertensives in other patients. Metolazone may provide as much diuretic potency on a once-a-day basis.

Potassium-sparing agents may add a few cents to the cost but save a good deal more by the prevention of diuretic-induced hypokalemia. All should be combined with another diuretic. The combinations of dyrenium (Dyazide®, Maxzide®) or amiloride (Moduretic®) are usually preferable to that of spironolactone (Aldactazide®) because the latter decreases testosterone synthesis. The dose of thiazide in one tablet of Dyazide® is half that of standard Moduretic®, which is preferable. In Europe, a "mini-Moduretic®" with half the standard thiazide dose is now marketed to overcome this objection.

Adrenergic Inhibitors

Of the centrally-acting agents, reserpine is easiest to use in a low dose of 0.05 mg/day that will provide almost all of its antihypertensive action with fewer side-effects than higher doses.[34] *Methyldopa*, still widely used despite adverse central symptoms and potentially serious hepatic and blood side-effects, acts like clonidine on central α_2-receptors without however (for unknown reasons) slowing the heart rate.[87] *Clonidine* and *guanabenz* provide all of the benefits of methyldopa with none of the rare but serious autoimmune reactions (as with methyldopa, sedation is frequent). A *transdermal form of clonidine* (Catapres-TTS®) provides once a week therapy likely minimizing the risks of clonidine-withdrawal. Guanabenz is similar to clonidine but may cause less fluid retention and reduces serum cholesterol by 5–10 percent. *Guanethidine* should be reserved for very rare patients resistant to all else. *Guandrel* is similar to guanethidine, but its duration of action is shorter, so fewer side-effects have been noted.

Of the α_1-*receptor blockers*, only *prazosin* (see p 140) is available in the USA, but others such as *indoramin* (Baratol®; Wydora®) are in use elsewhere (see p 141). Their advantages usually include freedom from the central nervous depression of centrally-acting drugs, the lipid perturbations of β-blockers, and a more appropriate physiologic action to lower peripheral resistance. Some patients develop troublesome side-effects: drowsiness, postural hypotension and occasional retrograde ejaculation. Tolerance, likely related to fluid retention, may develop during chronic therapy with prazosin, requiring increased doses.[69] Phenoxybenzamine and phentolamine are combined α_1 and α_2-blockers used only for pheochromocytoma.

A number of β-*blockers* are now available, 7 in the USA, and as many as 15 elsewhere (Chapter 1, Table 1-2). Of these, atenolol, acebutolol, and nadolol come closest to the ideal pharmacological profile (Fig. 1-7). Acebutolol, pindolol and oxprenolol with ISA may be better for those susceptible to symptomatic bradycardia or cold extremities or in the elderly.

Whenever the blood pressure is lowered by a nondiuretic drug (especially a vasodilator, including α-blockers), the hypertensive kidney may react by retaining more sodium.[26] The routine use of a diet moderately restricted in sodium may mitigate the volume retention, but if the drugs do not work or lose their effect, a diuretic may need to be added. ACE inhibitors and nifedipine, although vasodilators, appear to be exceptions to this rule because of their intrinsic diuretic properties.

Vasodilators

Hydralazine (see p 138) has been widely used as the third drug, its effectiveness enhanced and side-effects removed by concomitant use of a diuretic and an adrenergic inhibitor. Calcium antagonists will probably become main-stays of therapy for hypertension, because they avoid the risk of hydralazine lupus and seldom cause symptomatic tachycardia.[9] *Nifedipine* is the most effective antihypertensive of those now in use for severe hypertension. Other dihydropyridines effective on a once-a-day basis, such as *nitrendipine*, will soon be available. A mild diuretic effect of the dihydropyridines contributes to the long-term benefit. *Verapamil* and *diltiazem* are increasingly chosen as first-line antihypertensive agents, especially if angina is associated. *Minoxidil* is a potent vasodilator but causes profuse hirsutism so it is usually limited to men with severe refractory hypertension and renal insufficiency.

ACE inhibitors

Captopril is the most widely used. One or more without a sulfhydryl group such as *enalapril*, hopefully, will cause fewer side-effects (neutropenia, skin rashes, taste disturbances). These agents are on occasion almost miraculous especially in high-renin states, but for most patients they provide no better blood pressure control than other agents. A major advantage is the absence of any central nervous system side-effects so that **the patients usually feel very well,** especially in comparison with agents such as methyldopa or propranolol (see p 156). As many as half of normal to high-renin patients seem to respond particularly well to ACE inhibitor monotherapy, perhaps because the drug corrects an underlying defect in tissue angiotensin responsiveness.[93]

Step Care

When all of these factors are considered, an α_1 or β-blocker is now **increasingly chosen over a diuretic for initial therapy except in black, obese, or elderly patients where diuretic therapy still seems best.** ACE inhibitors or calcium antagonists will probably become first-line agents of choice, particularly when once-a-day formulations become available, because they basically leave the central nervous and autonomic nervous system responses unaltered, act specifically on peripheral resistance, and have few or no significant metabolic side-effects (see p 157).

Acute Severe Hypertension

For urgent therapy of acute severe hypertension (Table 11-5) the choice used to fall on an IV agent, but sublingual nifedipine is now almost standard therapy. It consistently reduces systolic and diastolic pressures by about 20 percent within 20–30 minutes.[4] Such a rapid reduction of hypertension may be safe even in the presence of cerebral symptoms;[40,57] **nevertheless it is prudent to consider whether rapid pressure reduction is really desirable in the presence of cerebral symptoms or papilledema or symptoms of myocardial ischemia.** Case reports indicating the precipitation of cerebral infarction by acute hypotensive therapy have consistently included therapies that cause excess hypotension,[47,73] whereas nifedipine has very rarely caused "overshoot" in the treatment of acute severe hypertension.[61] Nifedipine is especially useful in the therapy of hypertensive heart failure with pulmonary edema.

Parenteral agents such as nitroprusside are still extensively used. These all require careful monitoring to avoid overshoot. Nitroprusside reduces preload and afterload and has the risk of rebound hypertension. Diazoxide is best given by infusion and not as a bolus IV dose to avoid cerebral ischemia. Hydralazine and dihydralazine may cause tachycardia and are best avoided in angina unless there is concomitant therapy with a β-blocker. Labetalol does not cause tachycardia and gives a smooth dose-related fall in blood pressure; the side-effects of β-blockade such as heart failure and bronchospasm may be countered by the added α-blockade and ISA of labetalol. There is no IV preparation of prazosin, which does however have a rapid onset of action when given orally. Starting with an oral β-blocker seems to work well in some patients with acute severe hypertension even in the presence of papilledema.[61] At present, when **the ideal rate of reduction of hypertension requiring urgent therapy is not known,** the simplicity of sublingual nifedipine (10 mg) is increasingly seen as seemingly safe therapy, provided that there is no clinical evi-

TABLE 11-5

AGENTS FOR USE IN HYPERTENSIVE EMERGENCIES (CAUTION: SEE TEXT FOR RESERVATIONS)

Agent	Usual Dose	Side-Effects	Comments
Nifedipine	10–20 mg sublingually or orally	Few unless excess hypotension Risk of cerebral ischemia	Simple therapy, usually effective; needs further evaluation in presence of papilledema and hypertensive encephalopathy
Captopril	25 mg chewed*	Risk of renal failure	Excluded renal artery stenosis; not well tested
Nitroprusside	Infusion of 40–75 μg/min	Hypotension, must monitor constantly	Especially useful if pulmonary edema or encephalopathy
Diazoxide	100–150 mg IV for 5 min to 300 mg Infusion: 5 mg/kg at 15 mg/min	Difficult to control hypotensive effect; risk of cerebral ischemia	Better than single bolus
Hydralazine	5–10 mg IV every 4–6 hr	Less danger of hypotension than diazoxide Tachycardia, contraindicted in angina, ischemic strokes	Probably safer as infusion Tachycardia can be countered by propranolol 1–2 mg IV
Dihydralazine	6.25–12.5 mg IV slowly or infuse IV as 0.1 mg/min to total of 25 mg	As above, prefer infusion	As above
Labetalol	Infuse at 2 mg/min to total of 1–2 mg/kg	May worsen cardiac failure	Avoids tachycardia. Smooth and rapid dose-related fall in blood pressure
Reserpine	1 mg IM	Drowsiness, hypotension	Delayed effect (1–4 hr)

*See reference 92.

dence of cerebral or myocardial ischemia or clinically evident renal failure. When such complications are present, careful slow monitored reduction of blood pressure still seems best.

Systolic Hypertension

In systolic hypertension, the present trend is to reduce values to below 160 mmHg if possible. Younger patients may have an increased sympathetic tone that should yield to β-blockade. Older patients are likely to have a decreased vessel wall compliance, so for them one might choose a drug acting on the arteriolar wall, such as a calcium antagonist.[48] Decreased cerebral perfusion in elderly patients is a potential serious hazard so that, if nifedipine is chosen, an initial dose of 5 mg nifedipine may be better than 10 mg.[62] Where 5 mg capsules are not available (as in the USA), the contents of a 10 mg capsule may be extracted by a syringe and half given intraorally. Diuretics such as chlorthalidone are also effective in systolic hypertension in the elderly[81] and, presumably, are also effective with other agents such as β-blockers. With chlorthalidone the long action may cause inconvenient nocturia.

Hypertension in the Elderly

What constitutes hypertension in the elderly and indeed what constitutes an elderly population are moot questions. One recent European trial[37] treated patients over 60 with pressures above 160/95 mmHg initially by a diuretic plus potassium-sparer (Dyazide®) and then by added *methyldopa* (Aldomet®). Results were impressive with a reduction of stroke and cardiac mortality, nonetheless overall mortality was not affected. That trial showed that **elderly patients may well require therapy and perhaps should be regarded as a "high risk group."** Other agents advocated in the elderly are calcium antagonists, β-blockers (supposedly less effective in the elderly but several trials have shown benefit) and ACE inhibitors. In *severe hypertension* in the elderly, sublingual nifedipine seems as safe as in younger subjects,[48] but we recommend that therapy be started in such patients with a 5 mg dose (see preceding section). With nifedipine, as with any other effective hypotensive therapy, the risk of precipitating cerebral ischemia must be carefully evaluated despite the reported cerebral vasodilating effect of nifedipine.

REFERENCES

References from previous editions

For details see previous edition of Opie et al, Drugs for the Heart, American Edition. Orlando, FL, Grune & Stratton, 1984, pp 153–191.

1. Alderman MH, Madhaven S: Hypertension 3:192–197, 1981
2. β-Blocker Heart Attack Study Group: JAMA 246:2073–2074, 1981
3. Berglund G, Andersson O: Lancet i:744–747, 1981
4. Conen D, Bertel O, Dubach UC: J Cardiovasc Pharmacol 4:S378–S382, 1982
5. Dollery CT: Clin Sci 61 (suppl):413–420, 1981
6. Fuster V, Chesebro JH: Mayo Clin Proc 56:265–273, 1981
7. Fuster V, Gersh BJ, Giuliani ER, et al: Am J Cardiol 47:525–531, 1981
8. Freis ED: Sounding board: New Engl J Med 307:306–309, 1982
9. Gould BA, Hornung RS, Mann S, et al: J Cardiovasc Pharmacol 4 (suppl):369–373, 1982
10. Hjalmarson A, Hurlitz J, Malik I, et al: Lancet ii:823–827, 1981
11. The Joint National Committee on Detection, Evaluation and Treatment of High Blood Pressure: Arch Intern Med 140:1280–1286, 1980
12. Kaplan NM: Am Heart J 101:867–870, 1981
13. Kaplan NM: Am J Cardiol 51:621–627, 1983
14. Lancet Editorial: Lancet i:763, 1981
15. Lancet Editorial: Lancet ii:1316–1317, 1982
16. Laragh JH: Am J Med 55:261–274, 1973
17. Lee G, Low RI, Amsterdam EA, et al: Clin Pharmacol Ther 29:576–581, 1981
18. Lubbe WF, Podzuweit T, Daries PS, et al: J Clin Invest 61:1260–1269, 1978
19. MacGregor GA, Banks RA, Markandu ND, et al: Br Med J 286:1535–1538, 1983
20. Norwegian Multicenter Study Group: New Engl J Med 304:801–807, 1981

21. Pantridge JF, Adgey AJJ, Geddes JS, et al: In Pantridge JF, Adgey AJJ, Geddes JS, et al (eds): The Acute Coronary Attack. New York, Grune and Stratton, 1975, pp 42–78
22. Robertson RM, Wood AJJ, Vaughn WK, et al: Circulation 65:281–285, 1982
23. Rogers WJ, Segall PH, McDaniel HG, et al: Am J Cardiol 43:801–809, 1979
24. Rossi PRF, Yusuf S, Ramsdale D, et al: Br Med J 286:506–510, 1983
25. Ruberman W, Weinblatt E, Goldberg JD, et al: Circulation 64:297–305, 1981
26. Safar ME, Weiss YA, Corvol PL, et al: Clin Sci Mol Med 48 (suppl):93–95, 1975
27. Scheinman MM, Thorburn D, Abbott JA: Circulation 52:627–633, 1975
28. Schulze RA Jr, Strauss HW, Pitt B: Am J Med 62:192–199, 1977
29. Stumpe KO, Overlack A: Br J Clin Pharmacol 7 (suppl 2):189–197, 1979
30. Taylor SH, Silke B, Ebbutt A, et al: New Engl J Med 307:1293–1301, 1982
31. Timmis AD, Rothman MT, Henderson MA, et al: Br Med J 280:980–982, 1980
32. Todres D: Am Heart J 81:566–570, 1971
33. Velebit V, Podrid P, Lown B, et al: Circulation 65:886–894, 1982
34. Veterans Administration Participating Medical Centers: JAMA 248:2471–2477, 1982
35. Whitworth JA, Kincaid-Smith P: Drugs 23:394–402, 1982

New References

36. Alderman J, Grossman W: Are β-adrenergic blocking drugs useful in the treatment of dilated cardiomyopathy Circulation 71:854–857, 1985
37. Amery A, Birkenhager W, Brixko P, et al: Mortality and morbidity results from the European Working Party on high blood pressure in the elderly trial. Lancet ii:1349–1354, 1985
38. Beahrs MM, Seward JB, Giuliani ER, et al: Hypertrophic obstructive cardiomyopathy: 10 to 21 year follow-up after partial septal myectomy. Am J Cardiol 51:1160–1166, 1983
39. Beasley R, Smith DA, McHaffie DJ: Excess heart rates at different serum digoxin concentrations in patients with atrial fibrillation. Br Med J 290:9–11, 1985
40. Bertel O, Conen D, Radu EW: Nifedipine in hypertensive emergencies. Br Med J 1:19–21, 1983
41. Betriu A, Pomar JL, Bourassa MG, et al: Influence of partial sympathetic denervation on the results of myocardial revascularization in variant angina. Am J Cardiol 51:661–667, 1983
42. Betocchi S, Cannon RO, Watson RM, et al: Effect of sublingual nifedipine on hemodynamics and systolic and diastolic function in patients with hypertrophic cardiomyopathy. Circulation 72:1001–1007, 1985
43. Bonow RO, Dilsiziam V, Rosing DR, et al: Verapamil-induced improvement in left ventricular diastolic filling and increased exercise tolerance in patients with hypertrophic cardiomyopathy: Short and long-term effects. Circulation 72:853–864, 1985
44. Bounameaux H, Holditch T, Hellemans H, et al: Placebo-controlled, double-blind, two centre trial of ketanserin in intermittent claudication. Lancet ii:1268–1271, 1985
45. Bresnahan DR, Davis JL, Holmes DR, et al: Angiographic occurrence and clinical correlates of intraluminal coronary artery thrombus: Role of unstable angina. J Am Coll Cardiol 6:285–289, 1985
45a. Buffington CW: Hemodynamic determinants of ischemic myocardial dysfunction in the presence of coronary stenosis in dogs. Anesthesiology 63:651–662, 1985
45b. Chadda K, Goldstein S, Byington R, et al: Effect of propranolol after acute myocardial infarction in patients with congestive heart failure. Circulation 73:503–510, 1986
46. Coffman JD, Rasmussen HM: Effects of β-adrenoceptor-blocking drugs in patients with Raynaud's phenomenon. Circulation 72:466–470, 1985
47. Cove DH, Seddon M, Fletcher RF: Blindness after treatment for malignant hypertension. Br Med J 2:245–246, 1979
47a. Croft CH, Rude RE, Gustafson N, et al: Abrupt withdrawal of β-blockade therapy in patients with myocardial infarction: Effects on infarct size, left ventricular function, and hospital course. Circulation 73:1281–1290, 1986
48. Dais K, Jones J, Gooray D, et al: Treatment of hypertensive emergencies in geriatric patients with sublingual nifedipine. Circulation 72 (suppl III):III-50, 1985
49. Garson A Jr, Bink-Boelkens M, Hesslein PS, et al: Atrial flutter in the young: A collaborative study of 380 cases. J Am Coll Cardiol 6:871–878, 1985
50. Gersh BJ, Kronmal RA, Schaff HV, et al: Comparison of coronary artery bypass surgery and medical therapy in patients aged 65 years of age or older. New Engl J Med 71:217–224, 1985
51. Gersh BJ, McLaran CJ, Sugrue DD, et al: Electrophysiologic and clinical determinants of arrhythmia recurrence in survivors of out-of-hospital cardiac arrest. Circulation 72 (suppl III):III-160, 1985
52. Gilbert EM, Askins JC, Lutz JR, et al: Adverse outcome during long-term milrinone for advanced heart failure: A controlled pilot study. Circulation 72 (suppl III):III-201, 1985
53. Goodnight SH: Antiplatelet therapy for mitral stenosis Circulation 62:466–468, 1980

54. Hamilton A, Naccarelli GV, Gray EL, et al: Congestive heart failure with normal systolic function. Am J Cardiol 54:778–782, 1984

55. Hess H, Mietaschik A, Deichsel G: Drug-induced inhibition of platelet function delays progression of peripheral occlusive arterial disease. Lancet i:415–419, 1985

56. Hiatt WR, Stoll S, Nies AS: Effect of β-adrenergic blockers on the peripheral circulation in patients with peripheral vascular disease. Circulation 72:1226–1231, 1985

57. Huysmans FThM, Sluiter HE, Thien ThA, et al: Acute treatment of hypertensive crisis with nifedipine. Br J Clin Pharmacol 16:725–727, 1983

58. IMPACT Research Group: International mexiletine and placebo antiarrhythmic coronary trial. I. Report on arrhythmia and other findings. J Am Coll Cardiol 4:1148–1163, 1984

59. International Prospective Primary Prevention Study in Hypertension (IPPPSH): Cardiovascular risk and risk factors in a randomized trial of treatment based on the beta-blocker oxprenolol. J Hypertens 3:379–392, 1985

60. ISIS-1 Group: Randomized trial of intravenous atenolol among 16027 cases of suspected acute myocardial infarction. Lancet ii:57–65, 1986

61. Isles CG, Johnson AOC, Milne FJ: Slow release nifedipine and atenolol as initial treatment in blacks with malignant hypertension. Br J Clin Pharmacol, in press, 1986

62. Ito H, Arakawa M, Shibasaki T, et al: Acute antihypertensive effect of nifedipine by sublingual route in cases with clinically severe systolic hypertension. Drug Res 34:630–636, 1984

63. Julian DG: The practical implications of the coronary artery surgery trials. Br Heart J 54:343–350, 1985

64. Julian D, Pentecost BL, Simpson JM, et al: Intravenous (IV) hyaluronidase in suspected acute myocardial infarction (MI). Circulation 72 (suppl III):III-222, 1985

65. Kahan A, Foult JM, Weber S: Nifedipine and α_1-adrenergic blockade in Raynaud's phenomenon. Eur Heart J 6:702–705, 1985

66. Kaplan NM: Treatment of hypertension. In Clinical Hypertension, 4th edition. Baltimore, Williams and Wilkins, 1986, pp 180–272

67. Karchmer AW, Swartz MN: Infective endocarditis in patients with prosthetic heart valves, in Kaplan EL, Taranta AV (eds): Infective Endocarditis. American Heart Association Monograph Number 52, 1977

68. Karchmer AW, Stinson EB: The role of surgery in infective endocarditis, in Remmington JS, Swartz MN (eds): Current Clinical Topics in Infectious Diseases. New York, McGraw Hill Book Company, 1980

69. Khatri IM, Levinson P, Notargiacomo A, et al: Initial and long-term effects of prazosin on sympathetic vasopressor responses in essential hypertension. Am J Cardiol 55:1015–1018, 1985

69a. Kjekshus JK: Importance of heart rate in determining β-blocker efficacy in acute myocardial infarction intervention trials. Am J Cardiol 57:43F–49F, 1986

70. Konstam A, Benotti JR, Biddle T, et al: Multicenter comparison of milrinone and dobutamine in congestive heart failure. Circulation 72 (suppl III):III-201, 1985

71. Koster RW, Dunning AJ: Intramuscular lidocaine for prevention of lethal arrhythmias in the prehospitalization phase of acute myocardial infarction. New Engl J Med 313:1105–1110, 1985

72. Kupper W, Erelemeier HH, Hamm CW: Failure of long-term dobutamine infusion to maintain hemodynamic improvement in patients with severe heart failure. Circulation 72 (suppl III):III-405, 1985

73. Ledingham JCG: Management of hypertensive crises. Hypertension 5 (suppl 3):114–119, 1983

73a. MacMahon SW, Wilcken DEL, MacDonald GJ: The effect of weight reduction on left ventricular mass. A randomized controlled trial in young, overweight hypertensive patients. New Engl J Med 314:334–339, 1986

74. Mason JW, Billingham ME, Ricci DR: Treatment of acute inflammatory myocarditis assisted by endomyocardial biopsy. Am J Cardiol 45:1037–1044, 1980

75. McKenna WJ, Harris L, Rowland E, et al: Amiodarone for long-term management of patients with hypertrophic cardiomyopathy. Am J Cardiol 54:802–810, 1984

76. Medical Research Council Working Party: MRC trial of treatment of mild hypertension: Principal results. Br Med J 291:97–104, 1985

77. MIAMI Trial Research Group: Metoprolol in acute myocardial infarction. Eur Heart J 6:199–226, 1985

78. Mirowski M: The automatic implantable cardioverter-defibrillator: An overview. J Am Coll Cardiol 6:461–466, 1985

79. Muller JE, Turi ZG, Pearle DL, et al: Nifedipine and conventional therapy for unstable angina pectoris: A randomized, double-blind comparison. Circulation 69:728–739, 1984

80. Passamani E, Davis KB, Gillespie MJ, et al: A randomized trial of coronary artery bypass surgery, survival in patients with low ejection fraction. New Engl J Med 69:1665–1671, 1985

81. Perry HM, Hulley SB, Furberg CD, et al: Systolic hypertension in the elderly program (SHEP): Morbidity and mortality. Circulation 72 (suppl III):III-50, 1985

82. Porter JM, Cutler BS, Lee BY, et al: Pentoxifylline efficacy in the treatment of intermit-

tent claudication: Multicenter controlled double-blind trial with objective assessment of chronic occlusive arterial disease patients. Am Heart J 104:66–72, 1982

83.   Rae AP, Greenspan AM, Spielman SR, et al: Antiarrhythmic drug efficacy for ventricular tachyarrhythmias associated with coronary artery disease as assessed by electrophysiologic studies. Am J Cardiol 55:1494–1499, 1985

83a. Roth A, Harrison E, Mitani G, et al: Efficacy and safety of medium- and high-dose diltiazem alone and in combination with digoxin for control of heart rate at rest and during exercise in patients with chronic atrial fibrillation. Circulation 73:316–324, 1986

84.   Salathia KS, Barber JM, McIlmoyle EL, et al: Very early intervention with metoprolol in suspected acute myocardial infarction. Eur Heart J 6:190–198, 1985

85.   Soufer R, Wohlgelerenter D, Vita NA, et al: Intact systolic left ventricular function in clinical congestive heart failure. Am J Cardiol 55:1032–1036, 1985

86.   Spielman SR, Kay HR, Morganroth J, et al: Drug therapy in high risk patients following acute myocardial infarction: The results of the timolol, encainide, sotalol trial. Circulation 72 (suppl III):III-57, 1985

87.   Struthers AD, Brown MJ, Adams EF, et al: The plasma noradrenaline and growth hormone response to α-methyldopa and clonidine in hypertensive subjects. Br J Clin Pharmacol 19:311–317, 1985

88.   Suwa M, Hirota Y, Kawamura K: Improvement in LV diastolic function during intravenous and oral diltiazem therapy in patients with hypertrophic cardiomyopathy: An echocardiographic study. Am J Cardiol 54:1047–1053, 1984

89.   Swerdlow CD, Winkle RA, Mason JW: Determinants of survival in patients with ventricular tachyarrhythmia. New Engl J Med 308:1436–1442, 1983

90.   Topol EJ, Traill TA, Fortuin NJ: Hypertensive hypertrophic cardiomyopathy of the elderly. New Engl J Med 312:277–283, 1985

91.   Tresch DD, Wetherbee JN, Siegel R, et al: Long-term follow-up of survivors of pre-hospital sudden cardiac arrest treated with coronary bypass surgery. Am Heart J 110:1139–1145, 1985

92.   Tschollar W, Belz GG: Sublingual captopril in hypertensive crises. Lancet ii:34–35, 1985

93.   Williams GH, Hollenberg NK: Are non-modulating patients with essential hypertension a distinct subgroup Implications for therapy. Am J Med 79 (suppl 3C):3–9, 1985

94.   Wilson WR, Danielson GK, Giuliani ER, et al: Cardiac valve replacement in congestive heart failure due to infective endocarditis. Mayo Clin Proc 54:223, 1979

95.   Winniford MD, Gabliani G, Johnson SM, et al: Concomitant calcium antagonist plus isosorbide dinitrate therapy for markedly active variant angina. Am Heart J 108:1269–1273, 1984

96.   Yusuf S, Peto R, Lewis JA, et al: β-Blockade during and after myocardial infarction. Prog Cardiovasc Dis 27:335–371, 1985

97.   Yusuf S, Collins R: Intravenous nitroglycerin and nitroprusside therapy in acute myocardial infarction reduces mortality: Evidence from randomized control trial. Circulation 72 (suppl III):III-224, 1985

Index

Page numbers in *italics* indicate illustrations.
Page numbers followed by *t* indicate tables.

Diltiazem *(continued)*
  cardiac contraindications to, *39, 43t,* 46
  for cardiomyopathy, 47, 202
  in chronic stable effort angina, 46
  comparative properties of, *35t,* 36
  contraindications to, 39, *43t,* 46
  in coronary spasm, 46
  dose of, 46
  indications for, 46, *48t,* 49–50
  as peripheral vasodilator, 46
  pharmacokinetics of, 45
  in Prinzmetal's variant angina, 46
  in Raynaud's phenomenon, 46
  side-effects of, *39,* 46
  summary of effects of, *38*
  in unstable angina at rest, 46
Diphenylhydantoin as antiarrhythmic, 70
Dipyridamole
  aspirin combined with, 171–172
  for bypass grafts, 171–172
  platelet inhibition by, 171–172
  post-infarct, 197
  summary of, 172
  warfarin combined with, 172
Dirythmin. *See* Disopyramide
Dirythmin SA. *See* Disopyramide
Disopyramide, 64–65
  for cardiomyopathy, 65, 202
  comparative studies with, 78
  contraindications to, 65
  dose of, 64
  drug interactions with, 65
  for hypertrophic cardiomyopathy, 65, 202
  indications for, 64–65
  pharmacokinetics of, 64
  precautions with, 65
  QT-prolongation and, *76,* 81
  side-effects of, 65
  summary of, *60t, 62t,* 65
  therapeutic levels of, 64
  torsades de pointes and, 81
  verapamil and, 41
Disprin, 169
Diucardin, as diuretic, 116t
Diulo, 118
  as diuretic, summary of, 116t
Diuresis
  excessive, in edematous states, 123–124
  urinary electrolytes during, 112t
Diuretics, 111–127
  ACE inhibitors with, 122, 157–158
  arrhythmias and, 119
  benefit–risk ratio for, 111
  with β-blockers for hypertension, 10
  calcium antagonists as, 119
  carbonic anhydrase inhibitors as, 119
  combination, 122
  diabetes and, 120

  drug interactions with, 125–126
  high-ceiling, 111
  for hypertension, 8, 207, 208–210
  hyperkalemia and, 122
  hypokalemia and, 120
  hyponatremia and, 125
  lipidemia and, 186
  loop, 111–116; *see also* Loop diuretics
  metabolic side-effects of, 119
  minor, 119
  potassium-sparing, 121–122
  renal failure and, 125
  resistance to, 124–125
  side-effects of, 119–121
  sites of action of, *112*
  therapy with, 111–127
    potassium supplements in, 123
  thiazide, 116–121; *see also* Thiazide diuretics
  uses of, less common, 126
Diurexan, as diuretic, 116t
Diuril, as diuretic, 116t
Divistyramine for hyperlipidemia, 187
Dobutamine, 101–102, *104,* 132t
  clinical use of, 102
  in congestive heart failure, 201
  inotropic and vasodilator mechanisms, *104*
  intermittent, 145
  properties of, 103t
Dobutrex, 101–102
Dopamine
  dose of, 105
  inotropic and vasodilator mechanisms, *104*
  properties of, 103t
  side-effects of, 105
Dopaminergic agents, new, 105–106
Dopaminergic receptors, 104–105
Dopexamine, 105
  as vasodilator, 132t
Dreams, vivid, as β-blockade contraindication, 3t
  as β-blockade side-effect, 9
Dyazide, 122
  for heart failure, 120
  for hypertension in elderly, 213
"Dynamic stenosis,"
  effects of nitrates on coronary arteries and, 19
  "mixed" angina and, 7
Dyrenium, 121t
Dysrhythmias. *See* Arrhythmias
Dytec, 121t

Easprin, 169
Edecrin, 116
Edema, pulmonary. *See* Pulmonary edema